HEALTH EDUCATION

JOIN US ON THE INTERNET VIA WWW, GOPHER, FTP OR EMAIL:

WWW: http://www.thomson.com
GOPHER: gopher.thomson.com
FTP: ftp.thomson.com
EMAIL: findit@kiosk.thomson.com

A service of I(T)P

HEALTH EDUCATION

Effectiveness, efficiency and equity

Second edition

Keith Tones and Sylvia Tilford

Faculty of Health and Social Care
Leeds Metropolitan University
Leeds
UK

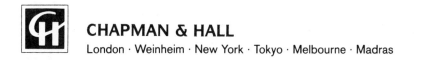

CHAPMAN & HALL
London · Weinheim · New York · Tokyo · Melbourne · Madras

Published by Chapman & Hall, 2-6 Boundary Row, London SE1 8HN, UK

Chapman & Hall, 2-6 Boundary Row, London SE1 8HN, UK

Chapman & Hall GmbH, Pappelallee 3, 69469 Weinheim, Germany

Chapman & Hall USA, One Penn Plaza, 41st Floor, New York, NY10119, USA

Chapman & Hall Japan, ITP - Japan, Kyowa Building, 3F, 2-2-1 Hirakawacho, Chiyoda-ku, Tokyo 102, Japan

Chapman & Hall Australia, Thomas Nelson Australia, 102 Dodds Street, South Melbourne, Victoria 3205, Australia

Chapman & Hall India, R. Seshadri, 32 Second Main Road, CIT East, Madras 600 035, India

Distributed in the USA and Canada by Singular Publishing Group, Inc., 4284 41st Street, San Diego, California 92105

First edition 1990
Reprinted 1991 (twice)
Second edition 1994
Reprinted 1995, 1996

© 1990 Keith Tones, Sylvia Tilford and Yvonne Robinson

© 1994 Keith Tones and Sylvia Tilford

Typeset in 10/12pt Palatino by EXPO Holdings, Malaysia
Printed in Great Britain by Clays Ltd, St Ives plc

ISBN 0 412 55110 1   1 56593 283 8 (USA)

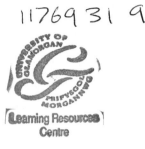

A Catalogue record for this book is available from the British Library

Library of Congress Cataloging-in-Publication Data available

∞ Printed on permanent acid-free text paper, manufactured in accordance with ANSI/NISO Z39.48-1992 and ANSI/NISO Z39.48-1984 (Permanence of Paper).

CONTENTS

ACKNOWLEDGEMENTS

We would like to acknowledge the contributions of Yvonne Robinson to the first edition of this book. We also wish to thank Health Education colleagues at Leeds Metropolitan University for their helpful comments and support during the production of this second edition.

Keith Tones
Sylvia Tilford

INTRODUCTION

Editor: Then you would regard education as an essential part of a progressive health policy?

Minister: There is no doubt about that ... one of the most noticeable characteristics of the dark ages was fatalism; men were over-whelmed by circumstances; they existed under a sense of impending disasters that they could neither see nor prevent. Men who feel as they did – that external circum-stances control their fate – despair of reform or progress; but let men once recog-nize that in large and increasing measure they are masters of their own destiny, and their life takes on a new, more hopeful, more purposeful aspect. Thus education is the instrument of reform, the giver of hope, the guide which directs the conscious individual effort without which health cannot be attained.

The above extract is part of a dialogue between the UK Minister of Health, the Rt Hon Ernest Brown, and the editor of the *Health Education Journal*. The date was 1943 and it featured in the very first issue of that journal.

Apart from being a kind of panegyric for an empowerment model of health education, it is notable for the high hopes for progress which characterized those heady days leading up to the launch of the welfare state. We still have high hopes for health education but since those immediate post-Beveridge days, we have been increasingly expected to actually prove that those expectations and aspirations are justifiable.

It could be said with some justification that the task of education is to safeguard people's right to learn about important aspects of human culture and experience. Since health and illness occupy a prominent place in our everyday experience, it might reasonably be argued that everyone is entitled to share whatever insights we possess into the state of being healthy and to benefit from what might be done to prevent and treat disease and dis-comfort. Health education's role in such an endeavour would be to create the necessary understanding. No other justification would be needed.

In recent years, however, questions have been posed with increasing insistence and urgency about efficiency – both about edu-cation in general and health education in particular. We can be certain that such enquiries about effectiveness do not reflect a greater concern to know whether or not the population is better educated: they stem from more utilitarian motives.

It is apparent, even to the casual observer, that economic growth and productivity have become a central preoccupation in modern Britain. Economic success is seen as depend-ing on the competitive urge which, among other things, should generate efficiency. It is, therefore, not surprising that health education should be required to prove itself – especially since both the education and health sectors have been subjected to critical scrutiny. In the first place, educational institutions are alleged to have failed to generate an entrepreneurial spirit; reforms have been urged which in-clude setting attainment targets by which efficiency may be measured. Again, in the health service, alarm has been expressed at the seemingly insatiable demands for health care and ensuing galloping inflation. Economies have been required – again in the interests of efficiency; performance indicators have been developed to assess progress.

Moreover, since publication of the first edition of this book, we have witnessed the appearance of the first genuine attempt in England to develop a health policy for the nation (DoH, 1992). Not surprisingly, it sets specific targets and the justification it provides for selecting those particular targets and the associated five key diseases is that they should not only be epidemiologically important but they should also be feasible and measurable.

Unlike many traditional educational disciplines, health education has consistently sought not merely to provide understanding about its substantive subject matter but has concerned itself also with such goals as attitude change and lifestyle modification. Indicators of successful health education have, for this reason, defined much more than gains in knowledge and understanding. Moreover, since health education is regarded as an arm of preventive medicine (at any rate by health professionals), it has been subjected to the same economic imperative as other branches of the health service. Furthermore, since health education occasionally, and usually unwisely, claims that prevention can save money by reducing the need for expenditure on curative medicine, it is not at all surprising that the question 'Does health education work?' really means 'Is it successful in preventing unhealthy behaviours and reducing health service costs?'. Such a perspective is, of course, as limited as the narrowly conceived view that economic growth and productivity is the most important recipe for human happiness. It is nonetheless important to recognize the impetus which economic philosophy provides in creating a demand that health education should prove itself.

We discussed the relationship between health education and health promotion in the first edition of this book. Since then the star of health promotion has continued in the ascendant – though its continuing popularity has not necessarily been accompanied by a reduction in the ambiguities and conflicting notions associated with the term. Paradoxically perhaps, the main philosophical and practical thrust of *The Health of the Nation* is much more consistent with a 'traditional' model of preventive health education than with the more radical ideology of World Health Organization (WHO) and Health for All by the Year 2000 (HFA 2000).

As we will see, arguably the most significant impact of the doctrine of health promotion has been its emphasis on the environmental determinants of health and illness and the consequent need for the development of 'healthy public policy' together with a continuing concern to foster empowered participating communities. It could indeed be asserted that after the Alma Ata Conference (see Chapter 1), which confidently asserted the centrality of health education in achieving health for all, health education has been somewhat marginalized in later developments, such as the Ottawa Charter, in the headlong drive to tackle health issues through the medium of policy and politics. As we will endeavour to show in Chapter 1, health education is viewed as making a major contribution to health promotion while not being synonymous with it. Indeed, an admittedly somewhat simplistic formula is used to capture the essence of the synergistic relationship between policy and education. It asserts that Health Promotion = Health Education × Healthy Public Policy.

This book then maintains its focus on health education and is concerned with its effectiveness and efficiency. Clearly we need to know whether our efforts are effective. We need to know whether, for example, programmes designed to reduce barriers to the utilization of mammography services actually increase service uptake while minimizing women's concerns and anxieties. We need to know whether an empowerment stratagem centring on local concerns over damp housing in an urban ghetto has had a positive effect on people's feelings of helplessness and influenced local politicians and decision makers. We need to know whether anticipatory guidance in the clinical setting has, for instance, helped diabetics cope with and manage their disease in the context of an empowering partnership with their health care providers.

At a simple level we can unequivocally answer the question, 'Does health education work?' with a simple affirmative: yes, it does! The reasons for such a confident assertion derive from the fact that there have been major changes in health-related behaviours over the past decade and, in many instances, an associated decline in premature death and the incidence of disease. In the USA, Britain and many other developed nations, there has been a substantial reduction in smoking and other risk factors implicated in coronary heart disease (CHD). In many countries there has been a significant improvement in cardiovascular health. Since the factors influencing these changes – cultural, behavioural and, arguably, epidemiological – must have been mediated by various forms of information, communication, persuasion and other educational activities, it would be churlish not to credit health education with the achievement.

For instance, Warner (1989) provides an update on the effects of the US antismoking campaign. He argues convincingly that:

In the absence of the antismoking campaign, adult per capita cigarette consumption in 1987 would have been an estimated 79–89 per cent higher than the level actually experienced. The smoking prevalence of all birth cohorts of men and women born during this century is well below that which would have been expected in the absence of the campaign. As a consequence, in 1985 an estimated 56 million Americans were smokers; without the campaign, an estimated 91 million would have been smokers. As a result of campaign-induced decisions not to smoke, between 1964 and 1985 an estimated 789 200 Americans avoided or postponed smoking-related deaths and gained an average of 21 additional years of life expectancy each; collectively that represents more than 16 million person-years of additional life each.

(*p. 144*)

Since the first edition of this book went to press, a new review of the effectiveness of health education was published by Liedekerken *et al.* (1990) at the request of the Dutch Health Education Centre. Its avowed purpose was to '... clarify the conceptual and methodological issues about the question of effectiveness and provide a state of the art review of effectiveness research'. It also sought to make recommendations for health education practice and policy. The book includes a useful brief review of 19 'subsectors' which provides a categorization of research by diseases and topics, settings and target groups. Interestingly, in seeking to respond to the question, 'Is health education effective?', the authors reach a similar conclusion to the one we reached in the introduction to the first edition. The conclusion: it depends!

Certainly, many people directly involved in programme development and evaluation are convinced that health education can be effective. Admittedly the cynic might contend that health educators must of necessity reach such a conclusion since they have an emotional (and political) investment in being seen to be successful. A recent WHO press release issued on 22 June 1992 is quite adamant.

Mass media campaigns, creative condom marketing programmes and the right messages from friends and co-workers have succeeded in slowing the spread of HIV, the AIDS virus, in projects around the world, a new analysis by the WHO reports.

In a review of 15 HIV prevention projects carried out in 13 countries, doctors and scientists from the WHO Global Programme on AIDS have confirmed the effectiveness of a handful of approaches in producing significant changes in people's sexual behaviour.

In Zaire, the most outstanding achievement is the dramatic year-by-year increase in condom use. In 1987 fewer than half a million condoms were distributed – mainly by government clinics – for a population of more than 30 million people. Sales of condoms totalled less than 100 000. But by 1991 condom sales had soared to over 18 million.

Condoms are also being promoted extensively in Thailand, where almost all new HIV infections are a result of heterosexual transmission. Many such infections occur among Thailand's estimated 100 000 sex workers and the men who buy their services. Thai health workers set themselves an ambitious goal – to back up sex workers' demands that clients use condoms by imposing a policy of '100% condom use' in the sex entertainment industry. The project worked with both the brothel owners and women, assuring each group that their income would not be affected if condom use became mandatory. They were also informed that non-compliance with the policy would be met with penalties for the brothel owner.*

The strategy is working. In Samut Sakhon in Thailand, client use of condoms is now nearing 100%. The number of condoms used by men who have sex with prostitutes in the province has gone up from less than 15 000 a month to over 50 000, and in Chiang Mai condom use has increased from 30% to 80–90% of sexual contacts. Encouragingly, the project has now been extended nationwide to 66 of Thailand's 73 provinces.

In the introduction to the first edition of the book we reminded readers of existing general reviews of published studies of the success of health education and noted that they all provided evidence of effectiveness. For instance, Gatherer *et al.* (1979) asked, 'Is Health Education Effective?'. He and his fellow authors then provided abstracts of research and an overview of evaluated studies. Bell *et al.* (1985) provide an annotated bibliography of health education research in the UK which includes many studies of effectiveness. Green and Lewis (1986) have been assiduous over the years in producing comprehensive and detailed lists of evaluated work together with critiques of research design which make it possible to judge the reliability and validity of the studies. It is, however, difficult to draw conclusions of a general nature from this kind of work – except that many of the interventions they describe have been effective in the sense in which the term has been used above. Gatherer's review, for example, reported that 85% of 62 reported studies demonstrated an improvement in knowledge while 65% of 39 studies indicated that there had been a change of attitudes 'in the desired direction'. Of 123 studies which sought to produce behavioural change, 75% actually succeeded in doing so. However, apart from elementary questions about research design such as whether the claimed changes could really be attributed to the health education intervention, there are more fundamental issues to be addressed. Foremost among these is the question of practical as opposed to statistical significance. For instance, how big were the changes in knowledge, attitude and practice? Were they big enough to justify claims of success? How big should they have been before we could argue a programme had been effective? Do the studies which apparently showed no change demonstrate the inefficiency of health education – or was it merely the case that the methods used and the available resources were inappropriate to the task? Or was the task intrinsically

---

*An interesting example of healthy public policy!

unsuitable for treatment by health education? Certainly, the observations of Gatherer *et al.* support the notion of ineffective delivery of the programme: 'The overall impression from much of the literature on health education is that too much of the health education practised is inappropriate for many, perhaps the majority, of the people for whom it is supposedly intended'.

It is, then, not possible to use reported research on effectiveness and efficiency – even when the research design has been impeccable – to reach conclusions about the success of health education. Before this is possible, we must be clear about the criteria by which a programme may be assessed and we must know a good deal about the circumstances associated with the design and delivery of the education. Two examples will serve to underline this assertion. The first of these describes a dietary intervention mounted in Spring, 1981, in a rural community in Finland (Koskela, personal communication).

Thirty Finnish couples were matched with 30 couples in southern Italy and an attempt was made to bring the Finns' dietary status more in line with the healthier status of the Italian group. They received intensive counselling and were provided with several '… strategic food items free of charge'. One dietitian visited six families frequently and also met them when they made a twice-weekly visit to clinics for blood pressure measurement. The intervention was manifestly effective: by the end of the counselling the Finnish families' diets approximated to the healthier Mediterranean type of diet. The proportion of energy derived from fats declined from 39% to 24%; the ratio of polyunsaturated to saturated fats increased from less than 0.2 to more than 1.0 (as compared with a shift in the P/S ratio from 0.24 to 0.32 recommended by NACNE (1983). The total serum cholesterol level also declined and there was a reduction in blood pressure in every subject. The intervention lasted six weeks and afterwards, subjects reverted to their normal (and presumably preferred) diets. The various physiological indicators followed suit along with their risk status.

The study appears to have been methodologically sound and the results genuine. Criteria of success were certainly consistent with a medical model – behaviour change associated with clinical improvement. Educational methods were appropriate and the choice of face-to-face counselling and behaviour modification techniques was consistent with learning theory. It was in most ways an efficient as well as an effective programme since it is hard to imagine how alternative educational strategies might have been used to achieve a better result. However, it is unlikely that such an approach would be widely used since the use of one dietitian per six families would almost certainly be considered too expensive. We cannot ignore the values underlying evaluation and the political factors which determine the priorities to be accorded to these. For instance it might well be the case that the alternative to the intervention described above would be to undertake the much more substantial costs involved in treating the disease which the intervention might well have prevented – probably because the necessary shift in resources from acute to preventive sectors would be politically unacceptable. The net result of the process of prioritization might well be a token mass media campaign which would be neither effective nor efficient.

The second example concerns the teaching of breast self-examination (BSE). This is a relatively inexpensive screening strategy designed to achieve early detection of potentially lethal abnormalities on the assumption that early intervention will result in a better chance of cure. A more expensive alternative device for detecting breast lumps in postmenopausal women is the technique of mammography. The study described here sought to compare the efficiency of BSE with mammography. Its starting point was that BSE is often ineffectively performed due to the use of inappropriate teaching techniques. Indeed, common sense, let alone learning theory, would suggest that the acquisition of the psychomotor skill involved in BSE will not be efficiently acquired by the use of, for instance, pamphlets or even filmed models. Pennypacker *et al.* (1982) utilized learning theory to create the proper conditions for the acquisition of the skill: they provided an opportunity for skills practice and provided immediate knowledge of results of successful examination of breast tissues. They employed not only silicon models of the breast to provide practice but also supplied television and computer-assisted display of information when women transferred their learning from the silicon models to their own breasts. As a result women not only acquired efficient scanning techniques but also learned to exert the right degree of pressure and discriminate normal from abnormal tissue. According to the researchers, the sample studied was more efficient than a mammography unit at detecting small lumps (a 5.8% hit rate compared with 5.3%). However, rather like the first study cited above, although the relative effectiveness (i.e. the efficiency) of the method was superior to competing techniques, the costs involved in the high technology, staffing and training would render it inappropriate for general use.

Apart from illustrating the complexity of determining efficiency and the political problems associated with basing decisions purely on the evidence of the relative effectiveness of competing strategies, the two studies allow us to make an important generalization. Provided that a given teaching method is based on sound educational theory, it is usually possible to achieve desired objectives. A good understanding of the psychosocial factors underpinning decision making and behaviour will help us design specific interventions which will be successful. However, the application of this understanding will often be severely curtailed by practical and political considerations. For instance there may be insufficient skilled personnel and resources to supply the conditions for efficient learning; the theoretically appropriate methods may be too time consuming or even unethical.

It seems clear, then, that health education can be effective but the important issue is about efficiency. In other words we need to know not merely whether health education has been successful but rather how successful it has been. Efficiency is thus concerned with the extent to which health education has achieved a given outcome by comparison with some alternative intervention. In the economic context outlined above, the criterion might be one of relative cost. In another context the yardstick might be the extent to which dietary behaviour has changed and the explicit or implicit comparison might be between individually directed health education or the introduction of labelling or other controls on food production and distribution. It is much more difficult to respond to the question of how efficient a given programme has been in achieving some desirable goal than it is to examine the issue of effectiveness. The answer to such a question will almost inevitably be 'it depends'. It depends, for instance, on the nature of goals, the criteria of success, the way in which the education is provided, the resources available. This is one of the issues which the book will seek to illuminate.

It might have been noted that the title of this edition of the book has acquired an appendage in the form of the word 'equity'. While we do not purport to provide a comprehensive discussion of this key issue for health education, we feel it provides a useful indicator of our own value position.

First of all, as we suggest in Chapter 1, it could be argued that the pursuit of equity and tackling inequalities in health are the major tasks facing health promotion. Although we have just presented in some detail two case studies of health education interventions which are concerned with conventional preventive medical outcomes, it will become clear that this book emphasizes the importance of broader empowering strategies which acknowledge the significance of those social, structural and environmental factors which ultimately determine our health status. Accordingly, we will argue that our evaluation goals must move beyond a narrow individualistic, preventive orientation. Above all, this book is concerned with the **meaning** of success. It is concerned to examine and explore the values and ideological issues which underpin different models of an approach to health promotion and health education – and the practices which result from such 'philosophical' concerns.

A natural consequence of this stance is what one might call a need for 'methodological equity'. Although the randomized controlled trial and the various experimental designs associated with more traditional research approaches have an important part to play, they are not the only relevant evaluation method. Indeed, we will comment that their use in some instances may be ethically, epistemologically and technically inappropriate for many of the purposes of health education research.

This book is concerned, then, with general questions of success. It will not provide a detailed compendium of exemplars of effectiveness, nor is it intended to be an evaluation primer – although in Chapter 2 it does seek to remind readers of major research issues and approaches to evaluation. The first issue it addresses has to do with the meaning of success. Chapter 1 shows how the measurement of effectiveness and efficiency must ultimately depend on how success is defined. The definition of success will, in turn, be based on ideology and philosophy. Since there are wide divergences of view about the purpose of health education, indicators of performance should logically be derived from a statement of the values underpinning programme goals.

The second issue is more technical and concerns the design of evaluations. Research design, despite its image, is not a mech-

anically scientific process involving the choice of an off-the-peg formula. It requires careful thought about the nature of the successful outcome, the use to which results will be put and the degree of insight which these results will provide into programme efficiency. It will remind us that there are different kinds of evaluation all having different capabilities for application to practice; it will also remind us that, like health education itself, there are important ethical issues to be considered in the research process.

The third issue concerns the role of theory. Reference has already been made to the importance of learning theory in determining the choice of teaching method. The whole book, in fact, is based on the premise that sound theory is essential to the design of effective, efficient and practical programmes. This contention is illustrated by the particular case of the choice of indicators. There are a wide variety of markers which might be used as measures of performance and selecting those which most readily reflect the nature and degree of success achieved by any given health education enterprise is no easy matter. Chapter 3 attempts to show how theoretical considerations should influence choice of indicator. It illustrates the point by describing how the Health Action Model and Communication of Innovations Theory provide a basis for reasoned choice of measures of outcome and both indirect and intermediate indicators of programme efficiency.

The remainder of the book seeks to illuminate the various issues discussed above within the general framework of five settings: schools, health service, mass media, workplace and community. Although some reference will be made, both directly and obliquely, to more specific methods, these will not figure prominently in our analysis.

Since terms such as 'setting', 'sector', 'context', 'strategy' and 'method' often feature in discussions about designing and implementing health education programmes – and sometimes may be used interchangeably – it may be useful to engage in some definition and clarification at this juncture. Moreover, given the observations made above about the centrality of values in any discourse about evaluation, it is important to recognize that such expressions as 'programme delivery' or 'strategic intervention' are themselves value laden and carry particular connotations. The following observations are more fully explored elsewhere (Tones, 1993).

First of all, the terms 'setting' or 'context' are relatively unambiguous: both refer to location and indicate **where** health education might take place. Some of the more popular settings include, for example, workplace, school, health care system and voluntary organization. Although 'setting' is currently favoured, we might just as well talk about 'context'. Indeed, the connotation of an inter-weaving of elements is particularly appealing since the peculiar mixture of organizational and interpersonal factors inherent in a given setting will influence the 'texture' of any health education programme provided in that setting.

Rather rarely the term 'sector' might be used – implying some kind of subdivision. Those who have been imbued with the spirit of the Ottawa Charter (Chapter 1), with its emphasis on 'inter-sectoral collaboration', might well prefer to use that particular word.

This discussion of terminological niceties is not as pedantic as it might first appear: choice of a particular term may – as mentioned above – signal some underlying ideological principle. For example, the word 'strategy' might be thought of as synonymous with setting or context. It might be said to be 'strategically sound' to use mass media to achieve the *Health of the Nation* objective of reducing the prevalence of cigarette smoking to no more than 20% by the year 2000. An alternative strategy might emphasize the importance of using the workplace as a locus for the efficient 'delivery' of health education.

Etymologically, though, the word strategy (or, more precisely, 'stratagem') does not only imply a military campaign but also incorporates the notion of 'trick'. Therefore for those whose ideological commitment is to build health education programmes on people's 'felt needs' and who seek to facilitate the achievement of self-empowered choice, these 'top-down' connotations of the term would strike a discordant note.

There would be much less disagreement about the meaning of methodology (i.e. a system of methods) when employed in health education. Methods are relatively specific (by comparison with strategies); they operate at the micro rather than the macro level. Very similar methods may be used in a wide variety of settings or contexts and may form part of or adjuncts to such strategies as mass media or community development. For instance, one or more different varieties of group discussion may form an integral part of strategies designed to stimulate community participation or be used as a follow-up to televised smoking cessation groups.

Whatever the terminology employed, it is clear that we are discussing initiatives which operate at different levels ranging from macro to micro – as may be seen in Figure A.

MACRO   **NATIONAL POLICY LEVEL**

STRATEGIC LEVEL
Mass media; community development; social action

SETTINGS
Schools; workplace; primary care; pharmacists; local authorities; voluntary bodies, etc.

METHODS
One-to-one; groups; role play; games; life skills, etc.

RESOURCES
Videos; leaflets; posters; educational broadcasts; worksheets, etc.

MICRO

Figure A: Levels of health education operation.

At the macro level we must include national policy and mass media. At the organizational or setting level we would identify key contexts for providing health education such as school, workplace, medical service, voluntary bodies and settings which are somewhat less easy to classify such as youth clubs. Clearly policy may be 'built in' to each of these intermediate levels.

Finally, at the micro level, a substantial array of specific methods together with ancillary audiovisual aids and learning resources may be deployed.

Two generalizations may be made at this point about settings. Firstly, any particular programme goals will be more effectively attained when different settings have congruent aims and operate synergistically. This principle will apply both to programmes which have a preventive orientation, such as the various CHD prevention programmes described in Chapter 8, and also to programmes having such goals as the achievement of empowerment or community participation. Secondly, there is a synergistic effect when health education is supported by policy: maximal efficiency will therefore occur when a coherent health education programme is supported by appropriate legal, fiscal, economic and environmental measures – and vice versa. Although this book does not directly address the effectiveness of social policy changes in enhancing health, the postulated synergism between education and social policy should always be borne in mind when considering the efficiency of either kind of intervention.

The education system has been widely seen as a major institution for the delivery of health education. Chapter 4 will assess the contribution it makes at a number of levels – from individual outcomes within the classroom to national policies and activities which support school activities. Both hospital and primary care services have been urged to develop the educational component of their activities – not least because, as we have seen above, educational inputs have been viewed as means of contributing to cutting health care costs. Chapter 5 will examine the philosophical approach adopted to education in a health care context, the success of education as exemplified by a small number of outcomes and will conclude with a general discussion of factors which enhance educational activity in primary care and in hospitals.

Chapter 6 seeks to provide a theoretical analysis of the use of mass media as a delivery strategy and identifies the features which distinguish this from all other strategies and settings discussed here. In general it supports the view that the proper application of social marketing principles will increase the chances of success while at the same time noting the fallacy of assuming that the process of marketing health is basically the same as that which is involved in selling commercial products. The chapter also reinforces the book's general contention about synergy and asserts that mass media are most effectively employed in the context of an integrated community programme. A larger and wider variety of specific evaluations have been included in this chapter compared with those chapters considering alternative delivery systems. This decision has been made because of the typically inflated aspirations entertained for mass media use. Attempts are therefore made to indicate the limitations of this particular strategy and also to show how different features of programme construction – the content of the messages, the target population and the intrinsic variations in the type of media used – can influence the chances of achieving success. It is hoped in this way to generate more realistic expectations of what mass media can achieve.

Chapter 7 examines health promotion in the workplace – a strategy which offers several interesting insights into the meaning of effectiveness and efficiency. The workplace provides excellent examples of the way in which different philosophies and models of health education give rise to widely divergent criteria of success. Moreover, the worksite illustrates the potential synergy between health policy and education in the form of, for instance, alcohol policy development and employee assistance programmes. In addition, evaluation of health education in the workplace provides us with some of the hardest evidence of effectiveness and efficiency.

The final chapter in this book focuses on the community. In doing so, it recapitulates themes explored in Chapter 1. More particularly, it compares and contrasts the essentially democratic, 'bottom-up' approach associated with community development with the 'top-down' approach exemplified by the strategic delivery of a number of well known international heart disease prevention projects. In making this comparison, we will also note that the notion of a simple dichotomy between top-down and bottom-up is not tenable in practice. However, we will be able to provide suggestions for a wide range of indicators of success which might be used in these different programmes and projects. We will also, in doing so, provide some evidence of effectiveness – and even efficiency.

No attempt is made in this book to relate the contents specifically to the UK scene – nor to review the international literature systematically. Rather it selects eclectically whatever examples suit the purposes of any given chapter. We choose from whatever source seems most appropriate to provide evidence in support of our arguments and assertions. However, because our experience is primarily of UK situations and the available evidence of

effectiveness and efficiency tends to have been generated in North America, most examples will be derived from Britain and the USA.

REFERENCES

Bell, J. *et al.* (1985) *Annotated Bibliography of Health Education Research completed in Britain from 1948–1978 and 1979–1983*, Scottish Health Education Group, Edinburgh.

Department of Health (1992) *Health of the Nation*, HMSO, London.

Editorial. (1943) *Health Education Journal*, **1**,1.

Gatherer, A., Parfit, J., Porter, E. and Vessey, M. (1979) *Is Health Education Effective?*, Health Education Council, London.

Green, L.W. and Lewis, F.M. (1986) *Measurement and Evaluation in Health Education and Health Promotion*, Mayfield, Palo Alto, California.

Liedekerken, P.C. *et al.* (1990) *The Effectiveness of Health Education*, Van Gorcum, Assen, Netherlands.

NACNE (1983) *A Discussion Paper on Proposals for Nutritional Guidelines for Health Education in Britain*, Health Education Council, London.

Pennypacker, H.S., Goldstein, M.K. and Stein, G.H. (1982) Efficient technology of training breast self-examination, in *Public Education About Cancer*, (ed. P. Hobbs), UICC Technical Report Series, UICC, Geneva.

Tones, B.K. (1993) Methods and strategies in health education. *Health Education Journal* **52** (3) 125–39.

Warner, K.E. (1989) Effects of the antismoking campaign: an update. *American Journal of Public Health*, **79** (2) 144–51.

WHO (1992) Aids prevention does work, says the World Health Organization. Press release, WHO/44, 22 June.

The fundamental purpose of the evaluation process is to determine the value or worth of an activity. In passing judgement on this activity, the evaluator comments on its success or failure in respect of some valued goal. Evaluation is concerned with effectiveness, i.e. it says whether or not the valued goal has been achieved. It also makes statements about efficiency by providing an indication of the extent to which the measures designed to achieve the valued goal have been effective, by comparing them with alternative and competing measures.

The implicit assumption underlying health education is, of course, that it is a worthwhile activity and is in some way good for people. It would, however, be wrong to assume that health educators have a common value system. Health education is no mere technical operation: health educators have different philosophies of professional practice which reflect their own values and define what it is they believe to be worthwhile about their professional goals. Although this situation is not peculiar to health education, those who seek to educate about health are subject not only to the intrinsic controversies of education but have also to address the problem of defining the nebulous notion of health. The difficulties involved in clarifying professional values are compounded by health education's lack of professional status. Although many people have challenged the desirability of professionalizing health education, the absence of the unifying framework of theory and practice which this process normally provides will tend to generate disagreement about aims and values.

This whole rather confusing scenario is further clouded by the recent emergence of the **health promotion movement**. For some, health promotion is an activity synonymous with health education; for others it is a related but substantially different process having different goals and values. Since health education is not a unitary process having a universally accepted philosophy and clear goals, it therefore follows that it is not possible to provide an unequivocal definition of what constitutes success without first examining the values upon which different approaches to health education are based. And since there still appears to be some confusion between health education and health promotion it would seem appropriate to try to resolve this demarcation dispute prior to considering the nature of different health education approaches. Accordingly this chapter will consider the ways in which health promotion relates to different models of health education and will subsequently examine the implications of this analysis for the definition of success and failure which is central to the process of evaluation.

THE MEANING OF HEALTH PROMOTION

A complete and comprehensive account of health promotion and its historical roots is beyond the scope of this book. However, for the reasons stated earlier, some further discussion is needed. This will involve separately analysing health promotion on the one hand as ideology and, on the other, as structure. In other words, the values underpinning dominant notions of health promotion will be considered; subsequently a model operationalizing the concept will be presented. This model will highlight its main component parts and, *inter alia*, demonstrate the relationship between health education and other major processes contributing to the promotion of health.

Before doing this, it might be illuminating to consider some of the different meanings associated with health promotion and, in particular, reflect on the contribution made by the Word Health Organization (WHO) to this debate.

A HISTORICAL PERSPECTIVE

Many publications have provided definitions of and perspectives on health promotion during the last few years (Anderson, 1984; Tones, 1985; Green and Raeburn, 1988; Minkler, 1989). It has been used to distinguish attempts to foster positive health or 'wellbeing' from initiatives designed primarily to prevent disease. It has been employed approvingly to describe media and marketing oriented attempts to 'sell health'. It also figured prominently in the influential series of publications produced by the US Department of Health, Education and Welfare (1978 and 1979) and the Department of Health and Human Services (1980) where it was contrasted with 'health protection' and 'preventive health services'. In this latter guise it was characterized by the specification of precise and specific *Objectives for the Nation* focusing on the primary prevention of disease. Indeed, the concept of health promotion is rather like virtue: it means all things to all people – who are united only in their agreement that it is rather desirable. Green and Raeburn (1988) describe rather nicely how a wide variety of different interest groups have laid claim to this essentially contested concept.

> Ideologues, professionals, interest groups, and representatives of numerous disciplines have attempted to appropriate the field for themselves. Health and education professionals, behavioral and social scientists, public administrators, town planners, futurists, holistic health and self-care advocates, liberals, conservatives, voluntary associations, funding agencies, governments, community groups, and many others all want something from health promotion, all want to contribute something, and all bring their own orientation to bear on it.
>
> *(p. 30)*

The stance adopted in this book may be said to follow the ideological canons of WHO (although there may be some departure from WHO's perspective in translating ideology into action). At all events, before considering the ideological dimension, we should perhaps remind ourselves of the various 'milestones' in WHO's progress towards the current formulation of health promotion.

Clearly the origins of health promotion may be found in WHO's original and classic definition of health (WHO, 1946) with its holistic emphasis and its accentuation of the positive. More recently, a major impetus was provided with the launch of 'Health for All by the Year 2000' (HFA 2000) at the 30th World Health Assembly in 1977. Interestingly, in the context of developing indicators of performance, this new movement included a more realistic definition of health than the classic 1946 version. As the then Director General of WHO pointed out:

> The challenging constitutional objective of the Word Health Organization: the attainment by all peoples of the highest possible level of physical, mental and social wellbeing, is now being transformed into the dynamic notion of a Health for All movement. With this change in emphasis, public health is reinstating itself as a collective effort, drawing together a wide range of actors, institutions and sectors within society toward a goal of a 'socially and economically productive life'. This social

goal ... moves health from being the outcome measure of social development to being one of its major resources.

(Mahler, 1986, p. 1)

A major event in the progress towards health promotion was the Declaration of Alma Ata (WHO, 1978). It made several important assertions which were later to be incorporated into health promotion. Above all, it declared that the existence of gross inequalities between advantaged and disadvantaged peoples was 'politically, socially and economically' unacceptable. Equity was the foundation for achieving HFA 2000. Economic and social development was therefore essential to the achievement of health. On the other hand, people themselves have not only a right but a duty to participate individually and collectively in the planning and implementation of their health care. **Primary health care** (PHC) was considered to be the key to achieving HFA 2000; and PHC was seen as not only more than primary **medical** care but ideologically different. Alma Ata broadened considerably the definition of health services by redefining agriculture, animal husbandry, food, industry, education, housing, public works, communications and other sectors as services essential for the promotion of health.

Alma Ata might with justification be viewed as a prototype for *Health Promotion* (WHO, 1984). A flavour of its ideological dynamic is provided by the following quotation from Kickbusch (1986) – a major figure in the proselytization of health promotion – which she describes as '... a new forcefield for health (which) integrates social action, health advocacy and public policy'. It incorporates:

... diverse, but complementary, methods or approaches, including communication, education, legislation, fiscal measures, organizational change, community development and spontaneous local activities against health hazards. It offers new

challenges to existing professional groups, commercial and corporate bodies, cultural norms and the inertia of health institutions ... it reiterates the Health for All components of intersectoral action and advocacy for health, stressing the need to go beyond health care and equity in access to a healthy life.

(pp. 437–8)

The Ottawa Charter (WHO, 1986; *Health Promotion*, 1986) provided an international clarion call for action towards a new public health. It embodied the principles of health promotion; its major thrust was for social change and political activity. Although it urged the development of personal skills its paramount recommendation was the need to 'build healthy public policy'. In so doing, it could be said that it marginalized health education – dislodging it from the centre stage position which Alma Ata bestowed on it. This point will be revisited later in the chapter.

Bearing in mind our interest in operationalizing the notion of health in the context of developing performance indicators and measurable educational objectives, we should at this point note that the Ottawa Charter was preceded by the development of 38 targets for achieving HFA 2000 in the European Region (WHO, 1985). These targets are clearly significant for our present purpose in that they could be said to provide the criteria whereby the success of health promotion might be judged. They are therefore reproduced in the Appendix.

Continuing the description of the development of health promotion, we should note two additional initiatives. The first represents the further pursuit of healthy public policy in the form of recommendations from the Second International Conference on Health Promotion in Adelaide (*Health Promotion*, 1988). The second and, perhaps the most influential, development has been the Healthy Cities Project which established a number of 'test beds' for health promotion in 11 European cities; this subsequently acted as a catalyst for similar developments in another 300 or more cities (Fryer, 1988; Kickbusch, 1989).

> The city with its own political mandate and often highly developed sense of civic pride is ... uniquely placed to develop the kind of citizen-responsive health promotion initiatives which are necessary to tackle the new health problems of the 21st century. As the most decentralized level which can marshal the necessary resources and which has wide-ranging responsibilities and networks it is in an ideal position to support the kind of intersectoral process which leads to creative, effective and efficient action.
>
> *(Morris, 1987)*

THE IDEOLOGY OF HEALTH PROMOTION

As we have seen, evaluation is concerned to assess the extent to which certain valued outcomes have been achieved. It is therefore important for us at this stage to give some consideration to the values which permeate health promotion – both 'orthodox' and 'unorthodox'. In short, we must consider the ideology of health promotion and, subsequently, the ideological basis of different 'models' of health education. First, though, some brief clarification of how the term ideology is being used here.

Although not as ambivalent and ambiguous a concept as health promotion, the term ideology is open to many interpretations. Indeed, one influential work on the subject (Eagleton, 1991) lists 'more or less at random' some 16 definitions in common use. These include: the process of production of meanings, signs and values in social life; the medium in which conscious social actors make sense of their world; the confusion of linguistic and phenomenal reality; a body of ideas characteristic of a particular social group or class; false ideas which help to

legitimate a dominant political power. The term will be used here simply to describe the complex of values and associated beliefs which provide people with meaning in their personal and professional lives and which, by way of example, would influence their preference for one or other 'model' of health education and their preferred way of working. Ideology would thus be used not only to justify adoption of a given model but might also serve as a basis for vigorously attacking competing models and associated practice!

The ideological basis of the WHO formulation of health promotion will have been evident in the Ottawa Charter and associated publications and pronouncements. The ethical and moral view of humanity enshrined in this perspective on health promotion may be summarized by the following principles and statements of belief:

1. Health should be viewed holistically as a positive state; it is an essential commodity which people need in order to achieve the ultimate goal of a socially and economically productive life.
2. Health will not be achieved nor illness prevented and controlled unless existing health inequalities between and within nations and social groups have been eradicated.
3. A healthy nation is not only one which has an equitable distribution of resources but one which also has an active empowered community which is vigorously involved in creating the conditions necessary for a healthy people.
4. Health is too important to be left to medical practitioners; there must be a 're-orientation of health services'. It is important also to recognize that a wide range of public and private services and institutions influence health for good or ill. Moreover, medical services frequently do not meet the needs of the public; they often treat people as passive recipients of care and are thus fundamentally

depowering. The main modus operandi of health promotion is one of enabling not coercing; the focus should be on cooperation rather than on compliance.

5. People's health is not just an individual responsibility; our health is, to a large extent, governed by the physical, social, cultural and economic environments in which we live and work. To cajole the individual into taking responsibility for his or her health, while at the same time ignoring the social and environmental circumstances which conspire to make them ill, is a fundamentally defective strategy – and unethical. It is, in short, victim blaming. For these reasons, the building of 'healthy public polity' is considered to be at the very heart of health promotion.

It would be interesting to know just how many of the signatories of the Ottawa Charter understood the policy implications of what they were signing or, if they did, whether they were fully committed to the ideological principles embodied in the Charter.

Green and Raeburn (1988) have argued that Canada's policy framework does in fact adopt an empowering approach congruent with Charter principles. On the other hand, the publications of the US Department of Health and Human Services to which reference was made earlier adopt a narrower, preventive perspective on health promotion. Green and Raeburn do, however, invite us to note that the reputation of this US conceptualization for focusing only on rugged individualism is somewhat undeserved. They point out that of the 15 prioritized areas for disease prevention and health promotion in *Objectives for the Nation*, two thirds are addressed to environmental measures or health care systems. On the other hand, the first serious attempt at a national health policy in England (DoH, 1992) is distinctly lukewarm in its commitment to the ideology of health promotion as formulated above. For instance, the five key

strategic areas selected for priority action are essentially 'vertical' programmes focusing on cardiovascular disease, mental illness, cancers, accidents and HIV/AIDS. It is true that reference is made to the significance of 'public policy' and 'healthy surroundings' and, moreover, the government's role in legislating for health is acknowledged. Reference is even made to the importance of 'decent local environment and housing conditions'. However, in the last analysis, broader socioeconomic influences on health and illness are effectively ignored; the prevailing concern is with individual lifestyle.

What is, of course, clear is that wholehearted commitment to the ideological principles of health promotion would require sweeping and substantial political change. In short, the existing power structure would be subjected to fundamental challenge. Under what conditions might such a challenge be successful? Clearly the reiteration of empty phrases such as the need for 'political will' will achieve nothing. If rhetoric is to be translated into reality, ideology must be operationalized. What follows is an attempt to provide a structural basis for this process of operationalization. It is therefore less concerned with presenting an ideology of health promotion than with depicting its 'anatomy'. The resulting model, described below, incorporates two main 'anatomical' features: health and social policy and education. These features are considered to operate synergistically.

THE ANATOMY OF HEALTH PROMOTION

Since the first edition of this book, a number of publications have provided analyses of the dynamics of health promotion. For instance, Tannahill has developed an elegant model in which health promotion is viewed as a number of different combinations of prevention, health protection and health education (Downie, Fyfe and Tannahill, 1992). The model to be discussed below, however, differs in its

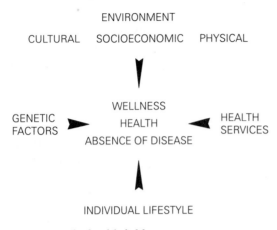

ENVIRONMENT

CULTURAL   SOCIOECONOMIC   PHYSICAL

WELLNESS

GENETIC   HEALTH   HEALTH
FACTORS   SERVICES

ABSENCE OF DISEASE

INDIVIDUAL LIFESTYLE

Figure 1.1 The health field concept.

concern to emphasize and explicate the contribution made by education; its structure represents a development of the familiar health field concept (Figure 1.1).

The health field concept was popularized in a working document on the health of Canadians which became widely known as the Lalonde Report (Lalonde, 1974). In fact, this derived from a conceptual schema outlined by LaFramboise (1973) which provided a simple map of 'health territory'. Health and illness are considered to result from the interplay of four key influences: genetic factors, the environment, lifestyle and medical services. Although this formulation was hardly novel, it acquired a special status when endorsed by a government agency!

Nonetheless, the health field concept identifies the key influences on health and, therefore logically, health promotion might be described as any deliberate or planned attempt to foster health or prevent and manage disease by achieving some judicious mix of the four 'inputs'. Since the genetic aspect is not effectively amenable to intervention (except perhaps by genetic counselling), the concerns of health promotion would in practice centre on the remaining three factors. Apart from the exhortation to 'reorient medical services' as part of a more general trend

to demedicalization, curative medicine has (rather churlishly perhaps) often been excluded from the health promotion field, leaving lifestyle and environment as the main areas of interest. This formulation of health promotion as **any** measure which promotes health is, of course, consistent with WHO's approach which accepted that health promotion was a '... unifying concept for those who recognize the need for change in the ways and conditions of living, in order to promote health' (WHO, 1984). Dennis *et al.* made a similar point in 1982, seeing health education as operating within a broad framework of policy.

Before considering how the health field concept might usefully be expanded, two incidental points should be made: first, health is defined both in terms of the prevention and management of disease and also as having 'positive' or 'wellness' aspects. Second, both health promotion and health education are considered to be planned activities. Of course, serendipitous events may result in health gain just as health learning may occur without any deliberate attempt to influence. However, the perhaps optimistic assumption is made in this book that the organization of learning experiences (i.e. teaching) and the intentional planning of policy initiatives are more likely to result in a positive outcome than reliance on happenstance. Clearly, it is assumed that the superiority of planned interventions will depend on the skills of the health promotion practitioner – although we must, however, regrettably accept that not all intentional attempts at health promotion will be in competent hands!

Figure 1.2 provides our 'anatomical' analysis of health promotion. The three central elements of the health field concept (i.e. those which are potentially amenable to influence) may be readily identified. They comprise, first of all, environmental influences, which are depicted as under the control of 'healthy public policy'. Second, we may note the impact on health of individual choice of

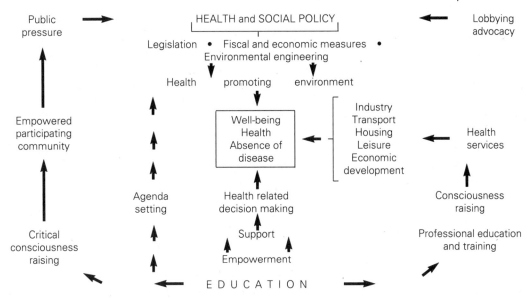

Figure 1.2 The contribution of health education to health promotion.

lifestyle and, third, an expanded health services input may be seen.

In addition, two deliberate strategies for producing change are featured in Figure 1.2. These are 'lobbying' and 'education'. Of the two, education is considered to have potentially the more powerful and multifaceted role. Lobbying may, nonetheless, make a major contribution to health promotion and its function is primarily that of bringing about 'healthy public policy'. Indeed, both education and policy are central to the achievement of individual, community and national health status. According to this conceptualization, it is possible to distil the concept of health promotion into an essential 'formula' – as follows: **Health Promotion = Health Education × Healthy Public Policy**. The nature of this multiplicative relationship will be explored below.

HEALTH EDUCATION AND HEALTH PROMOTION: A SYMBIOTIC RELATIONSHIP

As may be seen from Figure 1.2, health is substantially influenced by environmental factors: physical, socioeconomic and cultural. The influence may, of course, be positive or negative. One key aim of health promotion is to 'engineer' these various environmental factors in order to maximize opportunities for health and the avoidance of disease and disability. In so doing, 'healthy' decision making is potentiated: the healthy choice becomes the easy choice. The process of social engineering may literally involve environmental engineering – for instance, the construction of cycle tracks within 'healthy cities'. It may, on the other hand, require fiscal or economic measures. Legislation may or may not be involved in both of the instances cited above. Again, legislation, financial commitments and the like require the formulation of health policy – or broader social policies which have implications for health.

Healthy public policy, then, is necessary for environmental change. Clearly, a health promoting environment may operate at a macro level: for example, at national and international level. Additionally, the development and implementation of health policies will operate at local levels – and at the level of organizations; for instance, the importance of having smoking and healthy food policies within hospitals has long been acknowledged. Similarly, the notion of the 'health promoting school' centres on the implementing of environmental measures to support health teaching: for example, attempts by teachers to enhance the self-esteem of pupils may well be defeated in schools which appear to value only high academic achievers.

Returning to Figure 1.2, it will be apparent that education is shown as having a four-fold function. One of these relates to individual decision making; a second is concerned with the development and appropriate use of health services; two functions relate to the implementation of healthy public policy. These different functions are often associated with different 'models' of health education and will be explored later.

The two related processes of lobbying and advocacy are shown in Figure 1.2 as directed at influencing health and social policy. Lobbying is a traditional avenue for those seeking to influence policy. It is defined here as any attempt by individuals or organized interest groups to exert pressure on those having the power to introduce new policy or change existing policies. Advocacy is a particular variety of lobbying and, although the term is open to more than one interpretation, advocates have one trait in common: they actively seek to represent the interest of relatively under-privileged groups and thus redress, at least in part, imbalances in power.

Advocates have, by definition, greater power than their clients and particular skills which they put at their clients' disposal. The reality is, however, that even highly competent advocates may make little impact on dominant power structures. Indeed, in a recent critique of the notion of advocacy, Barić (1988) commented on the recently published Acheson Report on Public Health in the UK. This Report proposed the establishment of directors of public health who might reasonably have

been expected to have an advocacy function. However, these new public health specialists, unlike their forebears – the medical officers of health – were effectively forbidden from challenging authority even though to do so might well be in the public interest.

Both lobbying and advocacy figured prominently in the Ottawa Charter, along with 'mediation', as devices for influencing healthy public policy. The notion of mediation is useful since it reminds us that in the arena of conflicting demands for policy implementation, mediation between opposing interests is often a necessity. The result of such negotiation and bargaining is frequently compromise – as for instance when government negotiates 'voluntary agreements' with the tobacco lobby over restrictions in advertising.

Although there have been important instances of powerful bodies interceding on behalf of the disadvantaged and unhealthy – for example, the British Medical Association and the Church of England (Canterbury, 1985) have taken up the cudgels on behalf of a socioeconomic underclass – such efforts tend to merely dent the dominant ideology of prevailing power structures. For these reasons, we are here underlining the potential importance of health education as a means of creating public pressure to generate more fundamental change in health and social policy. Before examining this function, further consideration will be given to the importance of policy in health promotion.

THE PRIMACY OF POLICY IN HEALTH PROMOTION

Milio (1986), in an influential book on the subject, reminds us that, 'Most, if not all, of the variations in the modern illness profiles of men and women ... can be understood as responses to the differing environments which they ... typically experience'. She suggests two ways in which health promoting policy might be developed. First, a principle of equity might guide policy formation such that all groups of people might be exposed to the '... **same** excesses and deficits of **both** health-promoting and health-damaging circumstances'. Alternatively:

> Policy ... might be developed with a view of some attainable optimum in health, for instance, the level achieved by some groups (within the USA) or by certain other nations. Not only would all people be equally exposed to the pluses and minuses of environment, but the policy objectives would center on minimizing health-damaging circumstances and on minimizing or eliminating both excesses and deficits of health-promoting resources, such as selected food and energy supplies.
>
> *(p. 71)*

Healthy public policy is at the heart of an ecological approach to health promotion such as that embodied in the Ottawa Charter. In its list of prerequisites for health, the Charter demonstrates the breadth and scope of its conceptualization of health and social policy. It includes: food and education; shelter; a stable ecosystem and sustainable resources; peace; equity and justice. Central to the attainment of all these policy goals is the imperative of redistributing economic resources. If a reminder of the significance of the Charter's assertions should be needed, a particularly timely jog to the memory was recently provided by Doll in his Stallones Memorial Lecture (1992). In this he concludes that '... the principal environmental hazards worldwide are those associated with poverty of individuals within the market economy and of communities in the developing countries...'. In future, '... they will be the effects of overpopulation and the production of greenhouse gases'.

In a very real sense, then, economic policy is health policy. It is, therefore, especially appropriate that the World Health Organization has emphasized the importance of taking account of the health dimensions of economic reform (WHO, 1992) – especially in relation to developing countries. The notion of 'health conditionality' should be applied to all economic developments. In other words, the implications for health of any economic measure should be considered at the very start of the planning process and should be taken into account at the development and implementation stages of planning; '... the objective of economic decision making should from the beginning include the objective of protecting and promoting the quality of life' (WHO, 1992, p. ix).

Anderson and Draper (1991) have adopted an even more radical stance and called for a fundamental review of economic policy. They have, *inter alia*, called for a rethink in the way we define economic benefits. Of particular interest for this book, they have argued for the replacement of inappropriate indicators, such as gross national product (GNP), with new measures of economic success which are congruent with the goals of health promotion.

It was clear from the Black Report and the subsequent publication of *The Health Divide* that ill health and preventable death was associated with socioeconomic disadvantage; it was also clear that the gap between privileged and disadvantaged sectors of society in the UK had actually increased in recent times (Townsend and Davidson, 1992; Whitehead, 1992). Although the evidence on which both these reports was based is substantially unassailable, government felt it necessary to resist the implications of the reports on both financial and ideological grounds.

The financial basis for ignoring the uncomfortable evidence embodied in the Black Report and *The Health Divide* (and indeed, the whole overwhelming mass of international evidence leading to similar conclusions) is patently clear. As the UK Secretary of State's response to the Black Report in 1980 stated: '... additional expenditure on the scale which

could result from the report's recommendations – the amount involved could be upwards of 2 billion a year – is quite unrealistic'
(Townsend and Davidson, 1992, p. 31).

It would, indeed, be a brave government –
some might say suicidal – which would be
prepared to court electoral resentment at the
kinds of fiscal policy needed to redistribute
wealth. Governments of all political persu-
asions might feel it wiser to have recourse to
pious hopes of achieving some future economic growth which would allow them to
improve the status of the impoverished by
the familiar but dubious mechanism of
'trickle down'!

It is, of course, much more convenient
when ideology can be used as a basis for
inaction. The relevant ideological arguments
have been well rehearsed. They usually
centre on commitment to the values of robust
individualism and enterprise. It is considered
to be not only possible but actually a worthwhile and edifying experience to rise above
poverty and achieve success. Such points of
view are typically buttressed by assertions
that it is in fact possible (by employing
appropriate management skills) to live on
state benefits. An equally popular rationalization is that there is, anyway, no genuine
poverty in today's western democracies
(compared, say, with previous eras or with
the current situation in developing countries).
Reference will be made to the former claim
later in this chapter.

As for the latter point, we might note
Wilkinson's (1992) observations on the impact
of inequality on national mortality rates. He
notes the argument that poverty is relative
and, therefore, relatively small health gains
would be achieved in developed countries by
spending large amounts of money on a very
small minority of the really poor. However,
he goes on to argue convincingly that, in
wealthier countries, it is in fact **relative** deprivation which is associated with differential
health experience. He refers in particular to
the case of Japan:

In 1970 these two countries were much like
each other in terms of average life expectancy and income distribution, and in both
respects they were close to the center of the
field of OECD countries. Since then Japan's
income distribution has narrowed dramatically and is now the narrowest of any
recorded in the United Nations Human
Development Report. Over the same period,
Japan's life expectancy has increased at an
unprecedented rate and is now the highest
on record. [He goes on to suggest that] If
the United States or Britain were to adopt
an income distribution more like that of
Japan, Sweden or Norway, the indications
are that it might add two years to average
life expectancy.

A detailed analysis of policy and the social
context of health is, of course, beyond the
scope of this book. Nonetheless, an emphasis
on the primacy of policy has been justified for
two reasons: first as a reminder of its significance along with education in the development of effective health promotion. Second,
it signals the importance of education in
creating conditions where it might be possible
for government to exercise 'political will' in
reducing health damaging differentials in
socioeconomic status. Indeed, it may well be
the case that education will prove to be the
key ingredient for addressing the relationship
between health and perceptions of deprivation which figure in the scenario of relative
disadvantage to which reference was made
above. We will, accordingly, consider different approaches to health education and their
associated ideologies.

HEALTH EDUCATION: MODELS AND IDEOLOGIES

We earlier asserted that the synergistic relationship between healthy public policy and
health education provided the substantive
basis for health promotion. Figure 1.2 depicted the anatomy of this relationship and

showed health education as having four main functions. However, if we are to base our discussion of evaluation on a firm foundation, we must consider not only function but the values underlying function. For instance, we could say that health education has been successful if it raises awareness and leads to the implementation of policy: yet we identified in Figure 1.2 two varieties of awareness raising – agenda setting and critical consciousness raising. These two functions differ not only in their goals but in their ideological disposition. Again, we might say that professional education and training has been effective if professionals have acquired certain skills. However, supposing that those skills helped the professionals coerce and manipulate patients into unthinkingly complying with medical advice – could we really say that the enterprise had been successful? While the learning might have been efficient, the education would have been a failure when judged by the ideological criteria of health promotion. In short, the result would probably have been poor patient participation and disempowerment.

Again, in Figure 1.2, one of the functions of health education is shown as empowering and supporting individual choice – a goal which is clearly consistent with the principles of health promotion. Does this therefore mean that there is no place for persuasion?

These issues outlined above are all issues of ideology rather than technology. They are concerned with such questions as, what is the purpose of health education? What is the ethically appropriate stance for health educators? Clearly, 'technical' matters are also important. Whatever the ideology espoused, there are technically appropriate and inappropriate ways of seeking to achieve ideological goals. To embark on an ideologically immaculate health education enterprise without the necessary technical knowledge and skill is sheer incompetence – and unethical! A technical definition of health education is certainly relatively easy to provide. In fact,

before exploring the ideological intricacies of certain 'models' of health education, a technical definition will be offered as follows:

> Health education is any intentional activity which is designed to achieve health or illness related learning, i.e. some relatively permanent change in an individual's capability or disposition. Effective health education may, thus, produce changes in knowledge and understanding or ways of thinking; it may influence or clarify values; it may bring about some shift in belief or attitude; it may facilitate the acquisition of skills; it may even effect changes in behaviour or lifestyle.

The task of evaluating health education – as defined above – would then be to determine to what extent health or illness related learning had in fact taken place.

More typically, though, health education is not defined in such a neutral fashion. Indeed, attempts at definition are frequently characterized by dialectical dispute and divisive debate and the adoption of one definition or other reflects the ideological differences of its practitioners. It is hardly surprising, then, that typologies of health education have been based on philosophy rather than function, on values rather than on learning theory. However, before discussing some of the ideological bases for different 'models' of health education, it is worth reiterating the point that whatever the model adopted, the technical definition presented above holds true. The learning goals will be determined by ideology but the mechanisms of human learning remain the same.

A comprehensive account of contemporary models of health education is beyond the scope of this book. Several interesting analyses have been provided (for example, Draper *et al.*, 1980; Draper, 1983; French and Adams, 1986). More recently, Beattie (1991) has offered a 'structural map' which adopts a cross-classification device identifying two bipolar dimensions which are considered to account for major ideological stances in health promotion. The dimensions in question refer to 'focus of intervention' and 'mode of intervention'. The former has as its bipolar opposites an individually focused approach compared with a collective focus. Mode of intervention is characterized by either an authoritarian 'top-down' mode or, by contrast, a 'negotiated' or participative mode of functioning. Permutation of these two dimensions generates four preferred strategies: health persuasion techniques; legislative action for health; personal counselling for health; community development. These different strategies will doubtless be recognizable in the models to be discussed below.

Beattie has also provided an interesting historical analysis of the development of different ideological commitments over the years and it is worth noting that different 'philosophies' have underpinned health education according to the relative power of different ideologies.

It is clear then from even a cursory glance at models of health education that choice of model reflects underlying ideology. This is true whether the model in question has been explicitly, consciously and lovingly developed or, alternatively, is merely implicit in practice. Frequently these underlying values reflect either some dominant ideology or, conversely, represent a radical challenge to a dominant ideology. In recent years we have witnessed a kind of ideological progression from an individualistically focused and medically dominated health education towards a more 'enlightened' radical approach – which happens to be congruent with the ideological basis of the principles of health promotion outlined earlier. Rodmell and Watt (1986) have described the former approach as 'conventional health education' which they, with some justification, berate for its 'lifestylism' and victim blaming. However, the notion of some kind of steady progress – ideologically speaking – from authoritarian victim blaming to politically radical client

empowerment is an over-simplification (Tones, 1990). Similarly, an unsophisticated approach to analysing the nature of individually focused health education and various collective initiatives can lead to false dichotomies. This will hopefully become apparent after we have further considered different approaches to health education, of which the first is the celebrated – and frequently maligned – medical model.

THE PREVENTIVE MODEL

The term 'model' is often used in a rather too casual fashion. It is a theory driven construct which, ideally, encapsulates the essential elements of the theoretician's formulation of a particular aspect of reality. A good model will not only incorporate the essence of the construct, it will also represent reality in a simplified form. This simplification should, hopefully, clarify thinking and facilitate planning.

This book is concerned with two varieties of model: ideological models and technical models. In this chapter we are considering ideological constructions of reality: in other words, we are seeking to provide a simplified version of people's beliefs about the purpose of health education and the values loading those beliefs.

The first model to be proposed derives from that well established construct, the 'medical model'. The characteristics of this model are sufficiently well known not to need elaboration here. It may be summarized as having a mechanistic focus on microcausality; the body is viewed as a machine whose component parts are subject to attack from microbes or other pathogens. The prime function of medicine is to repair the machine when it malfunctions and to keep it in good running order. Health tends to be defined in terms of absence of disordered functioning.

Apart from its focus on object rather than person – its enthusiasm for investigating the component part at the most reductionist level

– the medical model has also been associated with another significant ideological imperative – the tendency for western medicine to lay claim to ever larger areas of human experience. As we have seen, the health promotion movement, with its emphasis on reorientation of health services and lay competence, has provided a fundamental challenge to this process of medicalization. In doing so it was, of course, following the rather more vitriolic example set by Illich (1976).

In case the ideological basis of what lay people in western society would regard as a perfectly normal way of thinking about health is not absolutely clear, it is worth recalling Doyal's (1981) lucid review of the ways in which health and illness are socially constructed. As she points out, the functional definition of health by medicine reflects a capitalist value system which '... defines people primarily as producers...' and is '... concerned with their "fitness" in an instrumental sense, rather than with their own hopes, fears, anxieties, pain or suffering'. Doyal cites Stark (1977) as follows:

> Disease is understood as a failure in and of the individual, an isolatable 'thing' that attacks the physical machine more or less arbitrarily from 'outside' preventing it from fulfilling its essential 'responsibilities'. Both bourgeois epidemiology and 'medical ecology' ... consider 'society' only as a relatively passive medium through which 'germs' pass en route to the individual.

The preventive model of health education, by definition, is concerned to contribute to the goals of preventive medicine and would thus be subject to the same ideological objections as the medical model proper. It would, however, be wrong to assume that the goals of health education and prevention were necessarily congruent with the dominant ideology of medicine (for which read **curative** medicine). Rather it represented a revisionist tendency, a point which merits a little further consideration.

The history of preventive medicine in the late 19th and the 20th centuries may be rather simply described as revealing a decline in the public health movement paralleled by the ascendancy of curative medicine. With the rising incidence of chronic degenerative disease, preventive medicine enjoyed something of a revival at the same time as the hegemony of curative medicine was increasingly being challenged – primarily by public health doctors. McKeown's (1979) critique is now well known and generally accepted. Professor Knox succinctly described medicine's contribution to the public health in a tribute to McKeown shortly after the latter's death:

> Before 1900, doctors probably did more harm than good; between 1900 and 1930, they broke even; only since 1930, by which time the major health improvements of the present era were established, was it clear that doctors were beginning to win.

Doctors such as Cochrane (1972) also began to ask rather awkward questions about the effectiveness of many routinely accepted medical procedures and writers such as McKeown also suggested that curative medicine was not only experiencing some difficulty with chronic degenerative diseases, it was also neglecting its traditional caring functions. He detected a '... new note of severity in contemporary criticism' of medicine and, rather mischievously, quoted Nancy Mitford's comparison of medical practice in the time of Louis XIV with the contemporary activities of curative medicine:

> In those days, terrifying in black robes and bonnets, they bled the patient; now terrifying in white robes and masks, they pump blood into him. The result is the same: the strong live; the weak, after much suffering and expense, both of spirit and money, die.
>
> *(Mitford, 1969)*

The justification for health education's contribution to preventive medicine may be summarized as follows:

1. Curative medicine has a limited capability for managing the major (western) burden of chronic degenerative disease and key infectious diseases such as AIDS. Moreover, its practice is characterized by accelerating costs and it incorporates not insubstantial iatrogenic 'side effects'.
2. Prevention is, therefore, better than cure. Since human behaviour plays a significant part in the aetiology and management of **all** diseases, education is needed to persuade people to behave appropriately.

Its functions in relation to the goals of preventive medicine are listed in Table 1.1.

After many years of neglect, the belated recognition of the importance of health education was greeted with a certain degree of satisfaction by health educators. Even so, the proportion of resources devoted by the UK health services to health education was still diminutive. Moreover, preventive medicine itself still occupied a relatively lowly position in the medical pecking order and its subsequent metamorphosis into community medicine did not necessarily improve matters. It remains to be seen whether the most recent change of name to public health medicine will signify a real rise in the status of public health.

Table 1.1 Health education and the preventive model

Level of prevention	*Function of health education*
Primary	
Concerned to prevent onset of disease; reduce incidence	Persuade individuals to adopt behaviours believed to reduce the risk of disease; adopt healthy lifestyle
	Persuade individuals to utilize preventive health services appropriately
	Concerned with **health behaviour**: those activities undertaken by individuals believing themselves to be healthy in order to prevent future health problems or detect them asymptomatically
Secondary	Persuade individuals to utilize screening services appropriately; learn appropriate self-care; seek early diagnosis and treatment
Concerned to prevent development of existing disease, minimize its severity, reverse its progress; reduce prevalence	Persuade individuals to comply with medical treatment and recommendations
	Concerned with **illness behaviour**: those activities undertaken by individuals experiencing symptoms in order to determine their state of health; subsequent adoption of measures designed to meet perceived needs
Tertiary	Persuade individuals to comply with medical treatment, including palliative measures, and adjust to limitations resulting from disease
Concerned to prevent deterioration, relapse and complications; promote rehabilitation; help adjustment to terminal conditions	Persuade patients to resume normal behaviours as appropriate
	Teach carers to respond appropriately to patient needs
	Provide terminal care counselling
	Concerned with adopting and relinquishing **sick role**

N.B. All three stages may involve provision of **anticipatory guidance**

At all events, the 1970s version of the preventive model of health education is currently experiencing a good deal of official support (ironically at a time when it is being subjected to vigorous criticism for its victim blaming tendency!). The reasons are quite clear: there is an assumption that money will be saved for the hard pressed medical services if people can be persuaded to adopt healthy lifestyles; there is some degree of consumerist challenge to the status and alleged restrictive practices of medicine. But above all, the approach is deemed to be ideologically sound in an individualistic enterprise oriented culture.

In the context of our earlier discussion of the ideological principles of health promotion, it is not surprising that the preventive model of health education has come under attack in recent years. In part, the critique has derived from a view that medicine has somehow 'hijacked' education as part of a process of professional medicalization (Vuori, 1980). Largely, however, dissatisfaction has centred on the preventive model's inherent victim blaming (Brown and Margo, 1978; Labonte and Penfold, 1981; Coreil and Levin, 1985). Historically the challenge is associated with Zola's celebrated 'river analogy' of medical care (Zola (1970) cited by McKinlay (1979)). This parable describes a doctor's increasingly frenzied rescue efforts as (s)he struggles to drag drowning people from the flood. The doctor remarks, 'You know, I am so busy jumping in, pulling them to shore, applying artificial respiration, that I have no time to see who the hell is upstream pushing them all in'.

McKinlay considered the individually directed approach of health education as a 'downstream' endeavour. He pointed out the ultimate futility of this kind of strategy and argued that we should '... cease our preoccupation with this short-term problem-specific tinkering and begin focusing our attention upstream'. Pursuing the nautical metaphor, and using a currently popular image, the preventive model of health education may be likened to the rearranging of the deck chairs on the Titanic.

Before considering an alternative 'radical' model, it may be useful to consider the technical educational implications of adopting a preventive model. In other words, it will be revealing in the light of discussion of technical models in Chapter 3 to consider briefly what would be involved in terms of communication, education and learning when the goals of preventive education are translated into practice.

The essential elements of the educational process are presented schematically in Figure 1.3. It has not infrequently been assumed that

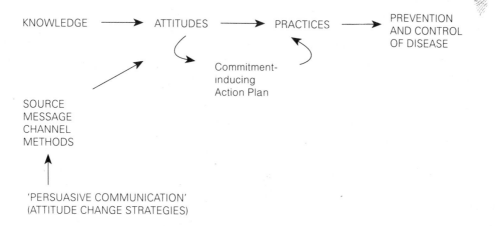

Figure 1.3 Prevention: the educational process.

if people are provided with health information, they will act on the knowledge gained
and behave 'rationally'. In this case rational
action is assumed to involve the adoption of
medically approved preventive behaviours.
Usually, though, it is understood that knowledge alone is insufficient to trigger preventive practices and that some device is needed
to motivate action and generate positive
attitudes. The K $\rightarrow$ P formula is thus converted into K $\rightarrow$ A $\rightarrow$ P (Knowledge –
Attitude – Practice). This formula, although
extremely simplistic, forms the basis for the
scheme shown in Figure 1.3.

The adoption of proper behaviours (which,
if there are enough of these, may be defined
as a healthy lifestyle) is considered to be
'proper' insofar as the behaviours lead to the
prevention of disease at primary, secondary
or tertiary levels, as indicated in Table 1.1.
The provision of knowledge is not important
for its own sake but only for its contribution
to the approved behavioural outcome. The
central focus is quite clearly the attitude
change strategy which is designed to galvanize the individual into action. The health
educator is therefore called upon to supply
whatever attitude change methods are available in the armamentarium. For instance,
'persuasive communication' tactics derived
from the Yale–Hovland school might be employed; attractive and credible communicators will be used to deliver the message
which will have been carefully structured to
achieve maximum attitude change. The right
level of fear appeal will have been calculated;
measures will have been taken to minimize
'reactance' and the audience will have been
carefully 'innoculated' against counter-
communications by the judicious provision of
a two-sided message (in which the counter-
argument will have been presented in an
attenuated form together with the information needed to refute it). An appropriate
communication channel will be selected –
possibly a form of group teaching with a
track record of successful attitude change.

This technique could, additionally, be delivered in the context of a mass media
campaign in accordance with the dictates of
social marketing theory (to which some
critical reference will be made in Chapter 8).

The nature and limitations of attitude
change strategies have been thoroughly
appraised both in general and, occasionally,
in the context of health education (McGuire,
1981; Zimbardo *et al.*, 1977; Kar, 1976; Flay
et al., 1980). Our present purpose, however, is
not primarily to consider the detailed
mechanism of communication and educational techniques but rather to contemplate
the ideological basis for selecting one set of
techniques over another – and, of course, to
comment on the implications of this choice
for evaluating effectiveness. We will therefore
turn now to an alternative philosophy and
discuss the main features of a more radical
ideological stance for health education.

THE RADICAL MODEL

The adjective 'radical' has been chosen as a
label for the model to be discussed now.
Bearing in mind Zola's exhortation to 'refocus
upstream', we might reasonably have called
it an 'upstream model' to distinguish it from
the preventive approach discussed above.
Acknowledging the primacy of social and
environmental influences on health, we might
alternatively have designated it a 'social–
structural' model of health education – or, in
recognition of a need for collective action to
influence health and social policy, we could
have used the term 'collectivist'. As it is, and
after etymological consideration, we have
employed the word 'radical' to indicate a
need to scrutinize the roots of health problems
and develop educational programmes accordingly. It might be argued that this is rather a
weak justification since advocates of the
preventive model would probably consider
the roots of ill health were to be found in an
individual's errors of omission or commission.
However, the notion of radicalism can also

serve to indicate a challenge to a dominant ideology (in this case, the preventive medical model).

That the origins of health and disease are social, cultural, environmental is a point that has already been made – and perhaps even laboured. If by way of example we consider what is arguably the most important of all public health measures – promoting good nutritional status – then individual dietary choice must always be considered in the context of proper access to supplies of healthy food. In an age of recurrent cycles of famine in developing countries, this observation is almost platitudinous! On the other hand, the issue is less clearcut in wealthy industrialized nations where we frequently witness a clash of ideologies in the explanation of poor nutrition. The debate is well illustrated – or even caricatured – by the pontifications of a former UK junior minister of health. It is, of course, a matter of epidemiological record that the diet in northern Britain is more unhealthy by and large than that of the (wealthier) south east of the country. The minister's advice to northerners was that they should act responsibly and eat prudently. The scarcely disguised implication of the exhortation was that failure to eat sensibly was due to ignorance at best and, at worst, fecklessness.

What is clear from research, however, is that the problem is not primarily due to ignorance. Moreover, if poor diet is related to any personal characteristic of the individual, that personality trait is not fecklessness. As we will see later, it would be more legitimate to ascribe unhealthy behaviours to general apathy and 'learned helplessness' resulting from chronic exposure to debilitating social conditions – and lack of money.

The importance of social and structural factors in determining whether or not individuals select and eat a prudent diet is certainly well documented. Charles and Kerr's (1986) research demonstrates categorically that women – the dietary 'gatekeepers' in most cultures – are well aware of the difference between healthy and unhealthy food. Although they might not possess detailed technical knowledge, they not only knew enough to produce nutritionally sound meals for their families, they were positively motivated to do so. They were, however, prevented from doing this by a series of barriers, of which one was quite simply the financial cost of healthy meals.

It is, of course, naive to argue that cost is the only barrier to the adoption of healthy behaviour in general and sensible eating in particular. It is nonetheless of paramount importance. Lang *et al.* (1984), for instance, demonstrated convincingly that in Britain, healthy food was both more expensive and less accessible for people living in disadvantaged circumstances. More recently the National Consumer Council (1992) commented that the cost of food in local corner shops was at least 20% more expensive than in (frequently less accessible) supermarkets. It noted too that 47% of families seeking help from the Family Welfare Association did not have enough money for food after paying for rent, fuel and other necessities. More than half were £10 per week short. The Council also argued that, contrary to popular belief, poor people often adopt a very rational course of action in managing their limited resources: they acquire more nutrients per penny than those who are better off. Unfortunately, in doing so, they exist on a diet high in sugar and saturated fats and low in fruit and vegetables.

VICTIM BLAMING AND RADICAL IDEOLOGY

We have already observed how the preventive model of health education relates to its bedfellow the medical model (though not always very comfortably). We also noted its relationship to the process of medicalization while commenting on the status of the medical model as the dominant ideology of health. In the context of our present discussion of radical ideology embodied in the radical model of health education, it is appropriate at this juncture to remark on the close ties between the values and beliefs underlying the individually focused preventive imperative and the key western ideology of capitalism.

In short, capitalism and the pursuit of profit are viewed as intrinsically unhealthy. For instance, concern for the environment is of secondary importance to profit; the workplace is frequently a source of illness (Watterson, 1986); the enterprise culture gives virtually free rein to the marketing of products irrespective of their effects on health. Indeed, it can be argued that health and wealth are in some fundamental way incompatible (Draper *et al.*, 1977). This point of view is, of course, central to Marxist tradition. As de Kadt (1982) succinctly points out:

> ... they see ideologies as weapons in the class struggle whereby, for example, hegemonic groups portray reality in such a way as to make those dominated conform to their fate, which may then give rise to 'false consciousness' on the part of the latter.

He goes on to cite the Communist Party Manifesto:

> ... the ruling ideas of each age have ever been the ideas of its ruling class.

Given the ideological cooperation of medical model and 'enterprise culture', it is not surprising that the dominant viewpoint in health is that individuals are responsible for their own health. Accordingly, a preventive model of health education stands accused of 'victim blaming' and collusion with the dominant ideology. Note, for instance, Navarro's often quoted attack on 'conventional' health education:

> ... rather than weakening, [health education] ... strengthens the basic tenets of bourgeois individualism ... far from being a threat to the power structure, this lifestyle

politics complements and is easily cooptable by the controllers of the system.

> *(Navarro, 1976)*

Given the nature and vehemence of this radical challenge to the twin dominant ideologies of 'conventional' health education and capitalism, it is hardly surprising that the individual focus of the preventive model of health education should be dismissed as 'victim blaming'. Later in this chapter, we will be mooting the possibility of some kind of 'reconciliation' between dominant and radical ideologies and calling for a critical reassessment of the often intolerant and doctrinaire assertions made about victim blaming. Before doing that, it may be beneficial to remind ourselves of the origin and meaning of the term, as coined by Ryan (1976).

Victim blaming, according to Ryan, is a tendency which relates not only to health and illness but is at the heart of many contemporary social phenomena such as crime, poverty and racism. In common with Navarro, Ryan views victim blaming as an ideological process which serves to justify inequalities in society, including inequalities in health. Inequality is not merely a regrettable byproduct of the pursuit of wealth but is an essential and enduring feature of capitalism. He describes John D. Rockefeller celebrating the virtues of inequality in Sunday school:

> The growth of a large business is merely a survival of the fittest ... The American Beauty rose can be produced in the splendor and fragrance which bring cheer to its beholder only by sacrificing the early buds which grow up around it. This is not an evil tendency in business. It is merely the working out of a law of nature and a law of God.

> *(p. 21)*

We should note that the crude social darwinism expressed by Rockefeller is not, according to Ryan, victim blaming proper. Victim blaming is espoused by liberal socially concerned professionals who are genuinely committed to deal with the effects of inequality and help its victims. Their victim blaming lies in the fact that they concentrate on the victims and seek to help them through variously individually focused enterprises. Their failure results from their not tackling the social origins of the problem.

For Ryan, the solution is dramatically simple: he encapsulates it in a subsection of his book entitled 'In Praise of Loot and Clout'. Power and money, in effect, provide the solution to the problem of inequality and its byproducts. In support of this contention he quotes the vaudeville star Fanny Brice's celebrated aphorism: 'I've been rich', she said, 'and I've been poor; and, believe me, rich is better'.

Ryan elaborates on the effects of poverty:

Being poor is stressful. Being poor is worrisome; one is anxious about the next meal, the next dollar, the next day. Being poor is nerve-wracking, upsetting. When you're poor, it's easy to despair and it's easy to lose your temper. And all of this is because you're poor. Not because your mother let you go around with your diapers full of bowel movement until you were four; or shackled you to the potty chair before you could walk. Not because she broke your bottle on your first birthday or breast-fed you until you could cut your own steak. But because you don't have any *money*.

(p. 157)

Ryan's scathing attack on essentially psychological (or rather psychoanalytic) remedies to social problems is undoubtedly timely. It is not possible to deny the central importance of poverty in the aetiology of social problems generally and health problems in particular. However, to argue only for a shift in the distribution of wealth as a solution to these problem is both politically problematic and technically naive, as we will later indicate. For the present, we will compare the educational requirements of the radical model with the educational process considered appropriate to a preventive approach and defined in Figure 1.3 earlier. In doing so, it may be revealing to consider possible similarities between the educational activities of those seeking to achieve the old public health and the proposals for educational action advocated by the proponents of the new public health.

There are indeed many interesting parallels between the first public health movement and the doctrine of health promotion. For instance, the sanitary reforms of the 19th century were associated with a general reforming zeal directed at the overall squalor, poverty and poor working conditions of the populace. Moreover, the reformers met with vigorous opposition and, as is the case today, their demand for state intervention was seen as ideologically unsound. We have already noted Rockefeller's recourse to social darwinism to support his Panglossian assertion that all is for the best in the best of possible worlds. In the 19th century, the writings of Herbert Spencer were used to show how poverty was part of the natural order of things (a role played today by appropriately selected economists). Again the perceived threat to profit stimulated angry reactions from commercial interests.

Health education was not recognized as such but health 'propagandism' and pamphleteering were in evidence – and greatly resented! Sutherland (1979) quotes a petulant article in *The Times* newspaper which declared that the people would '... prefer to take the chance of cholera and the rest than to be bullied into health' (p. 7). Incidentally, Sutherland also described a rather nice example of early 19th century victim blaming when he referred to the Manchester and Salford Sanitary Association's employment of working class women as indigenous health education aides to teach the 'laws of health' to the poor! We might also note the suggestion that one of the most significant influences on public health reforms was the perception by the wealthy that **they** were at risk from the unrest and diseases of the underclass – a matter of some significance for contemporary realpolitik! At all events, the pamphleteering of the 19th century would appear to have points in common with the radical health education process of modern times. The term which is most fittingly used for this process is critical consciousness raising (CCR); it was used in Figure 1.2 to describe health education's main radical thrust.

The term critical consciousness raising is inextricably associated with Freire's notion of *conscientização* ('... the development of the awakening of critical awareness', Freire (1974), p. 19). Freire contrasts critical consciousness raising with 'magical consciousness' which apprehends facts and fatalistically attributes them to some superior power. 'Naive consciousness', on the other hand, involves a more realistic perception of causality but accepts it uncritically. In other words it represents the 'false consciousness' of those who have accepted the rightful reality of a dominant ideology.

The purpose of CCR is to help people break free of false consciousness and it does so by using a four-step process:

1. Fostering reflection on aspects of personal reality;
2. Encouraging a search for, and collective identification of, the root causes of that reality;
3. Examination of implications;
4. Development of a plan of action to alter reality.

This integral process of planning and action rooted in critical reflection was referred to as praxis by Freire. The techniques and methods employed centred on group work ('culture circles') and used a 'dialectical' problem solving approach to discussion. A more comprehensive discussion of Freire's radical strategy is beyond the scope of this book. However, Minkler and Cox (1980) provide a succinct analysis of the approach with case studies of work in Honduras and San Francisco. Macdonald and Warren (1991) also offer a useful application of Freirean theory to primary health care.

Insofar as the radical model's main educational process is critical consciousness raising, then the essential elements would be as presented in Figure 1.4. It will be apparent that there are certain important differences

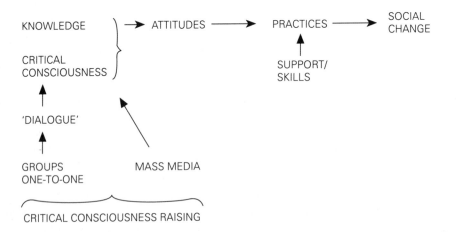

Figure 1.4 A radical approach: the educational process.

between Figure 1.4 and the schematic outline of the educational process associated with the preventive model. Although the basic 'K-A-P' formula may be discerned, the **quality** of the knowledge is distinctly different. As a result of the process of critical consciousness raising, those who have participated in the group dialogue will have not only a deeper understanding of their circumstances (as opposed to their personal risk) but also some important beliefs about self, i.e. their capacity to influence their circumstances. Again the implications of praxis are not at first glance dissimilar to the action planning built into the process of attitude change central to a preventive model. However, the commitment is to social rather than personal change.

Clearly educational methodology is different. Attitude change techniques are replaced by interactions in a face-to-face or group setting designed to challenge the status quo. Group teaching and face-to-face tactics may also be used to service the preventive model but their purpose is persuasion rather than enlightenment. Similarly, mass media may be employed but persuasive 'social marketing' would be replaced by an agenda setting or consciousness raising media function. In practice, of course, since mass media are frequently controlled by representatives of the dominant ideology, the utilization of media for consciousness raising is likely to be a subversive and 'underground' activity!

The implication of what has been said so far about the Freirean approach might lead to the conclusion that in challenging the dominant ideology and presenting an alternative meaning system, the radical model is in some way educating rather than persuading; is providing a 'true' picture of reality. This is not necessarily the case. As de Kadt (1982) notes:

In post-revolutionary situations, in countries with Marxist governments, *conscientisación* may be bound up with wider political activities and mobilization behind the party line. ... Freire insists that people must be allowed to discover things for themselves, that meanings must not be imposed for them on their world. Yet, of course, the discussion leader cannot but make available certain facts, give certain leads, encourage certain interpretations, which effectively turn the perception of the 'learners' in certain directions. This is above all true for the party militant, mobilizing the people for a particular social transformation. One type of consciousness is thereby replaced by another ... the new consciousness will also be a partial interpretation of reality. It may show little realism about the obstacles that stand in the way of changing present structures, or may provide little more than ringing generalizations and abstractions about the social arrangements to replace those at present stigmatized.

(p. 743)

Again, although on occasions Freire would aim to provide actual skills to those whose consciousness has been raised (after all, his original programme was concerned with adult literacy), there is no guarantee that the learners will have been equipped to change social circumstances. Apart from any possible misrepresentations of reality created by the teacher-activist, merely to raise consciousness in a general oppressive environment is considerably more unethical than victim blaming.

There are two alternative and, preferably, complementary strategies which might be adopted to handle the problem raised above. The first of these takes us back to our discussion of the Ottawa Charter. If consciousness raising is insufficient to bring about change at grassroots level, then attempts might be made to raise the consciousness of those who do possess power in a social system with a view to having them act as advocates for the disadvantaged. Given that this stratagem may not always achieve desired results, an alternative or additional approach would involve equipping learners

with a range of **empowering skills** which might improve their chances of influencing their environmental circumstances. This notion will receive further consideration in a later chapter when we examine community development. For the present, it serves as an introduction to the next health education model which we are to consider: a self-empowerment model.

EMPOWERMENT AND THE LIMITS TO CHOICE

One of the most significant values underpinning health education practice (at least, at a theoretical level!) is that of voluntarism. Tones (1987) argued that the principle of voluntarism was integral to what might be called an 'educational model' of health education. This derives in part from the views of philosophers of education, such as Hirst (1969), who considered that the cardinal characteristic of education was rationality and freedom of choice. The definitional criteria of education typically incorporate notions of an ethically acceptable goal and morally justifiable methods. The learner must fully comprehend what was happening to him or her during the educational process. Accordingly any kind of coercion – including persuasion – was by definition unacceptable.

Several 'official' health education pronouncements acknowledged this voluntaristic principle. The North American Society of Public Health Educators' Code of Ethics talked about informed consent and 'change by choice, not by coercion' (SOPHE, 1976). Green and Kreuter's (1991) oft quoted definition of health education incorporated the principle of voluntarism:

> In short, health education is aimed primarily at the voluntary actions people can take on their own, individually or collectively, as citizens looking after their own health or as decision makers looking after the health of others and the common good of the community.
>
> *(p. 14)*

At first glance, this 'educational model' might seem to be identical to the K-A-P formula – but without the 'A'! Indeed, it might also appear that the 'P' had been omitted too, since the concern appeared to be to provide knowledge and understanding while leaving the choice of action to the free will of the individual. This, of course, is not the case, as Figure 1.5 shows.

Indeed, a comparison of Figures 1.4 and 1.5 reveals that, if anything, the educational methods recommended for the voluntaristic

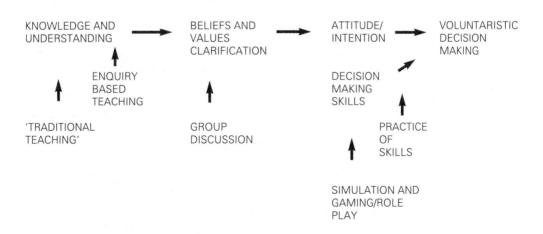

Figure 1.5 Voluntarism and the educational process.

educational approach are more sophisticated than those of the radical model. Clearly **understanding** is emphasized in relation to the knowledge (K) component but this would be supplemented by an insistence that learners go through a process of values and belief clarification before they are in a position to make a voluntaristic choice. The values clarification exercise would in turn require the use of group discussion, supplemented when required by an input of information involving either traditional teaching or individual student enquiry. If this educational process goes according to plan, students will have acquired necessary information, have gained a thorough understanding of all the relevant issues and clarified their beliefs and values and thus be in a state of readiness to make their decisions, either now or at some future time.

However, a more painstaking approach to education for choice would acknowledge the need for decision making **skills** (a rather vague notion but probably involving the acquisition of some sort of 'minimax' strategy for scanning alternative courses of action, calculating likely outcomes and comparing these with the values which have been previously clarified and then making an anticipatory decision designed to maximize benefits and minimize costs). Again this would require the use of 'informal' teaching techniques such as simulation, gaming or role play. A more refined version of the approach would go one stage further and build into the curriculum the possibility for practising decision making – typically in a simulated setting.

Now although this educational model is morally rather satisfying, it has its detractors. The first criticism might be levelled against an apparent assumption that education will have been successful provided only that the learners are in full possession of the facts, have an indepth understanding of the situation, have clarified their beliefs and values and acquired some practice in making decisions. In other words an implicit suggestion that it does not

matter what choice learners ultimately make so long as it is rationally based. Some of the exponents of the North American values clarification 'movement' were in fact taken to task over their apparent lack of interest in having a moral or ethical basis to their pedagogic concerns, apart from that of the process of values clarification itself. For example, Forcinelli (1974) took exception to the apparent amorality of the approach, noting that:

> … an educational system can produce a dishonest and potentially dysfunctional product and then merely say these are legitimate expressions of individual values. It is possible to conceive of one going through (a process of values clarification) and deciding that (s)he values intolerance or thieving.

It is, of course, legitimate to assert that the educational model described above can be applied to decisions about controversial issues, i.e. significant social issues on which different groups and individuals in society urge different and conflicting courses of action; and perhaps the prime example of such an approach in Britain has been the Humanities Curriculum Project (Stenhouse, 1969). Nonetheless, most projects which apparently operate in accordance with Figure 1.5 above would be firmly rooted, explicitly or implicitly, in quite conventional values. Many curriculum projects, for example, while emphasizing the importance of personal growth and fulfilment, actively promote respect and concern for other people's right to self-fulfilment. McPhail (1977) encapsulated this principle in the phrase 'considerate way of life' and this value would be intrinsic to all health education activities. It certainly underpins the supremely individualistic contribution to health promotion made by assertiveness training. Again, one of the most popular of the schools curriculum projects in Britain (Schools Council, 1977) not only urges a considerate way of life but also subscribes to a predominantly preventive medical paradigm.

It must therefore be acknowledged that the notion of freely choosing which seems to be at the heart of the educational model is, in fact, curtailed by moral imperatives. Its utility as a guide for health education planning is even more constrained by both a philosophical and common sense recognition that freedom of choice is a very rare commodity.

Clearly ignorance is a barrier to informed choice but ignorance is relatively easily rectified; certainly this particular obstacle poses no threat to the educational model. On the other hand a 'pure' educational approach would be unable to assist health educators to cope with two much more significant barriers to rational decision making: the first of these centres on individual limitations while the second reminds us again of the potentially unhealthy influence of environmental factors.

First, it is apparent that in many cases individuals are not free to choose: they may, for instance, lack the mental competence to make choices without damaging themselves or other people. Their freedom of choice may also be constrained by the presence of 'addictions' or other compulsive behaviours. As McKeown (1979) pointed out:

> ... it is said that the individual must be free to choose (whether he wishes to smoke). But he is not free; with a drug of addiction the option is open only at the beginning.
> *(p. 125)*

And, more subtlely, such aspects of personality as self-esteem or perceived locus of control will inevitably have an impact on genuine free choice.

As for the second problem for an educational model, the occasionally overwhelming obstacles to individual choice which are part and parcel of an oppressive environment should need no further elaboration.

There are three possible strategies which might be adopted to deal with these two barriers. The first of these draws on philosophical justifications for restricting individual choices. These are the principles of utilitarianism and paternalism. As we have seen, it is virtually axiomatic that individual freedom of choice must be curtailed when it is inconsistent with the 'considerate way of life'. The notion of utilitarianism thus asserts that people's freedom of action would be respected so long as it does not interfere with the **general** good. Utilitarian concerns may therefore be readily extended to restrain individuals' self-destructive behaviours on the grounds that the prudent in society should not be expected to pay for the excesses of the imprudent. It is actually not too difficult to demonstrate that most individual actions which do not conform to the dominant ideology have some sort of negative effect on the public good. The principle of paternalism states, quite simply, that it is quite legitimate for those possessing the necessary wisdom to act on behalf of those who, for whatever reason, are not capable of exercising choice – for the kinds of reason mentioned above.

The first course of action which might be taken to remedy deficiencies of the educational model would recommend the use of coercion to influence people's health and illness related behaviours. Traditionally this would involve a range of persuasive techniques. In other words, the principles of utilitarianism and paternalism are used to justify the adoption of a preventive medical model of health education. A rather more up-to-date solution, which has the advantage of apparently subscribing to the popular health promotion creed, involves implementing healthy public policy in such a way that the healthy choice becomes not merely the easy choice but the **only** choice!

The second course of action is quite simply stated. If the environment is the major barrier to health, then a radical model must be espoused – for the reasons stated earlier.

The third course of action seeks to remedy 'deficiencies' in the individual which militate against freedom of choice while at the same time employing strategies to manage environmental constraints. This is an 'empowerment model' of health education. Before discussing its ideological base and general features, however, we will give some thought to the characteristics of an empowered individual, i.e. the dynamics of self-empowerment.

THE DYNAMICS OF SELF-EMPOWERMENT

Earlier in this chapter, the centrality of empowerment to the ideology of health promotion was noted. Its contribution is represented schematically in Figure 1.6.

The underlying goal of health promotion is considered to be the achievement of equity, i.e. a fair distribution of power and resources. As we have seen, whether or not this goal is achieved depends on the environmental and social circumstances obtaining in a given country, city or neighbourhood. Physical environment, political system and a variety of socioeconomic features will either facilitate or militate against the achievement of health.

As regards empowerment, it can reasonably be argued that the state of empowerment

is fundamentally healthy and therefore worth pursuing in its own right. In Figure 1.6 its **instrumental** function is portrayed: an active, participating community (i.e. an empowered community) is a prerequisite for the development of healthy public policy.

A reciprocal relationship is deemed to exist between community empowerment and self-empowerment. An empowered community facilitates the development of self-empowerment in its members. On the other hand, although there is strength in numbers, an empowered community is no more than the sum total of its empowered members.

The relationship between people and their environment is also reciprocal. Clearly, the environment may exert a powerful controlling influence on people but people can also influence their environments. Two directions of popular influence on the environment are shown in Figure 1.6. An empowered community may exert pressure on government or other authorities in order to achieve the implementation of new health and social policy. Alternatively, a community might take direct action to improve its environment.

Individuals too may exert pressure for change through political channels – for

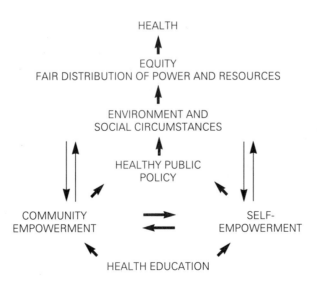

Figure 1.6 Health education, empowerment and health promotion.

example, by lobbying members of parliament or trade union officials. Again, at the micro level, individuals may battle against environmental circumstances in the pursuit of health. For instance, in the context of client contract behaviour modification, individuals might learn how to avoid environmental situations which trigger smoking or overeating; they might acquire skills in resisting social pressures to engage in unwanted sexual activities.

The major purpose of an empowerment model of health education in all this is primarily to raise awareness of key issues and provide those skills which are necessary for the development of both individual and community empowerment. Figure 1.7 identifies the major components of individual or self-empowerment. Embedded in this representation is the triangular relationship between

humans and their environment which figures prominently in social learning theory (and subsequently, social cognitive theory) and is associated with the work of Bandura (1977, 1982, 1986). One of these components is the environment itself – and the reciprocal relationship between the individual and the environment has already been mentioned. The second key element consists of a cluster of significant psychological characteristics. These are in turn related to the third element – the behaviours which act as a kind of interface between personality and the environment. These behaviours are described in Figure 1.7 as health and life skills. They comprise a wide variety of competences which facilitate environmental control, both directly and indirectly. A full discussion of life skills is not appropriate here but the

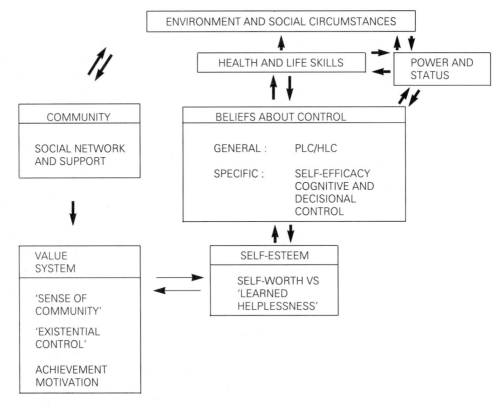

Figure 1.7 The dynamics of self-empowerment.

following list will serve to illustrate their nature.

1. How to communicate effectively.
2. How to make relationships.
3. How to manage conflict.
4. How to be assertive.
5. How to work in groups.
6. How to build strengths in others.
7. How to influence people and systems.

(Hopson and Scally, 1980)

The term 'health skill' is used here to refer to the application of life skills to specific health related situations; for instance, stress management skills or the use of assertiveness techniques to resist pressures to take drugs or to demand proper medical care from practitioners.

Although not normally used in this sense, life skills are also considered to incorporate 'self-regulatory' skills, i.e. techniques to help clients control various drives and urges or, more technically, to put them in charge of their own reinforcement (Kanfer and Karoly, 1972).

Central to the state of self-empowerment is a set of psychological attributes of which perhaps the most significant are beliefs about control. Langer (1983) provides a succinct definition of control as '... the active belief that one has a choice among responses that are differentially effective in achieving the desired outcome'. Various typologies of control have been provided by a number of authors and are discussed in further detail elsewhere (Tones, 1992). For instance, Sarafino (1990) compares 'informational' control (the possession of an opportunity to acquire information about, say, an aversive event) with 'decisional' control (the opportunity to make actual choice). Lewis (1986), in the context of providing anticipatory guidance for patients, refers to 'cognitive' control (the capacity intellectually to manage an event and thus reduce its threatening characteristics). This may be compared with 'behavioural' control in which the individual actually possesses some skill (e.g. a motor skill or health skill) which can provide some real, tangible control over events.

The notion of perceived locus of control (PLC) is perhaps the most widely known of the psychological constructs associated with beliefs about control. This key conceptualization is described by Rotter (1966) in a seminal article; the essence of the concept is clearly stated in Rotter's original definition:

> When a reinforcement is perceived by the subject as following some action of his own but not being entirely contingent upon his action, then, in our (US) culture, it is typically perceived as the result of luck, chance, fate, as under the control of powerful others, or as unpredictable because of the great complexity of the forces surrounding him. When the event is interpreted in this way by an individual, we have labelled this a belief in external control. If the person perceives that the event is contingent upon his own behavior or his own relatively permanent characteristics, we have termed this a belief in internal control.
>
> *(p. 1)*

It is worth noting that the emphasis is on **perceived** locus of control, i.e. a **belief** in capacity to control rather than actual possession of control capabilities. Moreover, these beliefs about control refer to reinforcement, that is, reward and/or punishment. For instance, an 'internal' differs from an 'external' in that (s)he is more inclined to believe that both the pleasant and unpleasant occurrences in life result from his or her own efforts. It is also important to note that these individual beliefs or expectancies are **generalized**: they refer to a general tendency to feel in control or, conversely, to feel powerless. They might therefore be usefully viewed as a personality trait or attribute.

The construct of locus of control merits a central place in any discussion of an empowerment model of health education; this is not only because of the pivotal role of control in empowered decision making but also because of its direct and indirect relationship to health. As indicated earlier, it is clearly possible to argue that a state of empowerment is *ipso facto* a state of health. It is equally clear that this assertion may be contested! However, it is much less contentious to argue that a complete feeling of powerlessness is unhealthy. Indeed, Seligman's (1975) notion of 'learned helplessness' could be described as the very antithesis of self-empowerment. In fact, Seligman provided a convincing argument that six major symptoms of learned helplessness had almost exact parallels in clinical depression.

More commonly, the relationship between locus of control and health is deemed to be mediated and investigation into the relationship between PLC and a number of health or illness related outcomes has been facilitated by the development of a number of psychometric scales. Rotter's original I-E Scale (1966) was later refined by Levenson (1973). It was not long before **health** locus of control (HLC) scales were also devised, largely by Wallston *et al.* (1976) and Wallston and Wallston (1978). Some reference will be made to the results of these investigations later in this chapter. For the present we will continue our review of key dynamics of self-empowerment by recording the importance of another significant control concept – that of 'self-efficacy'.

The construct of self-efficacy is associated with Albert Bandura (1977; 1982). Self-efficacy (or 'self-perceptions of efficacy') is, in effect, a belief. People who have self-efficacy expectations believe that they are capable of performing a given activity. The similarity of this concept to locus of control will be evident; the difference lies in the specificity of the former notion. Bandura's own elaboration of the concept is worthy of report:

Perceived self-efficacy is concerned with judgements of how well one can execute courses of action required to deal with prospective situations ... Self-percepts of efficacy are not simply inert estimates of future action. Self-appraisals of operative capabilities function as one set of proximal determinants of how people behave, their thought patterns, and the emotional reactions they experience in taxing situations. In their daily lives people continuously make decisions about what course of action to pursue and how long to continue those they have undertaken. Because acting on misjudgments of personal efficacy can produce adverse consequences, accurate appraisal of one's own capabilities has considerable functional value.

Self-efficacy judgments, whether accurate or faulty, influence choice of activities and environmental settings. People avoid activities that they believe exceed their coping capabilities, but they undertake and perform assuredly those that they judge themselves capable of managing.

(1982, pp. 122–3)

This relatively simple idea of self-efficacy is of especial importance to our analysis of control and empowerment. For instance, overestimates of capability will lead to failure and, if repeated, will limit future effort and damage self-esteem. Underestimates will, on the other hand, generally limit potential for learning and personal growth. Again, the stronger the perceived self-efficacy, the greater the level of perseverance and persistence and, typically, the greater the feeling of control. By contrast, low perceptions of self-efficacy are likely to produce negative self-evaluations, leading to lower self-esteem.

Self-efficacy has additional value for health education planning: it is not only a readily usable concept but also its very tangibility suggests techniques for enhancing beliefs about control. The prospect of changing deficits in global attributes such as self-esteem is at the very least rather complex; similarly, it would be difficult to provide an easy prescription for shunting 'externals' on to an 'internal' health career. On the other hand creating a self-efficacy belief in one's capacity to purchase condoms is more readily achieved by, for instance, situation specific assertiveness training. It would also not be unreasonable to assume that 'internality' represents the sum total of a lifetime's self-efficacy beliefs. Therefore, insofar as internality constitutes a desirable health promotion goal, it is potentially achievable by a consistent, continuing and coherent set of experiences designed to create experience of success.

Reference to Figure 1.7 will reveal the existence of a reciprocal relationship between the beliefs about control which we have outlined above and that cluster of feelings about self which is typically referred to as self-esteem. It will also be apparent that 'learned helplessness' has been included as a bipolar opposite of self-esteem. Earlier we suggested that it was the antithesis of self-empowerment. It would, however, be more accurate – given its association with the negative affective state of depression – to contrast it with (high) self-esteem. This latter concept itself is often employed in rather cavalier fashion and, given its frequent association with empowerment, it merits some further brief comment.

The empowered person, it is said, enjoys high self-esteem whereas learned helplessness is characterized by a sense of worthlessness. Coopersmith (1967), one of the earliest writers on self-esteem, quotes an even earlier observation by William James about the negative effects of low self-esteem.

A man ... with powers that have uniformly brought him success with place and wealth and friends and fame, is not likely to be visited by the morbid diffidences and doubts about himself which he had when he was a boy, whereas he who has made one blunder after another and still lies in middle life among the failures at the foot of the hill is liable to grow all sicklied o'er

with self-distrust, and to shrink from trials with which his powers can really cope.

(p. 2)

It is therefore clear that a good level of self-esteem is considered to be healthy, in several ways. First, it may with some justification be argued that realistically based high self-esteem is a significant feature of mental health. It may, in this context, be viewed as the obverse of learned helplessness and, thus, as a desirable 'medical' state. Alternatively, it provides a relatively tangible example of well-being and is worth pursuing in its own right.

Second, it would seem reasonable to assume that persons who value themselves are more likely to respond to the health educators' traditional 'look after yourself' message. After all, if you value yourself you will presumably believe you are worth looking after!

Less obviously, self-esteem is presumed to promote health in an indirect way. For instance, it is commonly assumed that people high in self-esteem are less likely to succumb to pressures to conform (Aronson, 1976) and more likely to have the courage of their convictions. There is also evidence to support the contention that self-esteem is positively associated with the ability to handle fear. This is not, of course, to argue for the use of fear appeal but merely to note that individuals frequently have to respond to communications which are intrinsically threatening. The 'approved' response is to deal vigilantly with the threat, seek out information and adopt an empowered decision. This somewhat idealistic strategy is, it appears, more likely to be pursued by those having a high level of self-esteem.

For instance, Dabbs (1964) showed that high self-esteem was significantly related to 'coping' and 'copers' tended to respond to fear in a realistic rather than a defensive way. Moreover, self-esteem was itself related to subjects' response to different levels of fear appeal designed to promote adoption of tetanus injections. Whereas low self-esteem subjects showed high compliance in both high and low fear of conditions, high self-esteem subjects showed compliance only in high fear conditions. The researchers presumed that high self-esteem people are more active and vigorous in dealing with their environments and more skilful in meeting danger. They were thus only motivated to take action when the threat was perceived to be very high. At first glance, it might appear that conformity shown by low self-esteem persons is actually desirable since the robust independence of those enjoying high self-esteem would not necessarily lead to compliance! It perhaps hardly needs saying that only convinced advocates of the preventive model should experience dismay at results such as these. It is one of life's little paradoxes that empowered people do not necessarily follow what educators feel is good advice!

There is, however, a further and perhaps more important set of observations about the indirect relationship between self-esteem and health choices. These centre on the fact that people having high self-esteem will experience greater dissonance (Festinger, 1957) if they fail to live up to their own expectations and moral imperatives (Aronson and Mettee, 1968). If someone believes that high fat consumption is unhealthy, values health and acknowledges that he or she consumes a good deal of fat, then dissonance will be experienced. Those having a high level of self-esteem will experience more discomfort than those having little self-respect. After all, people with low self-esteem will accept that such inconsistency is consistent with their normal behaviour. We should, however, not expect too much from these feelings of dissonance. As we will see in Chapter 2, there are many more psychological and social factors governing behaviour: in the last analysis the likelihood of action may depend on the outcome of conflict between dissonance and taste buds!

Two main inter-related factors appear important in determining self-esteem: one of these is the reaction of significant others to the individual; the other is the individual's success in achieving goals which are valued not only by self but by the social group.

A comprehensive discussion of tactics designed to enhance self-esteem is not possible here. We might observe that a judicious mix of appropriate socialization and life skills training would be central to the successful promotion of positive self-esteem. In the context of Figure 1.7 we should merely note that influencing the whole range of beliefs about control – especially by the provision of skills which enable individuals to control their environments – provides the most likely avenue to success. However, Figure 1.7 again reminds us of the potentially inhibiting or facilitating effect of the environment. In particular, we should note how people's actual power and status in a given social system can substantially influence their beliefs about control and their associated self-esteem. On the other hand, the reciprocity intrinsic to this analysis is again revealed in individuals' potential for acquiring status and power by means of both their belief in their capacity to do so and the possession of a number of necessary skills and competences.

Apart from self-esteem (i.e. the value we attach to ourselves), two other values related constructs may figure prominently in the model of self-empowerment portrayed in Figure 1.7. The first of these is nicely described by Lewis' (1986) term 'existential control'.

It is apparent to the casual observer that there are many people (perhaps even cultures) who clearly are not in control of their lives nor do they believe they are. Paradoxically, they appear to exhibit equanimity in this situation and, arguably, good levels of self-esteem. It would appear that the sense of well-being which is enjoyed is due to their capacity to impose meaning on their existence: even if they are not in control, they believe that someone or something **is** in control and they are happy with that arrangement. This somewhat Panglossian notion is closely related to Antonovsky's (1979) concept of a 'sense of coherence', i.e.:

> ... a global orientation that expresses the extent to which one has a pervasive, enduring though dynamic feeling of confidence that one's internal and external environments are predictable and that there is a high probability that things will work out as well as can reasonably be expected.
>
> *(p. 123)*

Coherence consists of three components: 'comprehensibility, manageability and meaningfulness'. The first of these describes the extent to which people consider that their worlds are predictable and make sense; the second refers to their perception that they have resources available to meet environmental demands. The meaningfulness component provides the closest parallel with Lewis' concept indicating the extent to which people's lives make sense emotionally. The term 'existential' has been used here since it has certain relevant linguistic associations, more particularly the perspective derived from existentialist philosophy that people are and should be free agents and impose meaning on an essentially meaningless world!

It will also be seen from Figure 1.7 that the term 'sense of community' has been included under the value system rubric and shown as a point of interface between individual and community. The relationship between community and individual will be further explored in a later chapter but we should at this point acknowledge that being a member of a relatively cohesive social group meets important needs for some people. Again, a community will provide a network of relationships which will support and validate individual beliefs and values. One of the most comprehensive analyses of the concept 'sense of community' was provided by Maton and

Rappaport (1984) who looked for the '... correlates and contexts of empowerment among members of a Christian, non-denominational religious setting'. Existential control seemed to be substantially related to a sense of community as defined by these researchers who refer to ' ... a sense of closeness with a loving God who actively transforms (i.e. empowers) members' lives... (i.e. increased compassion and humility and a desire to serve and help others)'. The researchers' summary of church members' verbalizations of their religious ideals provides a valuable illustration of one perspective on community empowerment and the sense of meaningfulness involved in existential control.

> ... a desire for increased closeness with God and for God to meet personal needs together with a desire to become more compassionate and self-sacrificing as people; the goal of developing deep trust and childlike dependence on God together with the need to retain intellectual honesty in dealing with doubts and personal responsibility for one's decisions; and a desire for the fellowship to be a 'family' which provides both interpersonal and material support for members together with a desire to involve everyone in decision making and to be able to change structures and traditions whenever they begin to rigidify and interfere with members' spiritual and personal growth.
>
> *(p. 42)*

One final point of explanation should be made about the relationship between empowered individuals and an empowered community. As will be seen from Figure 1.7, it is assumed that an individual needs skills to engage with and participate effectively in a community or social group. Similarly, it is acknowledged that appropriate health and life skills may be best provided within a community context.

A quite detailed analysis of the dynamics of empowerment has been provided so far. This reflects in part our concern to try to illuminate a concept which typically generates much heat but little light. A detailed analysis of the essential – and sometimes contested – elements of empowerment is also considered necessary in the context of a critical appraisal of real or imagined differences between the various models of health education discussed in this chapter. This will follow specifications for an empowerment model of health education which incorporates the 'radical' and 'educational' models mentioned earlier.

HEALTH EDUCATION: AN EMPOWERMENT MODEL

Figure 1.8 includes key elements of an empowerment model which is consistent with the ideological principles of health promotion and illustrates relevant educational methodology. It, therefore, could be said to replace the radical model as it incorporates key elements described above. It will also inevitably include a central educational process.

The elements which the empowerment model shares with the educational and radical approaches discussed earlier should be self-evident. If knowledge is power then an empowerment model should include not only the provision of relevant information but should emphasize the importance of critical appraisal encapsulated in the notion of critical consciousness raising. On the other hand, we have hopefully argued convincingly that CCR needs to be supplemented by empowering beliefs, feelings and skills. Consequently, the decision making competences which sophisticated 'educational' models would provide must be supplemented by the wide range of health and life skills which maximize genuine voluntaristic choice.

The term 'empowerment' rather than 'self-empowerment' has been deliberately selected in order to acknowledge the powerful effect of environmental factors in facilitating or hindering freedom of choice. It is assumed that the combination of consciousness raising and skills provision should maximize the

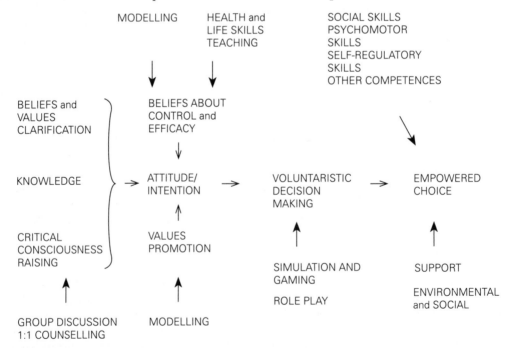

Figure 1.8 Empowerment: the educational process, including examples of key methods.

chances of managing environmental constraints. It is also assumed that the recipients of education will not only be the 'public' but will also comprise professionals and others who might act as advocates for environmental change according to the principles discussed at the beginning of this chapter.

One final point should be signalled: the outcome is shown not as 'approved' health or illness related behaviours, nor as radical social action. Both of these outcomes **may** result from the educational process but the prime goal is to maximize genuine voluntaristic choice, subject only to the moral imperative represented by the previously discussed notion of a 'considerate way of life'.

IDEOLOGICAL DIVIDES, FALSE DICHOTOMIES AND THE MEASUREMENT OF SUCCESS

So far, we have explored the ideological basis of health education and examined a number of models purporting to define different approaches to conceptualization and practice. We identified a preventive medical model and contrasted that with a radical model. We then, somewhat casually perhaps, incorporated that radical approach into an empowerment model. We also succeeded in enshrining the principle of voluntarism in this empowerment model and could thus be accused of annexing an educational model! This is not merely some meaningless sleight of hand; rather it reflects the fact that **any** model is just an attempt to impose meaning on complex realities. This particular attempt to simplify and make sense of the reality of debates about the 'true' purposes of health education has apparently resulted in the construction of two separate models: a preventive model with an authoritarian disease oriented focus and a radical, person centred empowerment model. However, even this distinction is far from cut and dried. For instance, it is probably the case that empowering people is more likely to achieve successful preventive medical out-

comes than an authoritarian approach employing coercive tactics. On the other hand, there is no logical reason why medical workers should not pursue preventive goals in a non-authoritarian client centred way.

We are not, of course, denying the existence of ideological divides in health education: there are undoubtedly often substantial variations in people's values and philosophies. It is, however, important to avoid reification; we must beware of false dichotomies and be sensitive to the fact that there may be several complex overlapping purposes in health education theory and practice. It is therefore our intention now to look for genuine conflicts in value and ideology and comment on false distinctions. A useful way of doing this is to revisit Figure 1.2 – the 'anatomical' overview which seeks to identify the various ways in which education may contribute to the goals of health promotion.

The presence of the various models of health education discussed so far may be discerned in Figure 1.2. For instance, reference to 'absence of disease' as part of the overall health goal inevitably acknowledges the importance of primary, secondary and tertiary prevention. However, given the ideological principles of health promotion adopted at the beginning of this chapter, it is not surprising that two features of the classic medical model are not represented. First, health education's traditional emphasis on persuasion has been replaced by an emphasis on the empowerment and support by voluntaristic choice. Second, the territorial claims of a medical model have succumbed to the challenge of demedicalization and 'reoriented' medical services are shown as just one part of a wider range of health promoting services.

We would, on the other hand, expect to see education making a contribution to the creation of healthy public policy. This function is indeed fully represented in terms of critical consciousness raising (CCR) and empowerment. We might, at this juncture, emphasize that these two processes are integral to the empowerment model of health education. We should also note that the process of empowering and supporting **individual** choice is congruent with this empowerment model, even though the choices may primarily be concerned with preventive outcomes.

However, although a simple radical model would clearly incorporate critical consciousness raising, it would be less concerned with community empowerment (although some lip service may be paid to the idea). Its goals would not be, first and foremost, to equip the community to make voluntaristic decisions; rather, they would be concerned with achieving social and political change. CCR has traditionally been associated with a radical challenge to the power base of society, usually capitalist. If social mobilization were to result in popular acceptance of capitalism and the status quo, radicals would be somewhat disappointed! Moreover, radicals would be expected to doubt both the efficacy and ethicality of pursuing **individual** empowerment and would reject life skills teaching as a form of victim blaming.

Reference to Figure 1.2 will reveal an educational process paralleling the 'mainstream' radical CCR/empowerment function. It has been labelled 'agenda setting'; it is superficially similar to CCR in its concern to raise health issues for public consumption and in its potential effect on health policy. We can identify two main operations. The first of these might merely consist of raising issues in order to facilitate decision making about policy matters. This function might be illustrated by the use of a television documentary to inform the public about any currently controversial issue. More typical, though, is the political use of agenda setting. In this latter mode, government may test the temperature of public opinion with a view to ascertaining the acceptability of new legislation. Since public policy measures are highly likely to result in some restriction of people's liberty or involve them in financial cost, psychological reactance is a predictable outcome.

Government is, of course, reluctant to court electoral unpopularity and can therefore use agenda setting tactics via mass media as a kind of 'softening up' process.

Agenda setting may well happen incidentally. Arguably, a series of mass media campaigns in Britain set the scene for the introduction of legislation making the wearing of seat belts in cars compulsory. While the campaigns achieved only moderate success in persuading individual drivers to voluntarily use seat belts, raising public consciousness about the problem of traffic accidents and the benefits of seat belts doubtless laid the foundations for legislation which restricted individual liberty without generating any serious electoral costs for the government of the day.

It could, of course, be argued that agenda setting and CCR are not qualitatively different processes. It could indeed be postulated that policy measures could be located on a spectrum of political acceptability. On the assumption that government can afford to be only one small step ahead of public opinion, this spectrum would reflect the public's latitude of acceptance. For example, government might be favourably disposed to measures designed to alleviate inequalities in health but consider that the increased cost in taxation would be met with furious opposition by tax payers and therefore deemed to be electoral suicide.

Clearly, it is possible to conceive of such a spectrum of acceptability; however it is more useful to consider the agenda setting and CCR functions as qualitatively rather than quantitatively distinct. As we have noted, CCR involves a radical challenge to dominant ideology and should be reserved for situations where such a challenge can be demonstrated. Consider for instance the abovementioned challenge to health inequalities. A left wing government might be ideologically committed to remedying inequalities but be persuaded that the cost of the radical measures would be electorally unacceptable; realpolitik might therefore dictate inaction plus some degree of agenda setting designed to produce a climate of public opinion conducive to some limited policy implementation. On the other hand, a right wing government might be totally opposed ideologically to state intervention irrespective of cost. Firm commitment to enterprise, the pursuit of profit and rampant individualism would be incompatible with radical healthy public policy.

In the interests of balance, we should perhaps provide an example of an alternative ideological clash. For instance, it is firmly established that the fluoridation of public water supplies is the most effective public health strategy for reducing the incidence of dental caries. Clearly any such policy constrains individual's freedom to drink non-fluoridated water. The scene is therefore set for an ideological confrontation between, on the one hand, the values of the medical model and, on the other hand, proponents of voluntaristic choice. The ideological concerns of right wing politicians may well be congruent with those of the medical lobby but, in the last analysis, perceptions of electoral gain may be the sole determinant of action. If agenda setting were to reveal general acceptability for the fluoridation, legislation would not be delayed by major ideological principle.

RADICALISM *VS.* INDIVIDUALISM: VICTIM BLAMING REVISITED

Returning to an earlier question about the existence of genuine differences between various models of health education, we do appear to have identified a categorically distinct ideological dimension in respect of one of the various educational functions shown in Fig. 1.2. By definition, the radical, CCR/empowerment function mentioned above exemplifies such a dimension since it consciously set out to challenge the dominant ideological positions. The singlemindedness of the stance adopted by the advocates of this approach has been contrasted with the

pragmatism of the 'agenda setting' function which, though sharing the goal of influencing public policy, lacks the purity of conviction of the former. This would therefore seem to be a useful point at which to consider the compatibility of the various health education functions examined so far. We might, for instance, ask about the possibility of compromise in the radical challenge to dominant values. This in turn raises two further questions: to what extent are radicals prepared to compromise and is compromise logically impossible?

Essentially the issue centres on whether or not meaningful change is possible without radical confrontation with a value system. It is an issue too complex to be addressed here in any depth but it is interesting to note that de Kadt (1982), in his discussion of ideological aspects of CCR, clearly believes that useful change has occurred without any fundamental change in capitalism, i.e. through a process of reform rather than by a 'radical transformation of the social system'. In support of his argument, he cites the emergence of legislation to curtail the unbridled pursuit of profit: safety at work legislation, legislation about health standards of products and, 'more timidly', environmental pollution.

Interestingly, de Kadt refers to the influence of moderate left wing writers such as J.K. Galbraith in achieving reforms. Whether or not these reforms are viewed as significant or minor and counterproductive, Galbraith has recently argued (1992) that compromise is the only way of changing the 'unacceptable face of capitalism'. In a lecture to the Institute of Public Policy, he commented on the success of previous left wing challenges to capitalism but advocated abandoning polarized attitudes. 'Ours is an age of constructive pragmatism... There can be no escape from thought into theology.' *Inter alia*, we must recognize that revolutionary challenge to capitalism is unlikely to be acceptable to the public; whether this be on account of self-interest or false consciousness is a matter of only academic importance.

In the context of this discussion about the efficacy and feasibility of espousing a radical ideology, we might usefully revisit the notion of victim blaming. It will be recalled that victim blaming refers to the prescription of individual solutions to socially determined problems. A radical ideology would assert that for this reason, only social/environmental solutions are acceptable – for instance by implementing appropriate health and social policy change. However, irrespective of any debate about compromise and the art of the possible, the radical solution in this instance is logically flawed. The assertion is naive in that individual learning will always be a necessary part of health education. First, there are instances where social or environmental measures are to a greater or lesser extent irrelevant. For example, patients need information, certain beliefs and attitudes together with actual skills if they are to manage their diabetes or their ostomies. Social/structural factors are important only to the extent that patients cannot afford to pay for the treatment or facilities are not available. Second, as we indicated in our comments on empowerment, individuals need a number of competences before they can engage in radical challenge: these cannot be magically supplied through some sort of community action.

Indeed, one of the important false ideological dichotomies in health education derives from a misinterpretation of the true nature of victim blaming. It centres on an ill thought out tendency to deride the empowering and supportive function adopted by health educators working with individuals or groups of individuals. The use of life skills, for instance, to facilitate and support personal choice may be condemned as a new form of victim blaming. The reality is that the only form of education which is not concerned with individual clients is the use of mass media – which more often than not are likely to be archetypically victim blaming! If we consider more politically correct activities such as the development of community coalitions or community development, we will find individually focused educational activities at their core. The formation of coalitions of community groups in order to create a power base from which to mount a radical challenge is an important strategy for remedying inequalities. However, the actual component educational activities involve work with groups and influential individuals such as community leaders.

Again, a classic element of community development consists of educational activities designed to empower small groups of individuals – especially women – in a neighbourhood context. In fact we might legitimately argue that consciousness raising without providing appropriate educational skills and competences may be self-indulgent posturing and as unethical as true victim blaming! It is therefore more meaningful to reserve the term victim blaming for those circumstances in which any kind of health promotion activity fails to take account of relevant social, structural or environmental factors.

IDEOLOGICAL DIVIDES AND PERSONAL PREJUDICES

We have so far discussed a number of health education models and their ideological peculiarities. These models are social constructions: they differentially represent people's beliefs about significant aspects of their world and the values they attach to them. If, therefore, we ask why people subscribe to one model or another we are enquiring into the beliefs and values they have acquired through the process of socialization. General experience and socialization will, for example, have created beliefs and prejudices about human nature and the purpose of life; professional socialization will have generated notions and feelings about the proper courses of action to adopt in any given occupational practice.

The results of both kinds of socialization may be observed in the ideological commitments espoused by health educators. Three dimensions of belief and value would seem to be especially significant in defining the purpose of health promotion and health education and, therefore, in defining the meaning of success. One of these might be described in terms of radicalism and conservatism; a second could usefully be described in relation to either a democratic view of people or, at the opposite pole, an authoritarian perspective. The third dimension, which we will now consider, concerns the beliefs and values associated with the medical model which is contrasted with an alternative, holistic view of health.

The nature of the medical model has already been quite fully discussed. Its major features include:

1. A mechanistic, reductionist disease oriented conception of health;
2. The territorial imperative derived from this notion and described by the term medicalization;
3. A tendency towards paternalistic authoritarianism.

As indicated earlier, ideological dimensions are not necessarily factorially unique. Insofar as medical practitioners do tend to be located at the authoritarian rather than the democratic end of the spectrum, then we might ascribe this phenomenon to the process of professional socialization which, rightly or wrongly, was derived from a belief that the effectiveness and status of doctors depended on patients adopting a passive role! Alternatively or additionally, those of an authoritarian disposition might have been attracted to this particular profession.

It is not uncommon, of course, to associate the medical model also with the first of the three dimensions mentioned above: that of radicalism versus conservatism. We have already noted Navarro's (1976) identification of medicine with capitalism and this is by no means an uncommon view. Clearly in many cultures – of which the USA would provide the archetypal example – medicine is virtually synonymous with the pursuit of profit. On the other hand, it would be unfair to tarnish socialist medicine with such an appellation. The essential nature of the medical model is more reasonably related to its narrow, mechanistic disease orientation. As such, any challenge derives from those who question its over-emphasis on physical aspects of health and the scant attention its pays to holistic approaches to well-being, 'positive health' and 'quality of life'.

Given the etymology of the word 'health', i.e. 'hal' or whole, an alternative holistic approach to definition is not surprising. As such, WHO's broad (1946) definition which also included an emphasis on well-being should be viewed as a major challenge to a dominant ideology. A detailed discussion of the nature of health has been considered outside the scope of this book. However, since some people have considered the distinguishing feature of health promotion as its pursuit of positive health or 'high level wellness', the following observations might usefully be made:

1. As Dubos (1959) has noted, health is like a mirage – it is unattainable but worth pursuing. Notions of positive health are even more ephemeral and evanescent. They too merit pursuit but may pose severe operationalization problems.
2. Notions of positive health are likely to be relativistic and often idiosyncratic. The word 'health' is often used to describe any personally held value, including moral and spiritual.
3. Notions of positive health – largely because of their vagueness – tend to irritate those who espouse the medical model! However, provided that the value position has been clarified and concepts have been operationalized, it is possible to construct indicators of performance and therefore assess the effectiveness and efficiency of strategies designed to achieve positive health objectives.

4. Several goals which derive from an empowerment model may legitimately be described as positive health outcomes, both for the individual and social group. Indeed, although it may have preventive benefits, empowerment itself could be described as a positive health state.

Before leaving the holistic notion of positive health, we should record that ideological jibes have not only been directed at positive health practitioners by adherents to the medical model. Radicals have rightly pointed out that in one important respect, devotion to the cause of fitness and well-being is as culpable as victim blaming disease prevention. Indeed, the derogatory term 'healthism' has been used to describe devotees' failure to ignore the general social and environmental factors influencing health, whether this be defined in positive or 'negative' terms (Crawford, 1980).

The two remaining ideological dimensions to which reference was made earlier should require little further elaboration. We have discussed in various contexts the nature of radical challenge to dominant ideologies, of which the critique of capitalism and the victim blaming tendency is a prime example. Again, insofar as the medical model represents the status quo, critics may legitimately be defined as radicals. On the other hand, acceptance of the status quo *in toto* characterizes extreme conservatism.

Just as people may well be normally distributed (statistically speaking) on a scale of radicalism versus conservatism, they may equally be located at some point on the third dimension – authoritarianism versus democracy. Those whose convictions result in their location at the authoritarian end of the scale would presumably believe that, since people are not to be trusted, it is legitimate to make decisions on their behalf. On the other hand, democratically inclined health educators would be convinced of the moral rightness of voluntarism and be committed to 'bottom-up'

programmes based on the felt needs of the population.

This analysis is, of course, not new. It has been debated in general psychology for some time. For instance, McGregor's (1966) analysis of two extreme styles of management centred on the notion that there were two extreme and opposing views of human motivation. He described these as 'theory X' and 'theory Y'. Theory X was based on an essentially authoritarian and 'top-down' perspective characterized by such beliefs as people are by nature indolent, lacking in ambition, self-centred, resistant to change and gullible.

Cattell (1965) reminded us of the ways in which personality attributes can generate prejudices which frequently underpin what are superficially rational arguments. He cited William James, stating that '... differences in intellectual conclusions among philosophers could be traced more to their differences in temperament than to any differences in facts available to them...' (p. 358). According to this viewpoint, ideological inclinations and the choice of health education model may be determined, at least in part, by temperamental factors. Interestingly, two of the personality traits which Cattell incorporated into his factorially determined system have parallels with the two dimensions under discussion here. They are radicalism versus conservatism and a factor most conveniently described as 'toughminded versus tenderminded'. Again, one of the better known personality typologies developed by Eysenck (1960) incorporates a two-dimensional model which seeks to explain various social attitudes including political orientation. These two dimensions are radicalism versus conservatism and toughmindedness versus tendermindedness. Thus communist tendencies would be consistent with toughminded radicalism while fascism would be characterized by toughminded conservatism.

It would undoubtedly be rash to apply these insights from personality theory to health educators' predilections for different models and ideologies, at any rate without support from substantial factor analytic studies. Nonetheless it is tempting to speculate that toughminded conservatives would more likely be enthusiastic advocates of the medical model whereas toughminded radicals would subscribe to movements seeking to challenge capitalist inspired victim blaming. Presumably tenderminded radicals would be well represented in advocates of holistic health and, perhaps, the gentler versions of community development.

At all events, whether it be personality traits or clusters of beliefs and values which influence theoretical preferences, we should recognize that values and subjective interpretation rather than rational and technical analyses actually determine choice of model. Suffice it to say at this juncture that the overview provided by Figure 1.2 aims to describe a variety of complementary policy and educational functions. These functions are ideologically consistent with the principles of health promotion outlined at the beginning of this chapter and with the empowerment model described subsequently. They are not congruent with a narrow medical model nor with those radical approaches which adopt authoritarian stances and seek to make the healthy choice the only choice. This assertion is, of course, itself a value statement and clearly readers are free to choose their own ideological interpretations. This chapter will conclude with a quite brief discussion of the meaning of success from the standpoint of devotees of different models and ideologies.

EVALUATION AND THE MEANING OF SUCCESS

Evaluation research seeks to provide answers to questions about the effectiveness of health promotion and health education. Its purpose is to measure success. Statements about success depend on the aims and goals of the health promotion or health education initiative. These aims and goals – as we have been at some pains to suggest – depend on ideological models. The **efficiency** of any given initiative is concerned with the degree of success achieved, i.e. with **relative** effectiveness, and involves explicit or implicit comparison with some alternative, competing initiative. The question of efficiency will be examined in a later chapter. Our present interest is to discuss what success would look like when viewed from the standpoint of different models.

For health promotion in general, success would have to be judged in relation to the key ideological principles listed earlier. In the last analysis we would look for evidence that people's lives were more socially and economically productive. We might look for evidence of greater equity – that Sir William Beveridge's 50 year old campaign to slay the 'five giants of disease, idleness, ignorance, squalor and want' was being waged successfully. We would look for signs of healthy public policy and empowered participating communities. It would, however, be unrealistic to use such broad outcomes as indicators of success: we would need some intermediate indicators, a point discussed in greater detail in a later chapter. For now we will merely consider in a relatively general way the effectiveness criteria for one of the two major components of health promotion – health education. More particularly, we will examine the criteria which would be used to assess success for an 'educational model'.

EFFECTIVENESS AND THE EDUCATIONAL MODEL

In its simplest form this model, as we have seen, consists of merely providing knowledge. Success is not only easy to define but easy to achieve. For example, evaluation of a programme of education about contraception would need only to demonstrate that the client group had understood and remembered the various facts, concepts and principles underlying the nature of contraception and contraceptive practice, together with related and subordinated notions such as the physiology of reproduction. A more sophisticated model, as illustrated earlier in Figure 1.4, would require evidence that additional competences had been acquired. An evaluator would now expect to find evidence that individuals had clarified beliefs and values relating to sexuality and, for example, acquired certain cognitive strategies to help them make decisions consistent with their values. The learners might also be assessed on their capacity to show their competence in making decisions in a simulated real life setting.

EFFECTIVENESS AND THE PREVENTIVE MODEL

It is quite apparent that it is more difficult to demonstrate success when obliged to use the criteria of a preventive medical model of health education, largely because desired outcomes consist of actions which typically require client groups to overcome a variety of personal, social and environmental barriers. By way of exemplifying the meaning of success for this particular model, it should be illuminating to make reference to the recent UK government policy document, *Health of the Nation* (DoH, 1992).

Although the ministerial preamble claims a commitment to '… the pursuit of "health" in its widest sense …', it is not surprising that the preventive model best defines the dominant ideology. In the light of our earlier observations about compromise between radical and conservative ideology, it is noteworthy that *Health of the Nation*, unlike earlier major official pronouncements, accepts the importance of public policy and the need for intersectoral collaboration and interagency working. Moreover, some reference is made to 'quality of life' in accepting that improvement to public health will be made not only by 'adding years to life' (i.e. increase in life expectancy and reduction in premature death) but also by 'adding life to years' (minimizing effects of illness and disability, promoting healthy lifestyles, physical and social environments and improving quality of life).

Again, in a section discussing the health needs of people in specific population groups, socioeconomic variations in health status are acknowledged. However, in respect of this latter acknowledgement of the possibility of broader social determinants of ill health, a passing reference is made to a complex interplay of genetic, biological, social, environmental, cultural and behavioural factors. It is noted that the variations in public health produced by this complex interplay '… are by no means fully understood', but more specific reference is made to individual risk behaviours: higher rate of smoking, poorer diets, heavier drinking and lower take-up of preventive health services 'in groups whose health is worst'.

Five key areas for action are listed in *Health of the Nation*. These are: CHD and stroke; cancers; mental illness; HIV/AIDS and sexual health; accidents. These are, of course, classic epidemiological targets but even in the two action areas where 'health' is mentioned, the focus is on disease. For instance, in the section appropriately headed 'mental illness', the only reference to mental health is about making an (unspecified) improvement to the mental health of mentally ill people. The objectives and targets of the chapter on sexual health (and HIV/AIDS) are concerned solely with the prevention of sexually transmitted disease and drug misuse.

We noted earlier that different degrees of radicalism were possible within any given health education/promotion programme and the term 'agenda setting' was employed and refer to reformist possibilities. In relation to smoking, *Health of the Nation* recognizes the need for using price controls on smoking in public places and controls on advertising and promotion. It also adopts a strategy of 'at least maintaining the real level of taxes on tobacco products' both in Britain and within the context of the European Community. On the other hand, it affirms that the decision whether or not to smoke is a matter of individual choice. Moreover, a complete ban on advertising tobacco products – directly or indirectly through 'brand stretching' – would seem to be still ideologically unthinkable!

These observations are not intended to denigrate what is a significant policy document: they merely reinforce earlier points about the primacy of ideology in determining the meaning of success. Success according to the preventive model and *Health of the Nation* is simple to illustrate. For instance, in order to achieve the 40% reduction of CHD and stroke in people under 65 by the year 2000, health education would be expected to contribute to a reduction in prevalence of cigarette smoking in men and women aged 16 and over to no more than 20% by the year 2000. Evidence from educationally sound programmes such as the North Karelia Project would seem to indicate that this kind of success can be achieved. Puska *et al.* (1985) reported a net change in the amount of daily smoking reported by men in North Karelia of 28% and by women of 14% over a six year period. Schwartz (1987), in a comparative report of the results of a number of community projects, recorded a decline in the number of male smokers in North Karelia from 44% to 31% compared with only a 4% reduction in the rest of Finland.

Health of the Nation has also established a series of objectives for dealing with another important set of preventive targets concerned with reducing the incidence of accidents. One of these specifies a one third reduction in road casualties by the year 2000 and this will serve as a second illustration of a major focus for a preventive model of health education. First we should note that a good deal of progress has been made in reducing accidental injuries: a fall of 23% has been observed between 1981 and 1991. It would

not be unreasonable to suppose that health education had made some real but unspecifiable contribution to that success. We do, however, have some more tangible evidence of the potential of safety education for influencing health behaviour.

Levens and Rodnight (1973) assembled evidence of the effectiveness of a series of carefully controlled area experiments in the use of mass media to promote the wearing of seat belts by car drivers and front seat passengers in Britain. They calculated that an appropriately structured mass media campaign could raise the level of seat belt use by a maximum of 16% from an initial 15% start point and do so within a period of three weeks. This result clearly demonstrates effectiveness; whether it demonstrates efficiency depends on what might be achieved by competing measures. In the case in point a much better result was achieved by legislation, i.e. by implementing healthy public policy. It is now rare in Britain for drivers not to wear seat belts. However, as was suggested earlier in the chapter, policy change would have been unlikely without the incidental agenda setting effect of individually directed campaigns. In fact this provides an excellent example of the interaction of education and policy. It also gives an indication of the potential of mass media in health education, something which will later receive detailed analysis.

EFFECTIVENESS AND THE RADICAL MODEL

Radical health education has one significant feature in common with the preventive model discussed above. It is concerned with action outcomes. A preventive approach looks for indicators of success in the adoption of behaviours and in medical or epidemiological outcomes which are considered to result from such behaviours – after a decent interval of time has elapsed! Success of a radical model would be measured in terms of social action. Again this action is not necessarily an end in itself but would be seen as a means of achieving healthy public policy in order to achieve the kinds of health promotion goals discussed previously, such as a redistribution of power and resources. We will consider here two examples of what proponents of a radical model might judge to be success. The first example concerns healthy diet.

A standard preventive model would seek to persuade individuals to adopt a prudent diet in order to minimize the likelihood of their falling prey to a number of dietary related diseases. The classic victim blaming approach would, in exhorting people to eat wisely, ignore the environmental circumstances which either promoted the consumption of unhealthy food or prevented people from adopting a healthy diet. A radical approach would set out to tackle those unhealthy environmental determinants of poor nutritional status. As Charles and Kerr (1986) have demonstrated in their research into the experience of 200 British women acting as nutritional gatekeepers for their families, ignorance of what constitutes healthy food is not the problem. Real barriers to choice included one or more of the following: accessibility and cost of healthy food; problems with food labelling or lack of it; relegation of the importance of providing healthy foods in the context of other social and domestic pressures; feelings of powerlessness.

Effective radical nutrition education would, therefore, be judged by such measures as (in descending order of radicalism): decrease in poverty; successful battle with food manufacturers seeking to promote junk food and empty calories in western countries and formula baby milk and diarrhoea medicines in developing countries; providing a full range of healthy foods (preferably subsidized) at retail outlets and in the context of institutional catering; proper food labelling. It is interesting to note that variations on the last two (relatively) radical proposals figure in *Health of the Nation*, indicating perhaps that reformist compromise is a real possibility!

Freudenberg (1981) provides our second exemplification of effectiveness in radical health education. The cases he cites include a range of intermediate and outcome indicators. Three examples are listed below.

1. In the context of critical consciousness raising about environmental issues, mothers in New Jersey were alerted to a cluster of child cancer deaths in an industrial area. As a result they formed an organization which exerted pressure on the state and, ultimately, forced it to undertake an epidemiological investigation.

2. In the context of occupational safety and health, the Carolina Brown Lung Association was formed. This set out to explain safety procedures to textile workers and taught them how to monitor dust levels in the workplace. They were also shown how to take action when legal standards were violated.

3. In the context of the women's health movement, groups of women were taught how to write papers and develop these as a course for women about women and their bodies. A Committee Against Sterilization Abuse was also formed. This action group resulted in the implementation of 'healthy public policy' in the form of new legislation requiring the provision of mandatory counselling and a 30 day waiting period between decisions about sterilization and performing the surgery.

Consideration of these examples of radical health promotion will reveal that a variety of different kinds of learning had taken place in addition to consciousness raising. Indeed it seems clear that empowerment figured prominently in all three instances. This serves to remind us of the difficulty of distinguishing health education models in practice. Nonetheless we will finally consider what success might mean for an empowerment model.

EFFECTIVENESS AND THE EMPOWERMENT MODEL

We have already noted that CCR and indeed, the radical model, form an integral part of the model of empowerment described earlier. It will also be recalled that the main difference between this and the radical model was the extent of the emphasis placed on the process of self and community empowerment. Not only was it argued that this process needed to be defined in terms of precise operations but we also sought to give a high profile to the principle of voluntarism. The implication of this for evaluation is quite simply that the ultimate indicator of success will be the extent to which individuals become empowered, either in general or in relation to particular courses of action. It does not matter if the course of action relates to some medically approved (or disapproved) behaviour or, alternatively, involves political action ('correct' or incorrect!) – the outcome measure should provide evidence of empowered decision making capabilities.

Clearly, in seeking to measure the success of empowerment strategies, health educators must rid themselves of the all too frequently self-indulgent rhetoric associated with empowerment and look for some solid indicators. These are not difficult to find and may be derived from Figure 1.6 which sought to describe key dynamic elements of empowerment – both self-empowerment and community empowerment. Since the matter of determining the nature and extent of effective 'interventions' to empower communities will receive careful consideration in the final chapter of this book, we will limit any observations here to indicators of individual empowerment.

In short, if health education has been successful, we should be able to demonstrate changes in one or more intermediate indicators of empowerment. These measures might, for instance, include beliefs about control, enhanced self-esteem or the acquisition of self-regulatory skills. One appropriate piece of evidence that an empowerment strategy had been successful might be an increase in internality. In actual fact, a variety of researchers have reported correlations between perceived locus of control and a number of health and illness related outcomes, suggesting that internality might well be a desirable goal for empowerment education. Strickland (1978), in a review of published work, made the following observation:

> '... the bulk of research is consistent in implying that when faced with health problems, internal individuals do appear to engage in more generally adaptive responses than do externals ... Findings suggest that the development of an internal orientation could lead to improved health practices for some individuals who have been inclined to believe that life events are beyond their responsibility and more a function of external control.
>
> *(p. 1205)*

At first glance, then, it would seem that we might use measures of internality to assess the effectiveness of programmes of empowerment education, especially since we have a number of more or less standardized psychometric scales at our disposal. Indeed, this might well be a feasible strategy, provided that we also take account of the many other factors which also contribute to empowerment – a point which will be made more explicitly in a later chapter. We would in addition need to have a substantial and long-lasting programme if we were to seriously expect a shift from externality to internality, given that locus of control results from a long period of socialization. A more realistic strategy might be to gauge effectiveness by looking for changes in self-efficacy beliefs and/or the acquisition of a set of competences and skills which are central to assertiveness. Both of these might ultimately be expected to make significant contributions to internality and empowerment more generally.

A review of the effectiveness of assertiveness training or of attempts to enhance self-efficacy is not appropriate at this point. However, by way of further exemplifying the nature of success for an empowerment model, we will comment on the effectiveness of providing anticipatory guidance in a clinical context and of enhancing feelings of control in institutionalized elderly people.

A large number of studies have provided an indication of the beneficial effects of providing patients with health education prior to their undergoing some more or less traumatic experience such as surgery. Arguably, the beneficial effects of the education or counselling derive in large part from the enhanced feelings of control they experience. One of the most impressive results of such 'empowerment' education is provided by an early and classic study by Egbert *et al.* (1964) in which an experimental group receiving anticipatory guidance required a significantly lower dosage of analgesics postoperatively and were discharged from hospital on average 2.7 days earlier than the control group. We might note here that the selected measures of success were in fact those associated with a preventive model rather than an empowerment model, which serves to make a point which will receive further consideration later: what might be considered to be appropriate outcome measures for one particular model will be regarded as intermediate indicators of performance for another model.

The final example selected to illustrate how the success of empowerment education within a general empowerment model might be judged concerns the significance of control in the institutionalized elderly. Unlike the previously reported study of Egbert *et al.*, the prime concern was to enhance quality of life: perceived, existential and actual control were all extremely important contributory factors. The research in question is, additionally, of interest in that it provides a nice illustration of a small scale health promotion programme, i.e. one which involved policy, environmental change and education.

Langer and Rodin (1976) deliberately attempted to enhance the independence and personal control of a group of nursing home residents. The elderly people concerned lived on one floor of what was described as a 'modern, high quality nursing home'. The residents were counselled about their existing opportunities to influence the ways in which the home was run – for instance, how they might influence menus – and, perhaps more importantly, given particular responsibilities. They were, for example, encouraged to arrange the furniture in their rooms and were given potted plants to care for. By comparison a control group occupying a different but similar floor in the home was merely provided with the plants and told that the nursing staff would look after them. Measures of activity levels and general happiness of the two groups revealed that the 'responsibility' group were more alert, active and contented than their counterparts. Moreover, a year and a half later the experimental group had maintained their gain in quality of life (Rodin and Langer, 1977). Similar results were recorded by Ryden (1984) who demonstrated that morale of a group of institutionalized elderly was significantly related to perception of situational control.

However, one of the most intriguing features of Rodin and Langer's research was the improvement in physical health of the 'empowered' elderly group compared with the control group: one of the more dramatic findings was that the death rate of the empowered group was half that of the residents who lacked the benefits of actual and perceived control over their lives.

CONCLUSION

In this first section of the book, we have discussed in some detail the meaning of health promotion and subscribed in general to the ideological stance underpinning WHO's conceptualization. We have considered the relationship of health education to this conceptualization and encapsulated it in a simple assertion that health promotion involves a synergistic relationship between health education and health policy. Above all, we have provided a quite detailed analysis of empowerment, viewing this as a central element in health education and health promotion.

We have, additionally, reviewed a number of so called 'models' of health education and, in doing so, have sought to compare and contrast differentiation made on the basis of ideology with more 'technological' distinctions. We have questioned the utility, and indeed the reality, of distinctions popularly made between models and noted areas of overlap and even false dichotomies. In practice many features of the different models may be reconciled in practice. On the other hand, it is hopefully clear that there are genuine differences in ideology inherent in this 'model making'; practitioners who opt for one or other model are, consciously or unconsciously, revealing what for them are important values and/or different ways of constructing their personal realities. In particular we have noted real differences associated with commitment to one or more features of a medical model; we have observed commitment to the principle of voluntarism; we have even speculated on the influence of personality in respect of people's location on tenderminded–toughminded and radical–conservative continua.

In this section we have explored the implications of subscribing to one or other model of health education for the evaluation of success. We have emphasized that, in seeking to answer questions about the effectiveness and efficiency to health education, we must first of all take account of these ideological and value considerations.

In the next section, our concern will be rather more technological than ideological. We will be seeking to illuminate the research process on which decisions about effective-

ness and efficiency are based. We will also be arguing that competent decisions about evaluation cannot be made without having an effective theoretical framework which helps us understand how people come to make health and illness related decisions. However, having stated that the 'technological' is likely to be our prime concern, it is interesting to note the extent of current debate about research methodology. Such controversy is grounded in personal and professional values and philosophies.

REFERENCES

Anderson, R. (1984) Health promotion: an overview, In *European Monographs in Health Education Research, No. 6*, (ed. L. Barić), Scottish Health Education Group, Edinburgh, pp. 4–126.

Anderson, V. and Draper, P. (1991) Economics and hostile environments, in *Health Through Public Policy*, (ed. P. Draper), Merlin Press, London.

Antonovsky, A. (1979) *Health, Stress and Coping*, Jossey-Bass, San Francisco.

Aronson, E. (1976) *The Social Animal*, 2nd edn, W.H. Freeman, San Francisco.

Aronson, E. and Mettee, D. (1968) Dishonest behaviour as a function of different levels of self esteem. *Journal of Personality and Social Psychology*, **9**, 121–7.

Bandura, A. (1977) Self-efficacy: toward a unifying theory of behavioural change. *Psychological Review*, **64** (2), 191–215.

Bandura, A. (1982) Self-efficacy mechanism in human agency. *American Psychologist*, **37** (2), 122–47.

Bandura, A. (1986) *Social Foundations of Thought and Action: A Social Cognitive Theory*, Prentice-Hall, New Jersey.

Barić, L. (1988). The new public health and the concept of advocacy. *Journal of the Institute of Health Education*, **26** (2), 49–55.

Beattie, A. (1991) Knowledge and control in health promotion: a test case for social policy and social theory, in *The Sociology of the Health Service*, (eds J. Gabe, M. Calnan and M. Bury), Routledge and Kegan Paul, London.

Brown, R.E. and Margo, G.E. (1978) Health education, can the reformers be reformed? *International Journal of Health Services*, **8** (1), 3–23.

Canterbury (1985) *Faith in the City: Report of the Archbishop of Canterbury's Commission on Urban Priority Areas*, Lambeth Palace, London.

Cattell, R.B. (1965) *The Scientific Analysis of Personality*, Penguin, Harmondsworth.

Charles, N. and Kerr, M. (1986) Issues of responsibility and control in the feeding of families, in *The Politics of Health Education: Raising the Issues*, (eds S. Rodmell and A. Watt), Routledge and Kegan Paul, London.

Cochrane, A.L. (1972) *Effectiveness and Efficiency*, Rock Carling Monograph, Nuffield Provincial Hospitals Trust, Oxford.

Coopersmith, S. (1967) *The Antecedents of Self Esteem*, W.H. Freeman, New York.

Coreil, J. and Levin, J.S. (1985) A critique of the lifestyle concept in public health education. *International Quarterly of Community Health Education*, **5** (2), 103–14.

Crawford, R. (1980) Healthism and the medicalization of everyday life. *International Journal of Health Services*, **10**, 365–88.

Dabbs, J.W. (1964) Self-esteem, communicator characteristics and attitude change. *Journal of Abnormal and Social Psychology*, **69**, 173–81.

De Kadt, E. (1982) Ideology, social policy, health and health services: a field of complex interactions. *Social Science and Medicine*, **16**, 741–52.

Dennis, J., Draper, P., Holland, S. (1982) *Health Promotion in the NHS*. Report from a Study Group, Unit for the Study of Health Policy, 8 Newcomen Street, London, SE1 1YR.

Department of Health (1992) *The Health of the Nation: A Strategy for Health in England*, HMSO, London.

Doll, R. (1992) Health and the environment in the 1990s. *American Journal of Public Health*, **82** (7), 933–41.

Downie, R.S., Fyfe, C. and Tannahill, A. (1992) *Health Promotion: Models and Values*, Oxford University Press, Oxford.

Doyal, L. (1981) *The Political Economy of Health*, Pluto Press, London.

Draper, P. (1983) Tackling the disease of ignorance. *Self Health*, **1**, 23–5.

Draper, P., Best, G. and Dennis, J. (1977) Health and wealth. *Royal Society of Health Journal*, **97**, 121–7.

Draper, P., Griffiths, J., Dennis, J. and Papay, J. (1980) Three types of health education. *British Medical Journal*, **281**, 493–5.

Dubos, R. (1959) *The Mirage of Health*, Harper and Row, New York.

Eagleton, T. (1991) *Ideology: An Introduction*, Verso, London.

Egbert, J.A., Battit, G.E., Welch, C.E. and Bartlett, M.K. (1964) Reduction of postoperative pain by encouragement and instruction of patients. *New England Journal of Medicine*, **270**, 825–7.

Eysenck, J.J. (1960) *The Structure of Human Personality*, Methuen, London.

Festinger, L. (1957) *A Theory of Cognitive Dissonance*, Row Peterson, Evanston, Ill.

Flay, B.R., DiTecco, D. and Schlegel, R.P. (1980) Mass media in health promotion: an analysis using an extended information-processing model. *Health Education Quarterly*, **7** (2), 127–47.

Forcinelli, O. (1974) Values education in the public school. *Thrust*, **2**, 81–4.

Freire, P. (1974) *Education and the Practice of Freedom*, Writers and Readers Publishing Co-operative, London (originally published in Portuguese, 1967).

French, J. and Adams, L. (1986) From analysis to synthesis: theories of health education. *Health Education Journal*, **45**, 2, 71–4.

Freudenberg, N. (1981) Health education for social change: a strategy for public health in the US. *International Journal of Health Education*, **24** (3), 1–8.

Fryer, P. (1988) A health city strategy three years on – the case of Oxford City Council. *Health Promotion*, **3** (2), 213–18.

Galbraith, J.K. (1992) Shifting gear, not direction. *The Guardian*, Wednesday 25th November.

Green, L.W. and Kreuter, M.W. (1991) *Health Promotion Planning: An Educational and Environmental Approach*, Mayfield Publishing, California.

Green, L.W. and Raeburn, J.M. (1988) Health promotion. What is it? What will it become? *Health Promotion*, **3** (2), 151–9.

Health Promotion (1986) **1** (4), whole issue.

Health Promotion (1988) The Adelaide recommendations: healthy public policy. *Health Promotion*, **3** (2), 183–6.

Hirst, P. (1969) The logic of the curriculum. *Journal of Curriculum Studies*, **1** (2), 142.

Hopson, B. and Scally, M. (1980) *Lifeskills Teaching Programme, No 1*, Lifeskills Associates, Leeds.

Illich, I. (1976) *The Limits of Medicine – Medical Nemesis: the Expropriation of Health*, Marion Boyars, London.

Kanfer, F.H. and Karoly, P. (1972) Self control: a behaviouristic excursion into the lion's den. *Behavior Therapy*, **3**, 398–416.

Kar, S.B. (1976) *Communication Research in Family Planning: An Analytic Framework*, UNESCO, Paris.

Kickbusch, I. (1986) Issues in Health Promotion. *Health Promotion*, **1** (4), 437–42.

Kickbusch, I. (1989) Health cities: a working project and a growing movement. *Health Promotion*, **4** (2), 77–82.

Labonte, R. and Penfold, S. (1981) Canadian perspectives in health promotion: a critique. *Health Education*, **April**, 4–9.

LaFramboise, H. (1973) Health policy: breaking the problem down into more manageable segments. *Canadian Medical Association Journal*, **108**, 388–91.

Lalonde, M. (1974) *A New Perspective on the Health of Canadians*, Government of Canada, Ottawa.

Lang, T., Andrews, H., Bedale, C. and Hannan, E. (1984) *Jam Tomorrow: A Report of the First Findings of a Pilot Study of the Food Circumstances, Attitudes and Consumption of 1000 People on Low Incomes in the North of England*, Food Policy Unit, Manchester Polytechnic.

Langer, E.J. (1983) *The Psychology of Control*, Sage Publications, Beverly Hills.

Langer, E.J. and Rodin, J. (1976) The effects of enhanced personal responsibility for the aged. *Journal of Personality and Social Psychology*, **34** (2), 191–8.

Levens, G.E. and Rodnight, E. (1973) *The Application of Research in the Planning and Evaluation of Road Safety Publicity*. Proceedings of the European Society for Opinion in Marketing (Budapest) Conference, 197–227.

Levenson, H. (1973) Multidimensional locus of control in psychiatric patients. *Journal of Consulting and Clinical Psychology*, **41**, 397–404.

Lewis, F.M. (1986) The concept of control: a typology and health related variables (unpublished manuscript scheduled for publication).

Macdonald, J.J. and Warren, W.H. (1991) Primary health care as an educational process: a model and a Frierean perspective. *International Quarterly of Community Health Education*, **12** (1), 35–50.

Mahler, H. (1986) Towards a new public health. *Health Promotion*, **1** (1), 1.

Maton, K.I., and Rappaport, J. (1984) Empowerment in a religious setting: a multivariate investigation, in *Studies in Empowerment: Steps Toward Understanding and Action*, (eds J. Rappaport, C. Swift and R. Hess), Haworth Press, New York.

McGregor, D.M. (1966) The human side of enterprise, in *Readings in Managerial Psychology*, (eds H.J. Leavitt and L.R. Pondy), University of Chicago Press, Chicago.

McGuire, W.J. (1981) Theoretical foundations of campaigns, in *Public Communication Campaigns*, (eds R.E. Rice and W.J. Paisley), Sage Publications, Beverly Hills.

McKeown, T. (1979) *The Role of Medicine: Dream, Mirage or Nemesis?* Blackwell, Oxford.

McKinlay, J.B. (1979) A case for refocusing upstream: the political economy of illness, in *Patients, Physicians and Illness*, (ed. E.G. Jaco), The Free Press, New York.

McPhail, P. (1977) *Living Well*, Health Education Council Project 12–18, Cambridge University Press, Cambridge.

Milio, N. (1986) *Promoting Health Through Public Policy*, Canadian Public Health Association, Ottawa.

Minkler, M. (1989) Health education, health promotion and the open society: an historical perspective. *Health Education Quarterly*, **16**, 17–30.

Minkler, M. and Cox, K. (1980) Creating critical consciousness in health: applications of Freire's philosophy and methods to the health care setting. *International Journal of Health Services*, **10** (2), 311–22.

Mitford, N. (1969) *The Sun King*, Sphere Books, London.

Morris, D. (1987) Healthy cities: self reliant cities. *Health Promotion*, **2** (2), 169–76.

National Consumer Council (1992) *Your Food: Whose Choice?* HMSO, London.

Navarro, V. (1976) The underdevelopment of health of working America: causes, consequences and possible solutions. *American Journal of Public Health*, **66**, 538–47.

Puska, P., Nissinen, A., Tuomilehto, J. *et al.* (1985) The community-based strategy of preventing coronary heart disease: conclusions from the ten years of the North Karelia Project. *Annual Review of Public Health*, **6**, 147–93.

Rodin, J. and Langer, E.J. (1977) Long-term effects of a control-relevant intervention with the institutionalized aged. *Journal of Personality and Social Psychology*, **35**, 897–902.

Rodmell, S. and Watt, A. (eds) (1986) *The Politics of Health Education: Raising the Issues*. Routledge and Kegan Paul, London.

Rotter, J.B. (1966) Generalized expectancies for internal versus external control of reinforcement. *Psychological Monographs*, **80** (1), 1–28.

Ryan, W. (1976) *Blaming the Victim*, Vintage Books, New York.

Ryden, M.B. (1984) Morale and perceived control in institutionalized elderly. *Nursing Research*, **33** (3), 130–6.

Sarafino, E.P. (1990) *Health Psychology: Biopsychosocial Interactions* (Chapter 10), John Wiley, New York.

Schools Council (1977) *Schools Council Health Education Project (SCHEP) 5–13*, Nelson, London.

Schwartz, J.L. (1987) *Smoking Cessation Methods: The United States and Canada, 1978–1985*, US Department of Health and Human Services, Washington, pp. 62–71.

Seligman, M.E.P. (1975) *Helplessness: On Depression, Development and Death*, W.H. Freeman, New York.

Society for Public Health Education (1976) *Code of Ethics*, SOPHE, San Francisco.

Stark, E. (1977) 'Introduction' to the special issue of health. *Review of Radical Political Economics*, **9** (1), 45–59.

Stenhouse, L. (1969) Handling controversial issues in the classroom. *Education Canada*, December.

Strickland, B.R. (1978) Internal–external expectancies and health-related behaviours. *Journal of Consulting and Clinical Psychology*, **46** (6), 1192–211.

Sutherland, I. (1979) *Health Education: Perspectives and Choices*, Allen and Unwin, London.

Tones, B.K. (1985) Health promotion – a new panacea? *Journal of the Institute of Health Education*, **23**, 16–21.

Tones, B.K. (1987) Health promotion, affective education and personal-social development of young people, in *Health Education in Schools*, 2nd edn, (eds K. David and T. Williams), Harper and Row, London.

Tones, B.K. (1990) *The Power to Choose: Health Education and the New Public Health*. Health Education Unit, Leeds Metropolitan University.

Tones, B.K. (1992) Health promotion, self-empowerment and the concept of control, in *Health Education: Politics and Practice*, Deakin University Press, Victoria, Australia.

Townsend, P. and Davidson, N. (1992) *Inequalities in Health: The Black Report*, Penguin, Harmondsworth.

Turner, B. (1992) An introduction to the sociology of the body, in *Health Education: Politics and Practice*, Deakin University Press, Victoria, Australia.

US Department of Health, Education and Welfare (1978) *Disease Prevention and Health Promotion*, Washington DC.

US Department of Health, Education and Welfare (1979) *Healthy People*, Washington DC.

US Department of Health and Human Services (1980) *Promoting Health, Preventing Disease: Objectives for the Nation*, Washington DC.

Vuori, H. (1980) The medical model and the objectives of health education. *International Journal of Health Education*, **23**, 1–8.

Wallston, B.S., Wallston, K.A., Kaplan, G.D. and Maides, S.A. (1976) A development and validation of the health locus of control (HLC) scale. *Journal of Consulting and Clinical Psychology*, **44**, 580–5.

Wallston, K.A. and Wallston, B.S. (eds) (1978) Health locus of control. *Health Education Monographs*, **6** (2).

Watterson, A. (1986) Occupational health and illness: the politics of hazard education, in *The Politics of Health Education: Raising the Issues*, (eds S. Rodmell and A. Watt), Routledge and Kegan Paul, London.

Whitehead, M. (1992) *The Health Divide*, Penguin, Harmondsworth.

Wilkinson, R.G. (1992) National mortality rates: the impact of inequality? *American Journal of Public Health*, **82** (8), 1082–4.

World Health Organization (1946) *Constitution*, WHO, Geneva.

World Health Organization (1978) *Report on the International Conference on Primary Health Care, Alma Ata, 6–12 September*, WHO, Geneva.

World Health Organization (1984) *Health Promotion: A Discussion Document on the Concepts and Principles*, WHO Regional Office for Europe, Copenhagen.

World Health Organization (1985) *Targets for Health for All*, WHO Regional Office for Europe, Copenhagen.

World Health Organization (1986) *Ottawa Charter for Health Promotion, An International Conference on Health Promotion, November 17–21*, WHO Regional Office for Europe, Copenhagen.

World Health Organization (1992) *Health Dimensions of Economic Reform*, WHO, Geneva.

Zimbardo, P., Ebbesen, E. and Maslach, C. (1977) *Influencing Attitudes and Changing Behaviour*, Addison-Wesley, Reading, Mass.

Zola, I.K. (1970) *Helping – does it matter? The problems and prospects of mutual aid groups*. Address to United Ostomy Association.

INTRODUCTION

While it is routine to reflect on the health education activities in which we participate, a commitment to evaluation requires that this reflection be formalized such that the worth of activities can be assessed and demonstrated. It has been commonplace in health education to deplore both the overall paucity of evaluation and the methodological shortcomings of that which has taken place. As the demand for, and commitment to, evaluation has increased so have the debates about its nature and purpose and the methodological approaches to be adopted in undertaking it.

Recently it has seemed that these debates have been somewhat livelier within the broader field of health promotion rather than within the more restricted one of health education – especially in those areas where the traditional focus has been oriented towards the evaluation of behavioural indicators (Kelly, 1989; O'Neill, 1988; Milio, 1990). This chapter will consider the nature of evaluation research both in general and with reference to health education before commenting on the current status of methodological debates.

While we do not seek to describe evaluation designs and research methods in detail we will provide some introductory discussions and comment on the factors which bear on the choice of designs. The final section of the chapter will comment on ethical and political issues in evaluation research and conclude with some reflections on the evaluation of health education within the wider context of health promotion.

WHAT IS EVALUATION RESEARCH?

As a process, evaluation is concerned with assessing an activity against values and goals in such a way that results can contribute to future decision making and/or policy. Quite simply, therefore, evaluation research describes the research processes which support evaluation where research is defined as any disciplined enquiry. This research activity may be directed to the process of an activity, the context in which it takes place and its outcomes – both immediate and long term. The attention given to the various elements will vary according to the purposes of an evaluation and the decisions made by the various stakeholders involved.

Much evaluation takes place as an integral part of routine health education practice and is undertaken by practitioners themselves. The results will be used locally for a number of purposes and may also be published more widely. In many instances, however, there is an external component to evaluation: this may be elicited by programme participants or it may be imposed by funders of activities. In the case of external evaluation there will be different viewpoints on the role of the evaluator which relate, as we will see later, to the methodological stance adopted towards the evaluation process. Earlier literature on the evaluation of social programmes tended to be concerned largely with evaluation as an independent and external element. This is now much less the case as a consequence of debates about the methodology of research and about relationships within the research process. Health education evaluation provides examples of the range of philosophical positions on evaluation.

Within the research literature there are debates about the extent to which evaluation differs from other research activity. Finch (1986) is of the view that evaluation involving empirical research raises a range of questions which are common to other types of research activity although the particular blend of these may be unique to evaluative studies. While we would endorse this position it may be helpful to note the aspects of evaluation which have contributed towards ascribing it a distinctive status (Smith, 1975).

1. Evaluation research is typically concerned to assess the achievement of desirable goals – both the processes involved and the outcomes – while general research has a wider range of purposes.
2. Evaluation research is more likely to be conducted for a client who may set the research questions and who may wish to use findings for defined purposes such as justification for continued programme support. The general researcher may therefore have somewhat greater control over the various stages of the research process although too much emphasis should not be put on this. As Jamieson (1984) has noted, the constraints on general academic research can be considerable while some major contractors of evaluation research, such as, for example, the Schools Council in England and Wales, applied relatively few constraints.
3. Where evaluation is essentially an externally managed process the evaluation elements of a programme may not be a priority to participants. Programme priorities can generate both conflicts of interest and conflicts over control of resources with the interests of the programme staff and researcher as inherently competitive. Programme staff can be predominantly service oriented and see data collection

procedures as disruptive. In addition evaluation may be perceived as both potentially worthless by programme participants if they already believe in the worth of a programme and potentially threatening if negative findings could lead to discontinuation of the programme. With the adoption of styles of evaluation where it is not externally located or where the evaluation and project teams negotiate fully from the start and there is a more equal participation in evaluation activities, the difficulties noted above will be less obvious.

4. Evaluation research findings can be used for a range of purposes: to provide feedback to activities and projects; for dissemination to others; for developing theory about activities and contexts studied; and for accounting purposes – assessing the worth in terms of effectiveness, efficiency and equity, etc. Some of these uses are specific to evaluation, others are shared with all research.
5. Because of the diversity of stakeholders in evaluation, there can be greater potential for conflict than in general research. Some areas of conflict have already been mentioned. In addition, each of the stakeholders may assess a project from different perspectives. In an extreme sample a health authority may proclaim the rhetoric of health promotion but may be predominantly concerned that evaluation demonstrate improvements in a narrow range of health indicators while the programme workers and participants may be fundamentally oriented towards achieving community empowerment. There can also be conflict over the emphasis to give to outcome in comparison with process measures and over the means of production, presentation and dissemination of evaluation findings.
6. The commissioned evaluation researcher may have less control over choice of research methods than in undertaking

general academic research and, if seeking to conduct an experimental style of evaluation, is likely to have less control over variables.

7. Most research is time bound. In evaluation which is externally funded or where a programme has a finite length, the time constraint may be particularly apparent.

8. Finally, a difference is commonly drawn between evaluation and general research in the use of findings. Jamieson (1984) sees the goals of the research report as the enhancement of understanding and knowledge via publication to the academic community while the evaluation report informs and/or influences decision makers. He emphasizes that these are not clearcut distinctions as much as relative emphases of the two areas of research.

EVALUATION OF HEALTH EDUCATION

Evaluation, it has recently been stressed (Candeias, 1991), should be seen not as an end in itself but as an integral part of all health education activities. While this may seem to be a truism the fact remains that much health education is still not formally evaluated or evaluation is seen to be narrowly focused on parts of programmes. The perceived shortcomings in evaluation may relate to resource issues but also to the philosophical approaches to the activity of those concerned.

Where the defined outcome of health education activity is behaviour change with the expectation that this will be related to health improvements, the focus of evaluation measures is going to be narrower and measurements somewhat easier than where empowerment goals are sought. Where the general focus is on outcomes associated with a preventive model of health education it has, however, increasingly been acknowledged that it may be important to address process as well as outcomes – either because response to formative evaluations may increase the

likelihood of achieving outcomes or because of some measure of commitment to enhancing wider participation in the evaluation process.

Process measures may be quantitative and/or qualitative. Commenting from a position of commitment to methodological pluralism (see below), McLeroy *et al.* (1992) noted that few process elements in quantitative evaluations actually include qualitative information on participants' perceptions of the programme. These writers have discussed the wide range of goals to which health education should be directed and the consequences of this for evaluation. The goals of health education should include, they say:

> … not only changes in health related behaviour but changes in the capacity of individuals, networks and organizations to address health problems. Whether labelled as capacity building, empowerment or other terms, what is missing from our literature are methods for measuring changes in problem solving ability at various levels of analysis.

They also note the importance of taking into consideration the wider social context in which evaluation programmes are embedded, a point which was emphasized previously by Parlett (1981).

As noted earlier, debates are increasingly taking place about the objectives and methods of research within the wider field of health promotion. These debates will be commented on briefly since they have implications for the practice and evaluation of the constituent activity of health education.

APPROACHES TO EVALUATION – METHODOLOGICAL CONSIDERATIONS

In common with other disciplines within the broad area of social and behavioural sciences, health education research has seen debates on epistemological issues leading to a range of proposals: choosing between competing paradigms; adoption of methodological pluralism;

seeking some new paradigm; or most recently, a more general challenge associated with postmodern theorizing. The discussion has, for the most part, organized around the consideration of opposing positions – at the level of epistemology in contrasting positivism with phenomenology or at the data level – quantitative with qualitative. The details of these debates have been discussed widely so brief comment will be offered here prior to commenting on the significance for evaluation research.

Put crudely, two contrasting research paradigms are commonly outlined: a positivist scientific approach which informs the natural sciences and those social sciences seeking to emulate them and leads to quantitative research and a phenomenological tradition which underpins qualitative research. The former position has a number of key elements: the assumption that objective accounts of features of the world can be generated; the attempt to describe general patterns and elucidate causal relationships and general laws; the proposal of unity of methods between the natural and social sciences; and the use of scientific method for testing of hypotheses. The contrasting position starts from the recognition that individuals routinely interpret and make sense of their worlds and the acquisition of knowledge comes from gaining access to these subjective understandings through defined processes.

The generation of qualitative data has been central to ethnographic enquiry within anthropology and increasingly influential in sociology. In its earlier history health education was largely dominated by research in the quantitative tradition – in part because, as a subject which drew on a number of contributory disciplines, it was influenced by the research tradition within each of them. For example, psychology, epidemiology and education were important early disciplines to which health education referred. At the time, these disciplines looked to natural science for their methodology and health education

followed suit. In addition, since the two broad paradigms have not in general been accorded equal status it has been the tendency of new disciplines, in establishing their credibility and a respectable research tradition, to adopt a scientific paradigm.

As the positivist tradition came under severe attack in disciplines such as sociology more research activity began to be underpinned by phenomenological approaches. For a number of reasons, including the growing emphasis on the analyses of the social context in understanding health and illness and the stronger influence of sociology and, to a somewhat lesser extent, anthropology, health education research began also, to varying degrees, to embrace the phenomenological tradition. Some researchers mainly committed to a quantitative tradition found it helpful to include some elements of qualitative data collection in surveys while others fully embraced a qualitative tradition (Tilford and Delaney, 1992).

The emergence of a general readiness to adopt pluralist approaches in social scientific research has been accompanied by differential acknowledgement of the epistemological difficulties in so doing. Bryman (1984), for example, in commenting on a series of accounts of research projects, noted the writers' practical justification for the particular methods used in studying organizations but the relative absence of epistemological comment. At the same time Silverman (1985), in his contribution to the methodological debate, challenged the assumption that the two paradigms are incommensurable or that they offer any worthwhile description of the major alternative directions in research. For example, he seeks to demonstrate some uses of quantification in research which is qualitative and interpretative in design: simple counting techniques can offer, he suggests, a means to survey the whole corpus of data ordinarily lost in intensive qualitative research. Some time ago Cicourel, with reference to sociology (1964), cautioned against abandoning quantitative data:

In a bureaucratic technological society, numbers talk. Today with sociology on trial we cannot afford to live like hermits, blinded by global theoretical critiques, to the possible analytical and practical use of quantification.

The combination of quantitative and qualitative methods in answering research questions has been seen by many researchers as both practical and unproblematic. This 'triangulation' of methodologies can be used in addition to triangulation of methods or of researchers. The term triangulation derives from an analogy with surveying where the use of two or more bearings, rather than one, enables a position to be located precisely. In research, reliance on one data type or source can, if errors are unrecognized, lead to inappropriate conclusions whereas use of more sources and/or types may enhance confidence in accuracy of results. Triangulation has been discussed in detail by Denzin (1978) and the notion has received much support, although reservations are also expressed. Adding up different sets or types of data does not necessarily provide a more complete picture – they could all be equally incorrect. Furthermore, as Hammersley and Atkinson note (1983), differences between sets or types of data may be just as important and illuminating. Where there is triangulation of data derived from methods associated with each of the opposing paradigms epistemological objections can be raised and Blaikie (1991) has cautioned against the easy acceptance of triangulation of methodologies.

In those disciplines whose focus of concern may be the need to understand individual interpretations within the constraints of social structures, some integration and synthesis of ideas from the two traditions seems to be called for. The realist position (Keat and Urry, 1975), for example, argues that social structures are real in the sense that they are partially independent of individuals and their perceptions. The role of meaning in social life is recognized without accepting that this dissolves the constraining power of social structures (Silverman, 1985) and research needs to address not one or the other, but both.

It is not possible to describe, within health education, a unified response to the paradigmatic debate. Many would wish to celebrate diversity in research activity while others might favour some unified position but see it as too soon in the history of the discipline for such a development. There is a degree of consensus that within the discipline as a whole, given the range of objectives of health education activities, methodological pluralism makes considerable good sense. There is rather less consensus that methodological pluralism within single studies is acceptable.

A new dimension to the discussion is being provided from discussions of postmodernism and health promotion. While discussion of postmodernism is beyond the scope of this book some brief observations can be made. According to such documents as the Ottawa Charter (1986), health promotion is oriented towards the achievement of equity, participation, intersectoral collaboration and so on. The implications for research of these health promotion goals have been discussed (Stevenson and Burke, 1991; Hayes and Willms, 1990; Kelly, 1989) and claims made that health promotion be seen as a postmodern project. Davies and Kelly (1993), for example, propose from their examination of Healthy Cities initiatives that some of the difficulties in developing a research programme stem from the failure to acknowledge the 'postmodern' nature of health promotion.

While there is a fair degree of confusion about the meaning of postmodern and a questioning as to whether it constitutes something distinct from 'modern' or simply describes a late stage in modernity, a number of features can be tentatively identified. In using the term postmodern a reaction to modernity is typically being registered; modernity as a composition of ideas and projects emerging from the Enlightenment (a label for a set of theories and attitudes developing just before and after the French Revolution) with its emphasis on equality, (limited) democracy, emancipation, the importance of rationality and efforts to solve problems through the use of scientific principles. Within the domain of health, modernity would be characterized by adoption of the medical model discussed earlier.

Despite the progressive goals of modernity, some disillusionment has developed in those societies which were the first to experience modernity. 'Postmodernists' criticize, according to Rosenau (1992), 'all that modernity has engendered: the accumulated experience of western civilization, industrialization, urbanization, advanced technology, the nation state, life in the "fast lane"'. Others would suggest a milder critique in proposing that the question of postmodernism is 'about the possible limits of the process of modernization' (Turner, 1990). Where knowledge is concerned postmodernists challenge the disciplinary boundaries of modernity which can be construed as attempts to bring order to a disorderly world and celebrate the breaking of boundaries. There can also be a rejection of conventional academic styles of discourse in favour of audacious and provocative forms of delivery (Rosenau, 1992).

One of the key observations to make about the discourse on postmodernism is that it is diverse, contradictory and beset with multiple definitions of the terms used. Where does this leave us? In order to relate health promotion to the postmodern discussions it may be helpful to draw on the distinction made by Rosenau (1992) between two broad orientations: the sceptical and the affirmative postmodernists. The former offer a wholly negative assessment of modernity and the postmodern condition. The 'affirmatives' accept the critiques of modernity but have a more optimistic view of a postmodern era. They are described:

as open to positive political action, or content, with the recognition of visionary,

personal non-dogmatic projects that range from New Age religion to New Wave lifestyles and include a whole spectrum of postmodern social movements. Most affirmatives seek a philosophical and ontological intellectual practice that is non-dogmatic, tentative and non-ideological. These postmodernists do not, however, shy away from affirming an ethic, making normative choices, and striving to build issue-specific coalitions. Many argue that certain value choices are superior to others.

(Rosenau, 1992)

Much of the discussion of health promotion as a postmodern project would seem to fit within this notion of affirmative postmodernism. While many would want to challenge the conception of health promotion as postmodern, we will simply note here the implications of postmodernism for the methodological debate. Given the support for diversity, it is not possible or appropriate to make definitive statements on postmodernism and research. While there is opposition to scientific styles of research and support for qualitative ones, this would be part of a broad eclecticism in modes of enquiry rather than a pursuit for a single paradigm within which to operate.

IMPLICATIONS OF THE METHODOLOGICAL DEBATE FOR THE EVALUATION OF HEALTH EDUCATION

As noted earlier evaluation research, while having relatively specific goals and operating within a number of constraints, is not a separate kind of research. As far as methodology is concerned the approaches adopted to evaluation mirror those in general health education research ranging from advocates of positivist evaluation using experimental and survey designs through to supporters of fully participative qualitative evaluation. Increasingly there has been support for evaluation which is methodologically pluralist. While it is difficult to generalize, much evaluation still remains essentially quantitative with small qualitative additions – either through the addition of open-ended questions in surveys or some limited qualitative process measures.

Aside from the epistemological debates there is the need to assess the implications for evaluation which arise from the nature of health education with its particular aspirations. If health education is seen to be a constituent of health promotion, defined broadly, and seeking to achieve the activities outlined in the Ottawa Charter it becomes important to ask how far it should, in its own activities, contribute to these goals, i.e equity, participation, concern with the subjective understandings of the communities in which research takes place and so on.

We would wish to emphasize the need to develop evaluation styles for health promotion research which seek to ensure participatory styles of evaluation where possible and appropriate. It is also important, however, to acknowledge the importance of pragmatism when we are seeking to evaluate health education in all its forms and contexts. The political sense of demonstrating success in quantitative and cost effective terms may be obvious when seeking to justify the use of resources or eliciting further funding. The danger comes when narrow evaluative goals are seen to be the most relevant or the only relevant ones in situations where a programme clearly has wider goals.

In practical terms evaluation needs to focus on four elements of health education programmes: the context of the activity; the planned content; the process of implementation; and the outcomes both immediate and longer term. Earlier evaluations focused heavily on the second and last of these but the third has increasingly been addressed while the first may still be relatively neglected, as noted earlier. Writers on evaluation distinguish the elements assessed in an evaluation in more than one way. A fairly common distinction, as noted earlier, can be between process, impact and outcome where impact is the overall effectiveness in terms of knowledge, attitudes and practices and outcome is changes in health variables. As will be clear from discussion elsewhere health educators need to be rather careful in allowing themselves to be evaluated according to such outcome measures.

A widely used distinction is that between formative and summative evaluation where formative focuses on the production of data in the course of an activity which can be fed back with the aim of improving it further while summative evaluation addresses the impacts and outcomes of activities. Formative evaluation can include both qualitative and quantitative elements. The language used to describe evaluation and the relationships involved in it reflects broad methodological approaches. Much evaluation literature informed predominantly by a quantitative tradition reflects a top-down approach in which programmes are said to be 'delivered' or 'implemented', will have 'impact' and generate 'outcomes' and where participants will typically be described as 'subjects'.

Where there is a stronger commitment to qualitative research the relationship between evaluators and programme participants is presented differently. Programme participants are described as 'collaborators' – knowledgeable people with a stake in the utility of findings (Glanz *et al.*, 1992) and with a unique and valuable perspective in answering the evaluator's questions. Participatory or partnership evaluation has been described by Argyros (in Reason and Rowan, 1981) as involving a participatory–collaborative relationship predicated on mutual benefits among coequal partners. The different partners contribute different things to the evaluation including technical and research skills, organizational ones, local knowledge, etc. Such an approach to evaluation is more likely to ensure trust between the various partners in an evaluative process.

While some participatory evaluations may be predominantly qualitative many do generate both quantitative and qualitative data. Even in cases where there is little commitment to participatory evaluation a measure of participation needs to be achieved if the products of the evaluation are to be owned by the participants and acted on appropriately.

Throughout the remainder of the book we will be referring to all types of evaluative studies informed by differing methodological approaches. In discussion of particular studies we will use the specific language adopted in them but in general the writer's preference is for the use of the softer language of the participatory approaches in discussions of evaluation in so far as this is appropriate.

DESIGNING EVALUATIONS

This section will review the main types of evaluation design used in health education and comment on the technical questions of reliability and validity of each. Reliability refers to the degree to which the results obtained by a measurement procedure can be replicated. Questions of validity address whether the observations made in a study correspond to an actual state of affairs. Various types of validity are described including external and internal validity: external validity addresses the extent to which findings can be generalized beyond a study population; internal validity addresses the appropriateness of research methods and the soundness of explanations, e.g. does what is interpreted as a cause actually produce the specified effects? Different research designs are variously reliable and valid.

A number of considerations will have a bearing on choice of design: the nature of the activity to be evaluated; the responsibilities and objectives of any funding agency; the overall philosophy of the evaluator; constraints including time and budgets; and the purposes for which evaluation is being undertaken. In categorizing designs it is quite common to find experimental, survey and ethnographic designs distinguished. Both

experiments and surveys would be seen to conform to the positivist paradigm – ethnography predominantly with the interpretivist. In practice, some surveys can include open-ended questions which generate qualitative data and ethnographies can include quantification.

In the following discussion we will examine the underlying premises of designs which predominantly locate to defined methodological positions. We will reflect the overall body of existing evaluation work in health education by looking first at experimental and survey designs. Of these two types, surveys of one kind or another constitute the larger proportion of evaluated work. We will start, however, by looking at experimental design since it is, conventionally, the route to developing the strongest evidence of effectiveness of health education programmes.

EXPERIMENTAL DESIGN

Experimental or intervention studies introduce a planned change and study its outcomes. The objective is to establish causal relationships between an intervention, typically described as the independent variable, and an outcome, the dependent variable. The relationship between the variables is expressed in advance in the form of a null hypothesis, i.e. that the independent variable under study has no association with, or effect on, the dependent variable. If this is rejected we have evidence that our hypothesized relationship does exist.

Such a decision is open to type 1 and type 2 errors. The former occurs when we wrongly conclude that the null hypothesis is false and the latter where we accept the null hypothesis when there is a real difference in the populations studied. An example of a study hypothesis would be: there is no association between participation in group discussion and decision making activities and attitude change.

If we are concerned to demonstrate the effectiveness of a particular health education intervention in achieving specified outcomes an experimental design provides the strongest design that can be used. It allows us, within specified limits, to rule out other causes of the outcomes. In more sophisticated designs we can also compare the relative impacts of subelements of a programme.

In their simplest form experiments use two groups: an experimental group receives the activity to be evaluated while the control group does not receive it. Individuals are randomly assigned (p. 61) to each of the two conditions in order to distribute other factors that might contribute to outcomes. Both groups typically undertake baseline measures followed by the intervention and then the measurement of outcomes. This can be presented in diagrammatic form:

Experiment

RO1	X	RO2	Experimental group
RO3	–	RO4	Control group

R = Randomization   O = Measurement
X = Intervention

An example of an evaluation study which conformed to this pattern is that by Basler *et al.* (1991) of nicotine gum assisted group therapy in a primary care setting with smokers identified as having an increased risk of coronary disease. The programme intervention consisted of use of the gum together with nutritional information, behavioural training for the promotion of self-management techniques and the prescription of a quit smoking date. The control subjects received no specific intervention but were offered the programme after the conclusion of treatment in the experimental groups. At a three month follow-up 63.9% of the experimental group were abstaining from smoking in comparison with 3.3% of the control group.

In some cases studies will be undertaken which contain the elements of an experimental design except that no pretest measures are carried out. This may be defended where a pretest may interfere with the impact of the intervention but has the disadvantage that there is less evidence that the intervention caused the outcomes. The impact of a pretest can be assessed using a Solomon 4 design. This includes four groups: two receive the intervention and there are two control groups but only one of the experimental and one of the control groups undertakes both the pre- and post-tests. The design is illustrated as follows.

Solomon 4

RO1	X	RO2
RO3	–	RO4
	X	RO5
	–	RO6

A hypothetical study using this design could evaluate the effect of a short programme of cancer education in secondary schools on knowledge, beliefs and attitudes towards cancer. The control group would have lessons on some other unrelated aspect of health education. The design would be as follows with pupils randomized into the four conditions.

Group 1	Pretest	Cancer education	Post-test
Group 2	Pretest	Control programme	Post-test
Group 3	–	Cancer education	Post-test
Group 4	–	Control programme	Post-test

If we compare the post-test measures for groups 3 and 4 the main impact of the intervention can be measured while post-test comparison of groups 2 and 4 measures the main impact of the pretest.

It is quite common in health education programmes to include a number of activities whose relative contribution to an overall outcome we wish to evaluate. For example, we may wish to assess the effects of differing educational methods, both separately and in combination. A factorial design can be used.

If X1 and X2 are two programme elements their effectiveness separately and in combination could be tested as follows.

Factorial design

RO1	X1	RO2
RO3	X2	RO4
RO5	X1X2	RO6
RO7	–	RO8

An example of such a design would be the investigation of the individual and combined effects of two teaching methods on the development of social interaction skills. Groups would be randomized into the four conditions.

Group 1 Pretest	Video demonstration	Post-test
Group 2 Pretest	Role play	Post-test
Group 3 Pretest	Video + role play	Post-test
Group 4 Pretest	–	Post-test

The results from group 3 may show an additive effect of the two separate interventions or even a multiplicative one.

More examples of specific designs for experiments can be followed up in general research texts. The above examples conform to what is typically described as 'true' experimental design. In some situations which are to be evaluated it may not be practicable, or be seen as ethical, to randomize individuals into experimental and control conditions. For example, we may wish to evaluate the effectiveness of the programme of cancer education mentioned above in schools and may have to work with existing classes. In this case we would seek to work with matched classes which would be randomized into the experimental and control conditions and we would have what Campbell and Stanley (1963) describe as a quasiexperimental design. This design is the nearest to meeting the full criteria for experimentation.

Other quasi designs are used and they are variously beset by shortcomings when compared with a 'true' design although they may be the most feasible in specific situations. A commonly used example is where one group only is used which acts as its own control. A series of measures may be taken prior to an intervention plus one or more post-test measures.

01	02	03	X	04	05	06

For example, we may wish to evaluate the impact of teaching about oral rehydration solution in a primary health setting. A series of measures could be made of the numbers of children under five years brought to a health centre with acute diarrhoea. The intervention would consist of discussing ideas about the causes and management of diarrhoea and teaching the skills of making and administering ORS. If the intervention is successful the numbers of children being treated should fall after the teaching. Clearly other factors than the intervention could have caused the effects and apparent success would need to be confirmed. For example, the incidence of diarrhoea could have dropped around the time of the intervention or an unanticipated consequence of the ORS teaching could be a change in the customary practice of parents to bring a child with acute diarrhoea to the health centre. The existence of a comparison group where the intervention did not take place strengthens such studies.

Strengths and weaknesses of experimental designs

There can be both practical and ethical barriers to the adoption of experimental designs even where their underlying philosophical rationale is accepted. We also have to raise questions about reliability and validity. Experiments are typically seen to have high reliability in comparison with other designs in that their procedures are clearly specified and are open to replication. They are also high in internal validity but since they are frequently carried out in artificial situations they may have reduced external validity.

Many quasi experiments may take place in community settings where the experimental community receives the intervention and the control or reference population does not. It can, however, be difficult in natural settings to prevent 'contamination' of the reference population. If this occurs the apparent impact of the intervention will be reduced. This was a problem in the North Karelia Project (Puska *et al.*, 1985) and has recently been discussed with reference to Heartbeat Wales (Nutbeam *et al.*, 1993). Although the selected reference population was relatively distant from Wales, the intervention country, the project had attracted interest and ideas and projects from it transferred rapidly with some consequential undermining of the quasiexperimental design. The writers make suggestions to overcome such difficulties: the fuller use of process measures in both study and reference populations and the use of outcome evaluation designs which do not rely on comparing change with a reference population.

The ethics of experimental design have been debated in general, and in particular, around the implementation of randomized clinical controlled trials – the experimental testing of new procedures and drugs within clinical medicine. The principle of randomization in such situations has been challenged and the rights of participants to have the opportunity to give informed consent have been claimed. When this right is built into a research protocol it may not subsequently be possible to recruit adequate numbers for satisfactory hypothesis testing. While health education experiments may not present quite such acute dilemmas as experiments in clinical medicine, the issues of consent have to be considered. They can easily be overlooked in work with children and other less powerful client groups.

In practical terms it can be difficult to plan and implement fully controlled experimental studies of health education activities. The use of laboratory type conditions can be both artificial and inappropriate and where interventions have been tested in such artificial situations we have to ask questions about the generalizability of findings to the real world. Even when experimental studies in health education have taken place in normal practice settings the outcomes which result from the extra efforts which typically go into an evaluated study may be a unrealistic guide to what can be achieved in routine practice. Finally, while experiments can establish statistical significance it may be more important to focus on practical significance.

SURVEY DESIGN

A survey is described by Marsh (1984) as an investigation where:

1. Systematic measurements are made over a series of cases yielding a rectangle of data;
2. The variables in the matrix are analysed to see if they show any patterns.

An extract from a case by variable matrix from a hypothetical survey of young people and alcohol is shown in Table 2.1. Respondents would all have responded to a standardized set of questions using a self-completed questionnaire or interview schedule.

Surveys can be either descriptive and enumerative or analytic and relational. The former generate counts: for example, the overall percentage of a population or representative sample who can list the causes of a specified

Table 2.1 Young people and alcohol

Variable	*Respondent 1*	*Respondent 2*	*Respondent 3*
Age	15	16	18
Sex	F	M	M
Units of alcohol/week	8	15	25
Alcohol knowledge	High	Low	Medium

disease. In our example above we would describe the average number of units of alcohol consumed per week by boys and by girls in specific age groups. Analytic surveys are designed to explore hypothesized relationships between variables. We could test the relationship between knowledge of alcohol and levels of use.

In contrast with experiments, surveys cannot establish definitively cause and effect relationships. Even in types of survey where an independent variable can be seen to have preceded the dependent one, as in cohort studies, it cannot be definitively shown that the effect may not have been caused by another third factor. Surveys can be carried out on whole populations and the population census is the best known example of such a survey. Most surveys, however, are carried out on representative samples and may either be of the one-off type or involve repeated measures. When more than one measure is taken it may be on the same sample or different representative samples may be selected on each occasion.

Data in surveys can be gathered by questionnaires, interview schedules or by observation. The three main types of survey are: one-shot designs in which information needed is collected in the course of one approach to a research population; time series or trend designs in which equivalent samples of a population are studied at different points of time and comparable information is collected on each occasion; and repeated contact designs which involve the collection of information from the same informants on two or more occasions. Each of these will be briefly considered and health education relevant examples provided.

One-shot designs

The most commonly used type of this design is the cross-sectional study (usually described as a prevalence study in epidemiology) where a representative cross-section of a population is studied. Information elicited typically refers to the present but retrospective data may also be obtained. Case control or retrospective studies are an extension of cross-sectional studies and are particularly used in epidemiological enquiry in analysing association between past exposure to aetiological agents and the presence or absence of disease. Cases are selected in which the subject of interest is present and matched with controls and comparable retrospective information elicited from each.

Health educators may be asked to promote the wearing of bicycle helmets and a case control study could examine the effectiveness of wearing such helmets and the contributory role of education. The study by Thompson *et al.* (1989) compared cyclists attending emergency departments with head injuries (cases) with cyclists attending with other injuries (controls). The study was a large one and the researchers were able to control for age, sex, income, education, cycling experience and severity of accident. The conclusion was that wearing of helmets was associated with over 80% reduction in head injury.

There are a number of difficulties with case control studies. Bias can result from the process of selection of cases and controls, e.g. eligible participants are not available or there are shortcomings in the matching of case and controls. These studies typically rely on retrospective information which can be difficult to recall accurately if anything beyond a short time scale is involved. Both recall and interviewer biases may occur: cases may recall more of their past health and health behaviour than controls and where interviewers are aware of which people are the cases and which the controls, the questioning of the former may be unconsciously more thorough.

Time series designs

The General Household Survey in the UK is an example of a time series design. Samples of 10 000 are selected annually and questioned about a range of subjects (including morbidity) in the last fortnight.

Repeated contact designs

These involve measures of the same population on a number of occasions. Depending on the field of study these studies are variously labelled as prospective, incidence or cohort studies in epidemiology and as longitudinal studies in such fields as education and developmental psychology. In epidemiology a population is followed up during which time some members are exposed to disease risk factors and some are not – the incidence of disease in the two groups is compared.

A recent study by McBride *et al.* (1992) of relapse to smoking after childbirth provides an example of a prospective study. One hundred and six women who had stopped smoking during pregnancy were surveyed at the 28th week of pregnancy and then six weeks and six months after the birth of their babies. The study aimed to understand the psychosocial factors which precipitated a return to smoking. Twenty-four per cent of the women had begun to smoke again after six weeks and 40% after six months. Predictors identified for a return to smoking were partner's smoking status; nature of social support; decrease in self-efficacy and the types of coping strategy used to resist smoking.

Prospective studies have some difficulties: where they are planned to continue for a long period loss of participants can occur and over time there may a drift in researcher practice in carrying out measures.

Planning surveys

There are a variety of texts which discuss in some detail the planning of surveys. We will comment on a few aspects which are relevant to later discussions.

While the population census is directed towards national populations it is usual, as noted above, for surveys to be orientated towards some defined subsection of the population appropriate to the research topic. A research population needs to be carefully specified such that it is neither too heterogeneous (including people from whom we do not require information for the purposes of addressing research questions) or too homogeneous (not including the full range of people from whom information is sought). For example, if we are interested in the attitudes to safe sex practices of 16–19 year olds in a region we do not include 15 year olds in the research population or confine enquiry only to public school pupils.

At times the whole population about which we wish to describe variables or offer explanations may be a small one. A study could in such cases collect data from the whole population. More usually we draw samples from the population of interest in such a way that we can, with specified degrees of confidence, apply findings to the reference population.

The ideal to be achieved for some surveys will be probability sampling where a probability sample is defined (Smith, 1975) as one where every unit has a chance of being selected which is different from 0 to 100% and that chance is a known probability. As a result of probability sampling we can accurately estimate the precision with which the sample represents the population from which it was drawn. The degree of precision to be expected from estimates can be laid down in advance of sampling and tolerance limits specified. The risks that such tolerance limits will be reached is presented in the confidence limits. The classic form of probability sampling is simple random sampling and is one where units from a reference population are drawn in such a way that all members have an equal chance of selection. It is clear that to sample in this way we must be able to identify all units in the total population – a complete sampling frame. Random sampling is not always possible and other forms may be used: systematic; stratified; cluster and multistage.

Systematic

The production of a specified proportion sample from a sampling frame, e.g. 1 in 20.

This is simple to do but there is a risk of bias resulting from hidden correlations between characteristics of a population and the numbering system in the sampling frame.

Stratified

Before selection takes place the population is divided into a number of strata such as age groups, classes, ethnic groups and random samples are then selected from each stratum. The sample size from each stratum may be in proportion to its population size or it may be disproportionate. We may choose disproportionate samples when the total numbers in specific strata are small.

Cluster

This is a sampling of complete groups or units. For example, a health survey of adults in a rural region could take villages as its clusters, select a random sample of the villages and administer the survey to all adults in the selected sample.

Multistage

This combines various types of sampling. For example, in the previous example where a region is very large it may be costly to sample randomly across the whole region. We can start from districts from which a random number is selected and then proceed to select villages within the districts.

Where the full population is not known, as, for example, in describing the current numbers sleeping rough in cities, purposive samples have to be selected. With such samples we do not have access to knowledge about sampling error since we lack a complete sampling frame.

Quota sampling, much used in market research and public opinion surveys, is a well known example of non-probability sampling. This is stratified sampling where the selection within strata is made on a non-random basis. For example, in a survey of voting intentions, interviewers will be given a list of categories and the number of people to interview in each of the categories. Categories could be occupational; age; sex; etc. The selection of respondents within the categories is left to the interviewer.

In qualitative research studies it is common to use snowball sampling whereby the initial participants in the study suggest further respondents.

Strengths and weaknesses of surveys

If we wish to elucidate casual relationships, surveys are less satisfactory than experimental designs. In health education, however, there are many circumstances where experiments would not be feasible or desirable and surveys will therefore furnish the next best evidence of causal relationships.

Surveys which are longitudinal are stronger than retrospective ones since hypothesized causal factors in the former precede effects. Where questions of reliability are concerned surveys are rated highly but may be challenged where validity is concerned, both on internal and external grounds. Because of the complexity of some of the concepts addressed in surveys they are often criticized for including weak operationalization. Marsh (1984) has defended surveys claiming that it is not the survey method itself which is the problem but poorly performed surveys.

ETHNOGRAPHIC DESIGNS

Ethnography is being used as a not altogether satisfactory heading for research design informed by an interpretivist methodology and leading to the generation of qualitative data. As a mode of enquiry its roots are in anthropology where it forms the dominant approach to data collection. It can include a range of methods including participant observation, unstructured and semistructured interviews, documentary analysis and focus groups. Where methods using questioning are involved the emphasis in ethnographic enquiry is not on providing these questions in an invariant form with the purpose of elucidating causal or other relationships but the use of questions which elicit from individuals and groups their own perceptions of situations and experiences.

The role of theory is different from experimental and survey designs. In the latter, theory structures the form of enquiry whereas in ethnographic research it is drawn from the findings. This 'grounded theory' may, in some cases, be tested out in later stages of enquiry but the theory is not seen as generalizable to other situations. Typically this style of research involves researchers and respondents in face-to-face relationships. It may, as in the case of anthropological fieldwork and some action research projects, involve participation in natural settings. People are seen as embedded in social contexts and the researcher attempts to interfere as little as possible beyond the recognition that to be present in a situation and taking on some negotiated role must perforce have an impact on that social situation.

In carrying out such studies researchers need to gain access to the situation of interest. This can be by agreement with participants or at other times the researcher may work covertly. Covert study has clear ethical implications although it has been justified, on occasion, in sociology where it has been maintained that overt access could not be negotiated and knowledge could not otherwise be obtained.

If carried out in community contexts, ethnographic field work can be time intensive. While in anthropological studies there may at times be a wish to document all features of a social group, researchers may alternatively start with a more restricted range of broad research questions. In the pursuit of data collection these questions may become more focused with emerging theory guiding the later stages of data collection.

Within health education qualitative research can be similar to that seen as anthropological fieldwork; documenting a community health project or using rapid anthropological assessment methods (p. 65) prior to planning a health education intervention. More commonly it is likely to be restricted to completion of a number of semistructured interviews with individuals or with focus groups. A number of problems are raised about data collection in natural settings including difficulties in gaining access to the situation or to parts of it such as, for example, access by men to women's activities; problems of selection of an appropriate focus for study in complex situations; bias in selection of information to report with criticisms being made of the tendency to report the exotic rather than the mundane; and doubts as to whether participants in situations can explicate them to outsiders.

The analysis of qualitative data is complex and does not form as distinct a stage in the research process as in the previous styles discussed. Approaches to analysis vary but the general aim is to draw themes from the data which may result in pattern models and the generation of theory. As already mentioned emerging theory can guide later data collection. That multiple interpretations of the same data can be derived has to be acknowledged. It is expected that researchers will be open and clear about their analytic procedures to enable others to assess their accounts. The use of respondent validation whereby participants can respond to findings is proposed as one way to expose bias although it is in itself somewhat problematic since participants may also be unable to see their situations objectively.

Where evaluation research has used qualitative methods a potential source of conflict arises where in final reports certain accounts appear to be given more weight than others. While many health education evaluations have increasingly incorporated qualitative elements into a predominantly positivistic study others have emphasized the switch in relationships which comes from focus on qualitative data. This has been summarized by Parlett (1981):

The evaluator assumes the position of being an orchestrator of opinions, an arranger of data, a summarizer of what is commonly held, a collector of suggestions for changes, a sharpener of policy alternatives. Illuminative evaluators do not act as judges and juries but, in general, confine themselves to summing up arguments for and against different interpretations, policies and possible decisions.

While participant observation and semi/unstructured interviews have long been common methods for collecting qualitative data there are some techniques which have recently been developed or have become more common. Examples are the use of focus groups and techniques of rapid anthropological appraisal.

Focus groups

Focus group interviews have been in use for some considerable time but have been adopted more widely in recent years. Originally used in market research to examine perceptions of and attitudes towards specific products, their use has broadened out. They have become particularly popular in data collection at village level in many parts of the world where they can be a natural extension of village meetings.

Focus groups are typically made up of eight to 12 people who share a common characteristic such as, for example, being mothers of children under five. They participate in a discussion on the topic of interest and this discussion is facilitated by a trained moderator (Eng *et al.*, 1990). Some researchers would stipulate that participants do not know each other in advance but this criterion, while used in product research, seems to be applied less often in health education.

Interviews are organized around a number of open-ended questions as in individual qualitative research interviews and the facilitator draws out contributions from all participants. To have a second facilitator acting as a recorder can be helpful but audio recording is a fairly important back-up, especially for times when discussion becomes animated and manual recording becomes difficult. Where the languages in use in discussions are not written ones, audio recording is essential. Examples of use of focus groups have been recorded by Brieger and Kendall (1992) as part of an exploration of village ideas about guinea worm disease in Nigeria, in Togo where health workers investigated the health practices of mothers of children under five (Eng *et al.*, 1990) and by Ong *et al.* (1991) in community needs assessment in part of Liverpool in the UK.

While there are disadvantages to the use of focus groups they are probably outweighed by the advantages. The failure to draw out ideas differing from the norm is a real danger in group interviews but in societies where the practice of one-to-one qualititative interviewing would be unusual, focus groups may be a much preferred way to elicit qualitative insights.

Where focus groups are used in the context of evaluating community development programmes the participation in the group discussions forms part of the ongoing development process. For example Eng *et al.* (1990) report how, in their work in Togo, the focus group, facilitated by trained local health workers, 'provided a starting point for building community participation and collective competence'. The use also had a number of positive developments for the health workers. Although already working in the communities, these health workers came to realize through the use of the discussions that they were ignorant of some experiences of village life. Through having to listen in new ways a shift in role from the customary one of expert adviser to non-judgemental listener and learner occurred and the focus group methods also enabled workers to bridge community perceptions and health programme prerogatives.

Rapid assessment

A variety of terms can be found in the literature which describe the use of rapid methods of data collection: rapid epidemiological assessment; rapid anthropological assessment; rapid rural appraisal; participatory rural appraisal; focused ethnography, etc. They have in common the objective of foreshortening the period from preliminary data collection to programme implementation but differ in the methodological positions with which they are associated. Overall, however, rapid appraisal techniques are predominantly qualitative.

While the term rapid is common, Brieger and Kendall (1992) prefer to use focused to avoid impressions of methodological laxity. They describe focused enquiry as looking indepth at one main feature of a culture while keeping an eye out for how that feature fits into a cultural milieu. At other times researchers may be attempting, through the use of a team approach, to provide a wide ranging account of a situation in a matter of weeks rather than the two or three years that may be required to complete an anthropological field study.

Rapid methods are not necessarily preferred to longer scale research studies but in some cases the need for some quick response to an emergent problem may be called for. In other cases rapid enquiries may lead on to major surveys or to extended anthropological studies. The usual debates around methodological approaches and the extent of participation by communities in the research process are found in discussions of rapid enquiry. Where the term anthropology or ethnography is used a phenomenological approach is to be expected although there is much evidence of pluralism where data collection methods are concerned.

The origins of much rapid appraisal research has been in countries of the 'south', initially in agricultural and development research rather than health research and often in rural contexts. A range of techniques have been used including those already common in qualitative research: semi/unstructured interviewing with community members and particularly with key informants; participant observation and focus groups. In addition, however, a variety of other methods have been developed which may be seen as more appropriate to data collection in some settings and which may also be valuable in building community participation where this is valued. In general these are visual rather than written methods. They include the development of maps – a shared activity between researchers and community participants. These may be social maps representing a number of features of a prevailing social structure, historical maps, resource maps indicating fields, grazing, water sources, etc. and body maps representing ideas of bodily structure. While maps may be represented on paper they may equally be drawn up on the ground using readily available materials.

Another widely used technique is the development of seasonal calendars which may incorporate a variety of verbal and pictorial features. A calendar might include such information as rainfall over the year, agricultural practices, water and food availability, work patterns, diseases, leisure activities and so on. Much valuable material may come directly from calendars but in addition the process of construction is a participative activity which can provide the stimulus for a whole range of discussions. The comparison of calendars drawn up by men and by women can, for example, be an effective and non-threatening way to begin examination of gender divisions. Calendars were used by Reed (1992) in studying ideas about malaria. Welbourn (1992) has commented on the increased empathy generated with villagers through the use of visual techniques and the ability to explore more sensitive issues that cannot normally be broached.

While these and other techniques, discussed in detail by Chambers (1992), can be used by researchers simply as methods of 'extracting' data from communities, they can also be used as an integral part of a participative empowering process and a distinction has been made in rural research between rapid rural appraisal and participatory rural appraisal. Participatory appraisal provides opportunities for people to conduct and present their own analyses and can strengthen commitment to and capacities for sustainable actions. Such approaches clearly require researchers to be ready to share research expertise and give up some or all of their traditional control. This has been a debated issue within anthropology and has clear relevance for health education research where there is a commitment to community participation and to empowerment.

In looking at the relationship between anthropology and rapid appraisal Cornwall (1992) sees the former as the parent of the latter but views it as an illegitimate child with a somewhat awkward family resemblance. A number of reasons are offered for the awkward relationship. The devolution of analysis to local people and to non-anthropologists can be uncomfortable and an apparent challenge to expertise. Two issues are seen to be at stake: the view that only the anthropologist is capable of processing and presenting information gathered in the field and reaching the closest approximation to a 'true' account. Those who are represented are seen as partial and blind to processes within their communities. The second concern addresses the use of knowledge. Analysis of ethnography often takes place outside the research context and communities may not be drawn into processes of respondent validation at the writing up stage. Cornwall suggests that not only are communities frequently excluded from analysis but they are also denied ownership of information for their own use. There are clear parallels between the debates about participatory appraisal within anthropology and those around participatory research in health promotion.

In conclusion, ethnographic enquiry is undertaken in order to generate intensive accounts and while it is hoped that findings might illumine similar situations the commitment to generalization of the previous research designs is not present. Because of the detailed involvement of the researcher and the types of methods used, ethnographic research would not be claiming nor would it be seen to score highly on reliability and internal validity.

META-ANALYSIS

In the following chapters we will be making a number of references to meta-analyses and evaluations. It is common to review informally a number of evaluations on a particular subject and draw conclusions. St Leger *et al.* (1992) have offered suggestions for improving this process.

1. Discard studies that are irredeemably methodologically unsound.
2. Where there are inconsistencies between studies, consider whether they might be due to any of the following: differences in aims and objectives; different procedures; incidental secular trends for studies separated in time; or differences in the underlying populations of studies separated in space.

Such informal meta-analysis entails 'using judgement, informed by the above criteria, to reach a plausible conclusion' (St Leger *et al.*, 1992). Panels of experts may be brought together to generate a consensus on studies in a specific area.

Formal meta-analysis is typically applied to experimental studies and aims to provide an integrated and quantified summary of research results on a specific question with particular reference to statistical significance and effect size (Rosenthal, 1984). Criteria are specified for inclusion in the analysis and each study is treated as a component of one large new study and subsequent to statistical analysis a single conclusion is reached for the aggregate. Meta-analyses have proved useful in health education in deriving some summary conclusions about effectiveness in specific areas of activity. In introducing a meta-analysis of controlled trials of cardiac patient education, Mullen *et al.* (1992), for example, say that the techniques were being used to address four questions.

1. What methods of education have been the subject of controlled trials?
2. What is the overall effect of patient education on adherence to the therapeutic regimen?
3. What are the relative effects of various methods of education?
4. What are the major gaps and innovations in the design of patient education for CHD?

THE POLITICS AND ETHICS OF EVALUATION

A variety of ethical and political issues have a bearing on all research activities, including those directed towards evaluation. It may be worth stating the somewhat obvious point that health educators have an ethical obligation to undertake evaluation of their activities. If we do not do so, we may not learn whether or not an intervention is effective in reaching specified goals – equally we may not know if we are causing harm.

A number of ethical considerations have been mentioned briefly in the discussion of particular research methods. This section will focus on a number of particular concerns with reference to evaluation research, namely: the relationship between sponsor and evaluator; the evaluator–programme participants relationship; methodology; and the production

and use of evaluation reports. At this point discussion will refer substantially to sponsored evaluation with a designated evaluator.

Sponsors will vary in the extent to which they have identified highly specific objectives for an evaluative study, indicated research methods to be adopted and specified the nature and uses of evaluation reports. Where there is a high degree of specificity in evaluation objectives, the evaluator, unless involved in the initial discussions, has restricted freedoms. The extent to which evaluators can expect to maintain some independence from sponsors has been discussed and claims for a degree of independence have been made. Simons (1984) argues that when an evaluation is funded by a specific body this does not mean that the evaluation is bought by that group and that the evaluator is seen as working for that group in the sense of providing them only with information that conforms to their values. She believes that there is a degree of consensus about the need for an initial contract between the evaluator and sponsor to secure procedures for undertaking a study, to prevent misunderstandings and to provide a basis for review in the case of disputes.

The relationship between a designated evaluator and participants of a health education programme is a crucial one and is strongly influenced by the preferred methodology. If an evaluation is to be informed by positivist methodology the methods to be used will be relatively clear from the outset, although negotiation may be needed around the design of data collection instruments, timing of data collection, writing up and presentation of findings. At each of these stages there is potential for conflict and ethical dilemmas to be resolved.

As an evaluation moves towards emphasis on gathering qualititative data and varying degrees of participation in ongoing activities, the richness of data obtained may be enhanced but so may the ethical difficulties. A central issue is the balance between the right to full knowledge about an activity and the rights to privacy of programme participants even in matters that pertain to the public good. This issue is succinctly analysed by Pring (1984) where he assesses whether the right to knowledge is a basic one which requires no further justification. He offers J.S. Mill's argument in support of this right in his discussion of freedom of discussion:

> If the opinion is right, they are deprived of the opportunity of exchanging error for truth; if wrong, they lose, what is almost as great a benefit, the clearer perception and livelier expression of truth, produced by its collision with error.

Pring supports the case for availability of information but argues that the right to know has to be established in particular cases and is not a basic one. Establishing such a case would require examination of both undesirable outcomes of acquiring knowledge and potential clashes with other values which could ensue from exercising the right to know. Values which would emerge in the evaluation context could be those of respect for others, trust and confidentiality. Where an evaluator undertakes a participatory role in programmes these matters can be particularly difficult. There is the question of whether, within a public arena, some areas of privacy can be maintained. Educational evaluators have commented, for example, on the feelings of teachers that the staffroom should be a 'private' area as far as data collection is concerned. Particular problems of trust and confidentiality can be triggered in using data from unstructured and semistructured interviews where interviewees can reveal matters that they would probably not do if presented with a structured questionnaire.

It is fairly obvious that negotiation between all parties prior to the onset of data collection can address some of the confidentiality versus the right to know issues but it is not a fully satisfactory solution. As Pring (1984) says, 'A contract has to be suffused with a spirit of respect for the other that can never be cap-

tured in a contract alone'. To the extent that evaluation can be distinguished from research in general we may argue that there is a greater prima facie case in the former for the right to knowledge. As Pring outlines, evaluations studies are concerned not so much with theory building or generalization as with a grasp of the particular and with improved practice and they could be seriously affected if particular episodes, interactions, relationships and differing perceptions which constitute the particular are omitted from the record. He suggests, therefore, that there are limits to how much negotiation is acceptable if the aims of the evaluator are to be achieved and this would need to be taken into account in any codes of practice.

The issues discussed so far will assume greater significance where the evaluator is aiming to take some independent stance in relation to the project for evaluation. Those whose preference is to facilitate participatory evaluation will have a different relationship with project participants and joint decisions will be made about content and methods of evaluation.

On completion of an evaluation, differences of opinion can occur over the type of report and the extent of dissemination. Again, problems are more likely to surface where an evaluation has been sponsored and it has been completed by an evaluator external to a programme. Those who wish to argue for some kind of independent position for evaluators would wish them to have some controls over the reporting of findings and would wish sponsors to publish results as they stand. Jamieson (1984) suggests that the publication of results becomes such a sensitive issue for evaluators because it is thought to involve moral issues concerned with censorship and the suppression of truth. He claims that the ethical issues are not so clearcut. Where illuminative evaluation has been undertaken we have to acknowledge the relativity of accounts and ask questions about any privileged status for the evaluator's report. More generally, he draws a difference between publication of evaluation results and those from general academic research. While publication of the latter is an expectation, he suggests that it should not be assumed that this is normal activity for the former. He does not argue that evaluations should not be published – more that because they are not undertaken, in general, with a view to informing the wider academic community but to assess the worth of a particular programme for its sponsors, publication lacks the same imperative. Although Jamieson acknowledges the artificiality of making too clear a distinction between evaluation and what he describes as 'academic' research, he is pushing the difference rather further than seems useful in health education.

In conclusion, we note the need for participants to have access to evaluation findings (when they have not participated in analysis and writing up) in an accessible form. Good discussion of this issue has been provided by Hunt (1993) with reference to housing and health research in Scotland.

HEALTH PROMOTION RESEARCH

Health education, as discussed in Chapter 1, is a major constituent of health promotion. At the beginning of this chapter we indicated that there was a developing debate about research and evaluation within this larger arena. While it is beyond the scope of this chapter to discuss these debates a few comments will be made since there are implications for health education research.

While concepts of health promotion continue to range from the narrowly circumscribed to the all-encompassing, to expect any definitive statements about health promotion research is premature. If committed to postmodernist analysis we might also retreat from such a project. Nonetheless if we take as a frame of reference the ideas about health promotion enshrined in documents such as the Ottawa Charter (1986) there are issues to be

addressed in the planning and evaluation of health promotion and these can be organized around the following three themes: the definition of health promotion research and its goals; methodological and practice issues; and the ownership and use of research and evaluation findings.

DEFINING HEALTH PROMOTION RESEARCH

At one level health promotion research may be addressing any of the constituent elements of health promotion as identified in the previous chapter. Much of this research might equally be described, depending on its nature, as epidemiological, psychological, sociological, social policy research and so on. While labels may not be important we may nonetheless wish to consider whether health promotion research is any more than the sum of its parts or whether it has distinctive characteristics.

At the simplest level there would be little challenge to a definition of health promotion research as that which is directed towards the analysis of factors influencing health and evaluation of activities oriented to the promotion of health. Such a statement is bland and does not obviously reflect the ideological commitment of WHO style rhetoric on health promotion. We might therefore wish to emphasize particular components of health promotion in defining health promotion research. We could expect such research to be oriented towards the analysis of the key components of the Ottawa Charter and to understanding of ways of achieving these outcomes of intersectoral co-ordination, community participation, equity, facilitation of healthy environments, development of personal skills and reorientation of health services. Such an approach would tend to reduce the relative importance of health education, irrespective of the philosophical model under which it is undertaken.

More generally we might wish to specify as health promotion research that which has a direct action component commensurate with health promotion goals. While the importance of action should be acknowledged it would seem to be restricting to exclude the kinds of health education research which might eventually contribute to development of health promotion actions but is initially carried out for purposes of simply enhancing knowledge.

Taking into account the varied contexts in which health promotion research and evaluation take place we may be happy to accept that the activities undertaken under its name may be highly varied. Assessed as a whole we would, however, expect to see the major goals of health promotion receiving substantial attention. For example, Milio (1990), in discussing research in relation to the new public health, claims that the response to the call for more attention by the major research establishments to health promoting living conditions has been slow and minor in comparison with biomedical, technological and health care economics research programmes. In addition we would expect to see health promotion goals to be given major consideration in identifying research topics. For example, research around young people's health could originate more frequently from their defined problems rather than those defined according to epidemiological criteria and be oriented to equity, participation and so on rather than highly focused analyses of narrowly specified behaviours. In addition, we may decide to monitor research activities addressing the full range of health issues defined by communities rather than those specified in such documents as *Health of the Nation*.

An alternative to attempting to define the subject of health promotion research would be to focus on its methodology and its general practices. As indicated in a number of places an activity that is seeking to enhance community participation and promote empowerment might choose to work within a research paradigm sympathetic to such objectives. The increased adoption of qualitative research approaches would provide support for the proposal that there is some effort within health promotion research to model in its processes some of its desired outcomes. It would be inappropriate, however, to be prescriptive in this respect unless we wish to rule out whole areas of research with value for the whole health promotion enterprise but which use non-participatory methods.

We have argued earlier for pluralism of methodology as the most appropriate way of seeking answers to the range of questions which health education seeks to address. In carrying out particular research methods we would expect to see full attention to relationships and to avoidance of negative consequences. Some of the writings of feminist researchers have been of particular value in reflecting on the conduct of research techniques – e.g. interviewing processes (Oakley, 1981), surveys (Graham, 1983) and experimental techniques (Jayaratne, 1983).

Finally we would expect to see the findings of health promotion research and evaluation used, whenever possible, to promote health. This means, for example, that research findings should be published and made available, possibly in a variety of written forms, to all those who have a stake in the research. One could also argue that health promotion researchers have some obligation to ensure that research findings are brought to the attention of those, politicians, health authorities, planners and so on, who might be expected to respond to them in the interest of promoting health of individuals and communities.

The importance of intersectoral collaboration to the achievement of health promotion is widely recognized and discussed. Less often addressed is the fact that much health promotion research and evaluation also requires collaboration across sectors and/or professionals. Such collaborators do not necessarily share research philosophies and successful activity is only likely to occur where there is understanding of different positions and the possibility of negotiating research strategies.

CONCLUSION

This chapter has discussed the nature of evaluation research, considered methodological positions to be adopted in practice and examined some of the main methods that can be used. Some brief discussion of politics and ethics of evaluation preceded some brief reflections on the nature and practice of health promotion research. Although there have been major developments in the extent and sophistication of evaluative studies in health education, criticisms continue to be made. Kok and Green (1990), in a discussion of co-operation between researchers and practitioners, said:

> Health promotion practitioners and administrators are not always interested in or receptive to evaluation research; furthermore they are often unaware of the conditions that must be fulfilled for valid research.

They conclude that more co-operation would be achieved if researchers learned more about practice and practitioners learned more about research. They suggest the effective way to improve health promotion is through practical research carried out co-operatively between researchers and practitioners. In later chapters we will be making reference to evaluation studies reflecting a diversity of philosophical positions on health education and on its evaluation.

REFERENCES

Basler, H.D., Brinkmeier, U. Buser, K. and Gluth, G. (1991) Nicotine gum assisted group therapy in smokers with an increased risk of coronary disease – evaluation in a primary care setting. *Health Education Research*, **7**(1), 87–96.

Blaikie, N.W.H. (1991) A critique of the use of triangulation in social research. *Quality and Quantity*, **25**, 115–36.

Brieger, W.R. and Kendall, C. (1992) Learning from local knowledge to improve disease surveillance: perceptions of the guinea worm illness experience. *Health Education Research*, **7**(4), 471–86.

Bryman, A. (1984) *Research Methods and Organisational Studies*, Unwin Hyman, London.

Campbell, D.T. and Stanley, J.C. (1963) *Experimental and Quasi-Experimental Designs for Research*, Rand-McNally, Chicago.

Candeias, N.M.F. (1991) Evaluating the quality of health education programmes. *HYGIE*, **X**(2), 40–4.

Chambers, R. (1992) *Rural Appraisal: Rapid, Relaxed and Participatory*, Institute of Development Studies Discussion Paper 311, University of Sussex, Brighton.

Cicourel, A. (1964) *Method and Measurement in Sociology*, Free Press, New York.

Cornwall, A. (1992) *Body Mapping in Health*, RRA Notes 16, pp. 69–76, Sustainable Agriculture Programme, IIED, 3 Endsleigh Street, London.

Davies, J.K. and Kelly, M.P. (1993) *Healthy Cities: Research and Practice*, Routledge, London.

Denzin, N.K. (1978) *The Research Act: A Theoretical Introduction to Sociological Methods*, McGraw-Hill, London.

Eng, E., Glik, D. and Parker, K. (1990) Focus group methods: effects on village agency collaboration for child survival. *Health Policy and Planning*, **5**(1), 67–76.

Finch, J. (1986) *Research and Policy: The Uses of Qualitative Methods in Social and Educational Research*, Falmer Press, Sussex.

Glanz, K., Brekke, M., Harper, D., Bache-Wiig, M. and Hunninghake, D.B. (1992) Evaluation of implementation of a cholesterol management programme in physicians' offices. *Health Education Research*, **7**(2), 151–64.

Graham, H. (1983) Do her answers fit the questions: women and the survey method, in *The Public and the Private*, (eds E. Gamarnikov, D. Morgan, J. Purvis and D. Taylorson), Heinemann, London.

Hammersley, M. and Atkinson, P. (1983) *Ethnography: Principles and Practice*, Tavistock, London.

Hayes, M.V. and Willms, S.M. (1990) Healthy community indicators: the perils of the search and the paucity of the find. *Health Promotion International*, **5**(2), 161–6.

Hunt, S.M. (1993) The relationship between research and policy: translating knowledge into action, in *Healthy Cities: Research and Practice*, (eds J.K. Davies and M.P. Kelly), Routledge, London.

Jamieson, I. (1984) Evaluation: a case of research in chains? in *The Politics of Evaluation*, (ed. C. Adelman), Croom Helm, London.

Jayaratne, T.E. (1983) The value of quantitative methodology for feminist research, in *Theories of*

Women's Studies, (eds G. Bowles and R. Duelli-Klein), Routledge and Kegan Paul, London.

Keat, R. and Urry, J. (1975) *Social Theory as Science*, Routledge and Kegan Paul, London.

Kelly, M. (1989) Some problems in health promotion research. *Health Promotion*, **4**(4), 317–30.

Kok, G. and Green, L.W. (1990) Research to support health promotion in practice: a plea for increased cooperation. *Health Promotion International*, **5**(4), 303–8.

Marsh, C. (1984) *The Survey Method; The Contribution of Surveys to Sociological Explanation*, George Allen and Unwin, London.

McBride, C.M., Pirie, P.L. and Curry, S.J. (1992) Postpartum relapse to smoking: a prospective study. *Health Education Research*, **7**(3), 381–90.

McLeroy, K., Steckler, A.B., Goodman, R.M. and Burdine, J.N. (1992) Editorial. Health education research: theory and practice – future directions. *Health Education Research*, **7**(1), 289–94.

Milio, N. (1990) Healthy cities: the new public health and supportive research. *Health Promotion International*, **5**(4), 291–8.

Mullen, P.D., Mains, D.A. and Velez, R. (1992) A meta-analysis of controlled trials of cardiac patient education. *Patient Education and Counselling*, **19**, 143–62.

Nutbeam, D., Smith, C., Murphy, S. and Catford, J. (1993) Maintaining evaluation designs in long term community based health promotion programmes: Heartbeat Wales case study. *Journal of Epidemiology and Community Health*, **47**, 127–33.

Oakley, A. (1981) Interviewing women: a contradiction in terms, in *Doing Feminist Research*, (ed. H. Roberts), Routledge and Kegan Paul, London.

O'Neill, M. (1988) Editorial. What kind of research for what kind of health promotion? *Health Promotion*, **3**(4), 339–40.

Ong, B.N., Humphris, G., Annett, H. and Rifkin, S. (1991) Rapid appraisal in an urban setting, an example from the developed world. *Social Science and Medicine*, **32**(8), 909–15.

Ottawa Charter for Health Promotion (1986) *Health Promotion*, **1**(4), iii–v.

Parlett, M. (1981) Illuminative evaluation, in *Human Inquiry: A Sourcebook of New Paradigm Research*, (eds P. Reason and J. Rowan), Wiley, London.

Pring, R. (1984) Confidentiality and the right to know, in *The Politics of Evaluation*, (ed. C. Adelman), Croom Helm, London.

Puska, P., Nissinen, A., Tuomilehto J. *et al.* (1985) The community based strategy to prevent coronary heart disease; conclusions from 10 years of the Karelia project. *Annual Review of Public Health*, **6**, 147–63.

Reason, P. and Rowan, J. (1981) *Human Inquiry: A Sourcebook of New Paradigm Research*, Wiley, London.

Reed, C.E. (1992) Malaria control through impregnated bed nets in South West Kenya. Leeds Polytechnic, MSc dissertation.

Rosenau, P.M. (1992) *Post-Modernism and the Social Sciences: Insights, Inroads and Intrusions*, Princeton University Press, Princeton.

Rosenthal, R. (1984) *Meta-analytic Procedures for Social Research*, Sage, Beverly Hills.

Silverman, D. (1985) *Qualitative Method and Sociology*, Gower, Aldershot.

Simons, H. (1984) Negotiating conditions of independent evaluators, in *The Politics of Evaluation*, (ed. C. Adelman), Croom Helm, London.

Smith, H.W. (1975) *Strategies of Social Research: The Methodological Imagination*, Prentice-Hall, London.

St Leger, A.S., Schnieden, H. and Walsworth-Bell, J.P. (1992) *Evaluating Health Services' Effectiveness*, Open University Press, Milton Keynes.

Stevenson, H.M. and Burke, M. (1991) Bureaucratic logic in new social movement clothing. *Health Promotion International*, **6**(4), 281–90.

Thompson, R.S., Rivera, F.P. and Thompson, D.C. (1989) A case control study of the effectiveness of bicycle safety helmets. *New England Journal of Medicine*, **320**, 1361–6.

Tilford, S. and Delaney, F. (1992) Editorial. Qualitative research in health education. *Health Education Research*, **7**(4), 451–5.

Turner, B.S. (ed.) (1990) *Theories of Modernity and Postmodernity*, Sage Publications, London.

Welbourn, A. (1992) *A Note on the Use of Disease Problem Ranking with Relation to Socioeconomic Well-being: An Example from Sierra Leone*, RRA Notes 16, pp. 86–7, Sustainable Agriculture Programme, IIED, 3 Endsleigh Street, London.

INDICATORS OF SUCCESS AND MEASURES OF PERFORMANCE: THE IMPORTANCE OF THEORY

3

In Chapter 1 we argued that the meaning of success in health education is dependent on the values and philosophies of practitioners. The measures used to indicate a successful outcome will in turn depend on the model of health education which is guiding practice. Indicators of effectiveness for a preventive model would consist of the adoption of appropriate behaviours and, possibly, the medical or epidemiological outcomes assumed to result from such behaviours. A radical model would look for outcomes which would indicate community action and possibly a change in public policy. Again, in the absence of a global measure of self-empowerment, appropriate outcome measures for a self-empowerment model might indicate enhanced self-esteem, increased internality and the acquisition of certain key social skills.

However, irrespective of the model of health education adopted, the use of **outcome indicators** will often be inappropriate. Indeed most programmes require a range of **intermediate indicators** of success. Moreover, in many instances even intermediate indicators may not provide the best way of evaluating a particular programme and an **indirect indicator** may be needed. Accordingly, this chapter will consider what it means to gauge the success of a health education venture by using 'distal' as well as 'proximal' indicators. More importantly, however, it will emphasize

the need for programme planners and evaluators to base their activities on sound theory. Without a sound theoretical model, the selection of intermediate and indirect indicators from what at first sight would appear to be a bewildering variety of alternatives would be a difficult and even arbitrary operation. For this reason, two theoretical models will be described. The first of these, the **health action model**, will be discussed in some detail in order to show how theoretical understanding can assist with making a rational rather than a less informed choice of intermediate indicator. Similarly, **communication of innovations theory** will be cited as a basis for selecting indirect indicators. Both theories will also assist with the process of generating a list of indicators for use in pretesting target groups and programmes.

The chapter will also draw the reader's attention to the importance of indicators of subjective dimensions of health and will comment on the recent interest in so-called **performance indicators**.

One especially important type of indirect indicator of successful media use is assessed by the techniques of pretesting and a discussion of this stratagem will be included. The importance of objectives in programme evaluation will also be raised and their relevance for standards of performance – including cost-effectiveness – will be discussed.

QUALITY AND ITS ASSESSMENT

Over the last few years there has been growing attention to the issue of quality and its measurement across all aspects of health, education and social care and Black (1992) has commented that observers of British health care could be forgiven for thinking that quality assurance was invented in the 1980s.

This focus on quality has occurred at a time of reforms associated with a growing consumerist ethos and pressures for greater accountability. In discussing, for example, the pressures for changes in education in the 1980s in a number of European countries, Moon (1990) said: 'The theme of quality reverberates through political advocacy for new directions and new approaches'. In the UK the document *Working For Patients*, which instituted the major reforms of the National Health Service, had two key objectives:

1. To give patients, wherever they live in the UK, better health care and greater choice of the services available;
2. Greater satisfaction and rewards for those working in the NHS who successfully respond to local needs and preferences.

The seven measures which were proposed for achieving the targets included improvement in the quality of service and audit of quality across the health service.

Quality assurance can be described as an evaluative activity in which quality of provision in a service is assessed against standards developed for the structure of that service, the processes within it and its outcomes together with efforts to make changes as and when necessary. If we confine discussion at this stage to health care settings the initial attention to quality tended to be a concern of health systems in the USA and Europe rather more than of those in developing countries. As Forsberg *et al.* (1992) point out, attention in the developing world has tended to date to be on the extension of services to previously unmet groups. The

lesser attention to issues of quality had led, however, to the extension of unevaluated services to new areas or groups. There is now a growing interest in quality assurance in developing countries.

In developing tools for quality assurance it is necessary to define the dimensions of quality and develop standards against which that quality is to be assessed. Maxwell (1984) suggested six aspects of quality of health care: access to services; relevance to need for the whole community; equity; social acceptability; effectiveness; efficiency; and economy. Black (1992) identified one fewer in defining a high quality service as one which provides effective care, that meets everyone's needs and that is delivered equitably, humanely and efficiently.

Within the NHS, systems of audit exist to monitor quality – both medical and clinical. Audit is defined as the monitoring and assessment of health care to ensure it is of as high a quality as research findings suggest can be expected (Black, 1992). *Working for Patients* defined medical audit as the:

> ... critical analysis of the quality of medical care – including procedures used for diagnosis and treatment, the use of resources and the resulting outcomes for the patient.

This audit can take place at three levels: at the individual consultant level where a consultant reviews the work of a unit with junior staff; peer review where members of a discipline review each other's work; and external audits, carried out at district, regional or national levels (St Leger *et al.*, 1992). Clinical audit has a wider remit – it includes medical audit and is a critical analysis of the quality of all professional care. On the basis of an audit changes designed to increase quality may be instituted. A quality assurance process, therefore, is a framework for a systematic and continuous monitoring and evaluation of agreed levels of service and care provision.

QUALITY OF HEALTH PROMOTION

Given the continuing debates around the nature of health promotion it may be premature to define rigid criteria for auditing quality although Catford (1993) has recently suggested that there should be a common set of criteria that can be used to assess performance and quality. At a certain level of generality we can probably agree on dimensions of quality to be assessed. At a more specific level, as earlier discussion in Chapter 1 has shown, what will be used as criteria of quality within these dimensions will depend on philosophical approach, whether we are addressing elements of health promotion or the whole of it, client groups and so on. Catford, while stating that health promotion is a diverse field, appears to be working broadly within the health promotion concepts and principles advocated by the WHO. He offers some 'vital signs of quality':

1. Understanding and responding to people's needs fairly.
2. Building on sound theoretical principles and understanding.
3. Demonstrating a sense of direction and coherence.
4. Reorienting key decision makers.
5. Connecting with all sectors and settings.
6. Using complementary approaches at both individual and environmental levels.
7. Encouraging participation and ownership.
8. Providing technical and managerial training and support.
9. Undertaking specific actions and programmes.

These statements, at differing levels of specificity, provide a basis for debating quality measures in health promotion – the list may be amended, some items replaced and others added. Some would clearly be

	Structure	Process	Outcomes
Acceptability	Designated space meeting agreed criteria	Assessment of staff attitudes	Uptake of clinics
Need	Practice based mobile clinics	Client participation	Reports of needs met
Effectiveness	% attenders	Patient and professional satisfaction	Health measures e.g. BP cholesterol
Efficiency	Patients seen per hour	Ratings on counselling techniques	Cost in relation to behaviour changes
Equity	Availability of interpreter services	Use of AV and written materials in minority languages	Impact on inequalities in health statistics

Figure 3.1 Assessing quality of health promotion clinics in general practice: selected indicators.

operationalized more easily than others. All of the above statements would fit into one or other of the three areas of activity on which quality assurance processes focus: the structures within which an activity in question occurs; the processes undertaken; and the outcomes. Figure 3.1 could be used for generating audit measures for assessing health education or health promotion. If, for example, we wished to audit health promotion clinics in general practice we could suggest measures that might be used in each of the cells.

PERFORMANCE INDICATORS

As part of a general strategy to encourage more efficient use of resources, performance indicators (PIs) were introduced to monitor performance within the NHS. They were essentially attempts to introduce more central control of health expenditure and effective scrutiny of performance (Small, 1989). PIs were intended to be practical and useful tools for management. The original approach was to develop a range of crude indicators of performance from routinely collected data on the basis of which comparisons could be made between districts, between types of service and between specialisms. Some examples of PIs are: length of stay in hospital; annual throughput per hospital bed; cost per day; ratio of trained to untrained staff, etc. PIs can be of three types: clinical, manpower, financial and estate management. The first set of indicators was used on a trial basis in 1982 and the complete set published in 1983 and revised in 1985. It has frequently been stressed that while helpful to compare performance across authorities, the published reports were not intended to be seen as league tables.

What is the relationship between PIs and quality? They are indicators of input and overall levels of activity and may have a bearing on the structure and process elements of quality assurance but don't actually measure the impact of inputs on the health of populations. The underlying assumption is, of course, that indicators are in some way related to positive outcomes. This has been one of the main criticisms voiced about performance indicators. This focus on inputs and levels of activity can encourage reduction of costs and increased productivity without at the same time requiring related assessments of impacts on health and other outcome indicators. There have also been criticisms of the number of indicators and their comprehensibility as well as questions about the accuracy of summary statistics resulting from their use (Allen *et al.*, 1987).

Finally, there are problems in making comparisons within and between health districts since institutions within districts or districts as a whole operate in environments where there are different levels of need and demand (Small, 1989).

PERFORMANCE INDICATORS AND HEALTH EDUCATION

A great deal of health education activity is not easily reduced to lists of performance indicators but some can be useful taken alongside other measures. They can be particularly useful where there is a strong basis of knowledge which relates specific inputs to outcomes. For example, as will be seen in a later chapter, there is evidence that more criteria associated with effective patient education are achieved in hospitals which have trained co-ordinators (Pack *et al.*, 1983). An easy to measure PI for a health district would therefore be the number of hospitals with patient education co-ordinators. There is evidence that written material in booklet form is an effective way to reinforce education in hospital settings and is associated with patient satisfaction. A simple indicator would record the percentage of patients who have received such booklets.

Used selectively where there is good evidence of a link between input and outcome, performance indicators can be useful measures.

INDICATORS OF WELL-BEING

Before reviewing this chapter's discussion of indicators of success, it is important to give some consideration to measures which might be used to indicate well-being. Reference was made in Chapter 1 to the concern felt by some people involved in health promotion that there should be a greater emphasis on promoting positive health in order to counterbalance the predominant orientation towards cure and prevention of disease – a viewpoint which is, of course, entirely consistent with the WHO's seminal concept of 'well-being'.

As Hunt and McEwen (1980) point out in their rationale for the development of the Nottingham Health Profile, the philosophical shift from logical positivism and empiricism combined with the changing nature of disease and disability in contemporary society has lead to a concern to devise more subjective measures of well-being and quality of life. In the context of this book, such indicators are the positive analogues of the traditional medical outcome measures such as mortality, morbidity or individual clinical measures such as level of serum cholesterol or number of decayed, missing and filled teeth. A brief comment will therefore be made about the kinds of subjective indicator which have been used and are available to the evaluator.

Briscoe (1982), writing from a social work perspective, comments that '... subjective measures of well-being are therefore needed in order adequately to assess – and hence treat – a wide spectrum of psychosocial dysfunction'. The reference to 'dysfunction' and 'psychosocial' should incidentally remind us that it is difficult completely to distance oneself from negative aspects of health. Hall (1976) underlines this point in his observation that two of the best buys in subjective indicators are the Housing Nuisance Index and the Health Symptom Index!

Hall describes the development of a variety of subjective measures of quality of life in Britain between 1971 and 1975. Clearly the most problematical aspect of measuring quality of life is defining it. Hall cites Tom Harrisson, the founder of Mass Observation, who said, 'You cannot, yet, take a census of love in Liverpool or random sample the effect that fear of the future has on the total pattern of contemporary life in Leeds'. Nonetheless, Hall describes the result of the Social Science Research Council's 1975 survey in which respondents were asked to define 'quality of life'. The results are particularly revealing – not only for the construction of subjective indicators but also for the way they provide an insight into perceptions of health and well-being. For instance 23% of the sample of 932 people of all social groups referred to 'family, home life, marriage' while 19% made rather more vague references to being contented or happy. A further 17% and 18% valued decent living conditions and money respectively. Health was relegated to a 10% response rate while more abstract and altruistic aspects of quality of life, such as equality and justice, were mentioned by only 2% of the sample. These findings confirm the view that many people's notion of positive health or well-being derived from whatever happens to be their salient value system and/or from a meaning of health which is consistent with the medical model perspective – lack of disease or social impairment.

Measures of quality of life, therefore, included people's level of satisfaction with the various 'life domains' mentioned above: more particularly, housing, health, standard of living, etc. In addition, more global measures of well-being were used. These sought to measure personal competence and trust in others and positive and negative affect (using, for example, Bradburn's (1969) Affect Balance Scale).

By contrast, the Nottingham Health Profile (Hunt and McEwen, 1980) adopted an approach which focused more on personal than social well-being. The Profile consists of six sections referring to emotional life; experience of pain; energy levels; social integration; physical mobility; and sleep patterns.

While this brief glimpse of indicators of quality of life reveals the richness and variety of possible measures by comparison with traditional epidemiological indicators, we should still remember the cautionary note about using certain classes of outcome indicator as measures of health education success. Although positive health indicators will probably be more appealing to health educators than illness related measures, they may prove to be equally, if not more, problematic. Like mortality and morbidity, quality of life will be affected by a wide variety of social and environmental influences beyond the control of even the most thorough programme. It would therefore be just as unwise to use well-being as an indicator of success as it would be to employ 'medical' indicators.

THE IMPORTANCE OF INTERMEDIATE INDICATORS

At first glance it would seem sensible to determine the effectiveness and efficiency of health education programmes in terms of the ultimate desired outcomes. For various reasons that is rarely possible and sometimes not desirable. The three most important situations in which intermediate indicators are needed are described below.

The first and most obvious instance of the inappropriateness of an outcome measure is where the link between an epidemiological or medical outcome and some precursor event is probabilistic or may have been inadequately established. For example, the assumed causal link between a human attribute or behaviour and a disease process may be unproven. The association between type A behaviour and coronary heart disease (CHD) (Rosenman, 1977) would fall into this category and it would therefore be unwise to judge the effectiveness of a health education pro-

gramme designed to produce a shift towards type B characteristics in terms of a reduced incidence of acute myocardial infarction.

Again, the link between a given behaviour and a medical outcome might have been epidemiologically established to the satisfaction of a majority of experts but the specific behaviour in question might operate only in the presence of other factors or at any rate be potentiated by them. The classic instance of such synergism is provided by the aetiology of CHD. It would clearly be foolish to expect a programme which was confined only to increasing levels of exercise to have a measurable effect on the incidence of CHD within the target population. Similarly it would be wrong to judge the effectiveness of a practice nurse's 'broad spectrum' risk factor counselling in terms of an individual's subsequent experience of CHD since she clearly cannot influence the patient's genetic predisposition or previous history. Furthermore, a health education programme might have been singularly successful in influencing exercise patterns but, because the exercise regime had not been tailored to the particular physiological needs of each individual, it might well have been insufficient to strengthen the cardiovascular system significantly. It could not therefore be expected to affect the natural history of the population's coronary disease in any way. The failure would have been one of epidemiological and physiological diagnosis: in other words, the educational 'operation' had been successful but the patients died.

And also, in the context of a preventive model, health educators would be rash to allow themselves to be assessed by epidemiological or medical indicators. The endpoint indicator for the preventive model would thus be the adoption of a healthy behaviour or lifestyle and/or changes in existing unhealthy practices. This kind of behavioural outcome would thus be an intermediate indicator within the context of a broader community health promotion programme seeking to improve health and prevent disease.

The second situation in which health education must look for an intermediate indicator is analogous with the one just discussed in that it relates to the kind of all-embracing approach to health promotion discussed in Chapter 1. It will be recalled that the ultimate health outcome (achievement of health and/or prevention of disease) depends on a kind of synergy between educational input and changes in policy. For instance, anti-smoking legislation and related educational/publicity initiatives may arguably have a much greater combined impact than either one operating singly (note Warner's (1981) claim that the joint effect of cigarette price increases and associated publicity in the USA was to 'decrease consumption by 41.5% below what it otherwise would have been'). It would thus be fatuous to expect health education to achieve substantial social change in the absence of supportive public policy which makes the healthy choice the easy choice. It would equally be unrealistic to expect major policy changes to happen in the absence of a health education programme which seeks to raise consciousness about the need for such changes.

In both of the situations described thus far we must therefore assess separately a variety of subprogrammes which are individually necessary but not sufficient to achieve an ultimate health promotion outcome. Even so, within each of these subprogrammes we will often be unable to use outcome measures because of an inevitable time lag between educational input and the attainment of the desired goal. This 'sleeper phenomenon' is the third of the three situations referred to earlier and will now be considered.

One of the more common difficulties faced by evaluators is that posed by the gap between the completion of a given educational programme and the desired outcome. An obvious instance is the delay which would inevitably be expected between changes in behaviour, consequent reduction in risks and the final epidemiological outcome. This phenomenon was illustrated by an earlier example which described the links between exercise and the incidence of CHD. It has been argued, however, that health education should not be evaluated according to such criteria and so the following example is of greater interest. This considers the time gap between the delivery of health education and the opportunity to put what has been learned into practice.

Consider the case of a school-based programme of cancer education. Let us assume that the prevailing model of health education is preventive and the goal is secondary prevention. The purpose of the teaching is to contribute to the achievement of early diagnosis and thus to persuade individuals to seek early medical advice whenever one of the classic early warning signs and symptoms of cancer present (cough or hoarseness, change in appearance of wart or mole, etc.). Clearly such symptoms are unlikely to occur and require attention for perhaps 20 or 30 years or more after the teaching has taken place. Any meaningful evaluative study of the effectiveness of the educational input would thus require a cohort study if the causal chain between education and behavioural outcome were to be established. Such a study would be too costly to contemplate even if all the extraneous inputs of information and influences occurring over 20 years or more could be controlled. Intermediate indicators of the acquisition of knowledge, beliefs and attitude would have to suffice.

The kind of time lag examined above is perhaps self-evident. Less obvious is the time lag imposed by the dictates of sound educational theory and practice. For instance, recognition of the ways in which the various processes of socialization contribute to the development of a health career – the development over an individual's lifespan of health related behaviours and the psychosocial factors underpinning these – should lead educational planners to devise a 'spiral curriculum'. This seeks to provide appropriate teaching at significant points on the health career such that a topic is not merely taught at only one point in time but is rather revisited and handled in a manner appropriate to the developmental requirements of the student. The adoption of a health career approach should thus ensure that a planned and cumulative series of educational inputs have been provided prior to the moment when an individual is expected to make a given health choice. The concept of a smoking career exemplifies this process since research on the natural history of smoking has made it clear that a single lesson or even a series of lessons on smoking will neither prevent recruitment nor facilitate genuine decision making about whether to smoke or not. A programme must be started long before early secondary school age and the time when experimentation starts in earnest. Such a programme will require not only differential provision of biological and social knowledge related to the children's developmental age but also expert teaching which will equip young people with social interaction skills so that they might be 'inoculated' against various pressures to smoke. Each element in the smoking career is necessary and intermediate indicators are needed *en route* to check that each stage of the programme has been effective. (This should, ideally, be part of the process of formative evaluation, to which reference was made in the previous chapter.)

A sound programme of health education will thus require not only co-ordination of inputs throughout the health career but also co-ordination across the range of inputs provided at any one time. In other words both longitudinal and cross-sectional integration are a prerequisite for most complex programmes since the influences of health related behaviours are many and varied and are brought to bear in a cumulative way over time. This complex of psychosocial and environmental influences is illustrated in Figure 3.2 and describes the multifactorial nature of drug misuse.

A detailed discussion of the nature of these causal factors and their interplay is beyond the scope of this book (Tones, 1986; 1987) but two things should be apparent from Figure 3.2 in addition to the complexity of the factors contributing to drug use and misuse. First, the multifactorial nature of many health problems requires a multifactorial educational programme if success is to be a real possibility. Second, each subprogramme will generate intermediate indicators. In the context of Figure 3.2 these will include: knowledge of the nature and effect of drugs; the acquisition of skills to resist social pressures; the acquisition of alternative forms of gratification; the modification of beliefs about drug misusers; enhancement of self-esteem, and so on.

The importance of being fully cognisant of the multifaceted influences on the behaviours involved in the use and abuse of substances should not be underestimated. Indeed, it is worth noting the relevance of this observation for both the 'educational diagnosis' and evaluation of 'vertical' disease focused programmes. For instance, let us consider the five key areas targeted in the UK government's strategy for health in England (DoH, 1992). These five key areas (selected on the basis of '... both the greatest need and greatest scope for making cost-effective improvements...') comprise coronary heart disease and stroke, cancers, mental illness, HIV/AIDS and sexual health, and accidents. Each of them might be the focus of a health promotion programme; each programme might be evaluated in terms of outcome measures such as a reduction in the incidence of accidents among children under 15 or by a decline in the overall suicide rate. However, to develop five separate 'vertical' programmes would not necessarily be the most efficient nor the most economical strategy since a number of 'horizontal' influ-

Indicators of success and performance

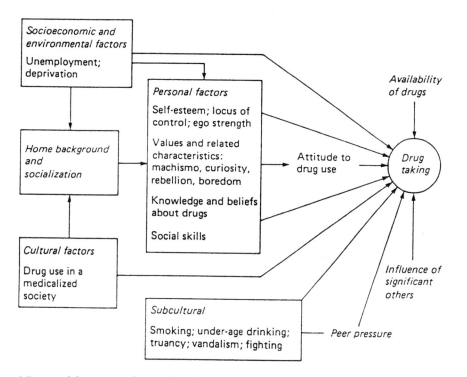

Figure 3.2 Misuse of drugs: psychosocial and environmental influences.

ences underpin some or all of the five disease related outcomes. The five key vertical areas are shown in Figure 3.3 together with these underlying 'strata'.

First of all, it is clear that some of the five key areas have risk factors in common (for example, diet and smoking in the case of cancers and cardiovascular disease). At a more fundamental level, certain attributes of the at-risk population predispose them to adopt a lifestyle which puts them at risk from the diseases and disorders defined by the five key areas. A 'horizontal' health and life skills programme which addresses this underlying lifestyle is more efficient because it is literally more radical, i.e. it gets at the roots of the situation. A yet more radical programme

consonant with the philosophy of health promotion will also seek to tackle the environmental and sociostructural factors under pinning lifestyle by incorporating healthy public policy.

Figure 3.3 also reminds us of the reciprocal determinism of environment and life skills: healthy public policy facilitates healthy lifestyles; life skills are needed to influence the implementation of healthy public policy. Additionally, it enables us to look for different intermediate indicators of success at each horizontal layer.

A further instance of the importance of not being seduced by superficial manifestations of deepseated health problems is provided by Jessor and Jessor's (1977) work on 'problem

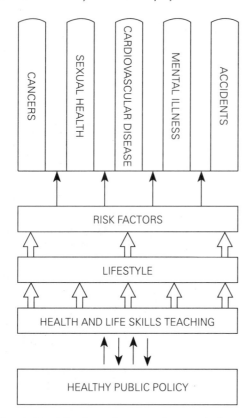

Figure 3.3 A horizontal approach to vertical problems.

relates to activities which are traditionally the main concern of health educators. These 'health compromising' behaviours would include sexual behaviours leading to sexually transmitted infection or unwanted pregnancy, substance misuse and a variety of other 'risky' behaviours. Segment III is concerned with 'psychopathology' – for instance, depression or suicide.

Overlap in the categories can be readily identified. Area 'a' in the venn diagram could include car theft and drunk driving; area 'b' might be illustrated by dietary disorders such as anorexia and bulimia. Area 'c' would represent some awesome combination of all three: perhaps suicidal ram-raiding while under the influence of hallucinogens and without wearing seat belts.

Clearly these different problem behaviours can be directly related to the five key areas emphasized in *Health of the Nation*. Again, Jessor's analysis reveals the wisdom of avoiding the vertical programmes which might result from too narrow a response to deepseated difficulties.

Figure 3.4 provides a further reminder of the reciprocal determinism of the individual and the environment. This is not untimely as in the recent past we have frequently witnessed attempts to explain antisocial and 'delinquent' behaviour either in terms of broader social factors, such as poverty or

behaviour' in adolescents. Adolescence is widely recognized as a period of transition which is likely to be more or less problematic. However, it is not uncommon to concentrate on the 'symptoms' of adolescents' attempts to cope with the developmental tasks imposed on them by the culture in which they live. Quite frequently we ignore the fact that what are superficial behaviours – healthy or unhealthy – derive from more fundamental developmental pressures. Figure 3.4 below is a simplified version of Jessor's model of problem behaviour.

Figure 3.4 shows three overlapping varieties of dysfunctional behaviour. Segment I has been labelled antisocial behaviour, such as vandalism and 'twocking' (taking vehicles without the owner's consent)! Segment II

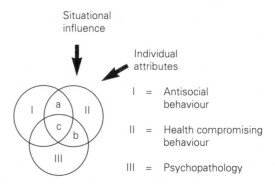

Figure 3.4 Problem behaviour in adolescence (after Jessor and Jessor, 1977).

unemployment, or in terms of individual lack of 'responsibility', often allegedly due to failures of parenting. Preference for one of other stance seems to be determined by ideological orientation or even narrow party political preference.

As with our analysis of the five vertical programme areas, indicators of effectiveness are stratified in that we might identify ways of measuring broader social factors or, more superficially, individual attributes. For instance, it seems probable that a strong network of community control and social support would minimize the likelihood of problem behaviours and thus we could have recourse to network analysis. On the other hand we could resort to the more familiar terrain of measuring coping skills and beliefs about control to gauge the effectiveness of our anticipatory guidance or life skills teaching.

THE IMPORTANCE OF THEORY

It should by now be clear that there is a wide range of measures which might and should be used to evaluate any given health promotion programme. Obviously such measures should not be selected randomly and it is perhaps the main contention in this chapter that in order to make a judicious selection of indirect, intermediate and outcome indicator, we must have a sound theoretical framework. Apart from any other more technical reason, we need such a framework to enable us to justify our choice with confidence when confronted with the often unreasonable demands of managers and politicians!

A sound theoretical framework will, then, provide a substantial basis for practice. The main requirement for such a framework is that it should help explain how people make health related decisions, individually or *en masse*. It will attempt to define the ways in which social and environmental factors influence these decisions and will provide insight into the nature of both inter- and intrapersonal dynamics governing behaviours. If we have some understanding of the constellation of factors influencing human behaviour in health and illness, we will be in a better position to devise strategies and formulate methods which will achieve our health education goals – no matter what our philosophy or what model we choose to follow. Again, if we understand the existing relationships between, for example, knowledge, beliefs, skills, attitudes, social pressures and environmental constraints, we should have some insight into the likely effects of a given educational programme and might thus select our indicators of success in a more rational and meaningful way. For instance, we might on the basis of theoretical understanding expect a conventionally taught and essentially didactic lesson on drugs to produce an increase in knowledge but little else. We would not expect it to affect attitudes or any of the other factors which Figure 3.2 suggests will influence drug misuse. We would therefore have a limited expectation of what the lesson might achieve and what it might contribute to a more comprehensive drug education programme. We would also know that the only appropriate indicator to use would be one which measured recall of information.

MACRO LEVEL THEORY: THE COMMUNICATION OF INNOVATIONS

Both health promotion and health education are concerned to promote change. In the last analysis health education, as pointed out earlier, seeks to promote health and illness related learning, i.e. a relatively permanent change in disposition or capability. Before considering theories which seek to explain and predict individual learning, we will briefly review change at the macro level – the level of the social system. One of the best researched and most useful of such theories is communication of innovations theory (Rogers and Shoemaker, 1971).

Although this theoretical approach is not by any mean the only theory which seeks to describe the ways in which large numbers of people (populations or communities) come to change their customary practices and adopt new behaviours, it has a particular appeal in that it has been thoroughly researched and many reported studies include analysis of the adoption of health related innovations.

According to the authors, it is based on seven major research traditions and, at the time of publication, drew upon 1084 publications in anthropology, sociology, education, communication and marketing.

According to Rogers and Shoemaker, an innovation is:

> ... an idea, practice, or object perceived as new by an individual. It matters little, so far as human behavior is concerned, whether or not an idea is 'objectively' new as measured by the lapse of time since its first use or discovery. It is the perceived or subjective newness of the idea for the individual that determines his reaction to it. If the idea seems new to the individual, it is an innovation.
>
> *(p. 19)*

Self-evidently, our concern here is with health innovations.

A community (or, more accurately, a social system) may be geographic, i.e. a group of people in a defined place, or less typically 'relational'. In the latter instance the social system will be defined in terms of interactions which are not geographically rooted; for instance a 'population' of doctors, teachers or nurses widely distributed throughout a relatively large area and, accordingly, not having an opportunity for face-to-face primary contact. The issue of geography and 'neighbourhood' will receive further comment in Chapter 8.

Five generalizations may be made from the findings of communication of innovations theory. They are concerned with the rate of adoption of innovations and with the impact of certain important variables on the rate of adoption. These variables include:

1. the characteristics of potential adopters;
2. the rate of adoption;
3. the nature of the social system;
4. the characteristics of the innovation;
5. the characteristics of 'change agents'.

CHARACTERISTICS OF ADOPTERS

Adopters of an innovation are presumed to move through a series of stages similar to those embodied in the 'K-A-P' formula. In other words, awareness of the innovation is followed by arousal of interest prior to trying out the new practice and, ultimately, adopting it. Individuals differ as regards the length of time they take to progress through each phase. Accordingly, those that Rogers and Shoemaker termed 'laggards' will take an inordinate amount of time before committing themselves to action whereas 'innovators', who are presumably more exposed to communication, for some reason express immediate interest and eagerly espouse novelty. Table 3.1 lists the different adopter categories.

As may be seen, those who adopt first of all are labelled innovators; they are closely followed by early adopters who are in turn succeeded by the early majority. Bringing up the rear are the late majority and, last of all, the laggards.

RATE OF ADOPTION: THE S-SHAPED CURVE

When the proportion of those who adopt the innovation is plotted against time, a characteristically 'S-shaped' curve results. The shape is determined by the differential rate of adoption of the population. A steep curve indicates a rapid rate of adoption; a flattened curve shows a slow rate of adoption. This is shown graphically in Figure 3.5.

There are two key points worthy of note by programme evaluators. The first lesson to be learned from communication of innovations

Table 3.1 The communication of innovations: major adopter categories (adapted from Rogers and Shoemaker, 1971)

Adopter category	Characteristics
Innovator	2.5% of population: eager but a 'deviant'; probably mistrusted by the safe majority
Early adopter	13.5% of population: respectable but amenable to change; good candidate for opinion leader or community aide
Early majority	34% of population: according to Rogers and Shoemaker their motto might be 'Be not the last to lay the old aside, nor the first by which the new is tried'!
Late majority	34% of population: the sceptics reluctant to change until benefits of innovation have been clearly proven
Laggards	16% of population: the diehard conservatives! Will doubtless incorporate a subgroup who will never change and appear to be against everything most of the time

It will be noted that these adopter categories represent ideal types and their distribution is viewed by Rogers and Shoemaker as matching the normal or Gaussian curve

theory is that it can take a very long time before the last laggard has yielded to the force of change! Indeed, Rogers and Shoemaker cite early examples of diffusion time lag and readers may be interested in the following somewhat esoteric facts. It apparently took some 40 years before the tunnel oven was adopted in the English pottery industry, 14 years for the adoption of hybrid seed corn in Iowa, 50 years before US schools adopted the idea of the kindergarten and five or six years to adopt modern maths in the 1960s (p. 16).

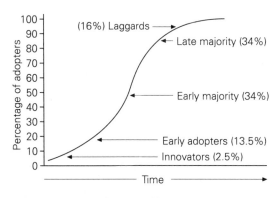

Figure 3.5 The S-shaped diffusion curve and adopter categories (after Rogers and Shoemaker, 1971).

It is clearly wise not to expect instant success and, more technically, to take account of the fact that it will be increasingly difficult to influence later adopters and shift a residual hard core within the broader category of laggards. In other words, a law of diminishing returns will operate in health education programmes seeking to influence large groups of people. Evaluators should, on that account, build some form of compensation into their calculations. Green and Lewis (1986) have argued that this ceiling effect, originally noted by Hovland *et al.* (1949) in the field of mass communications, may be countered by means of an 'effectiveness index' derived from the following formula:

$$EI = \frac{(P_2 - P_1)}{(100 - P_1)}$$

where EI = Effectiveness Index, P_1 is the percentage of the population adopting the innovation prior to the educational intervention and P_2 is the percentage adopting at a given time after the programme.

And so, a relatively small change in the group of diehard 'resistants' may be a cause for congratulation whereas a similar or even greater degree of change in an unexposed and virgin population might well require a change of programme and personnel.

THE SOCIAL SYSTEM

Only a brief observation will be made about the remaining factors influencing rate of adoption. The first of these is the nature of the social system itself and in this respect it seems reasonable to accept Rogers and Shoemaker's view that certain 'traditional' communities will take longer to adopt **any** innovation whereas, on the other hand, a 'cosmopolitan' social system will be more open to change, perhaps because it lacks the culturally created caution of the former or has better communication systems – or both.

CHARACTERISTICS OF THE INNOVATION

We may paraphrase Rogers and Shoemaker's list of the features which maximize an innovation's likelihood of adoption. Ideally it should have the following characteristics: relative advantage; compatibility; complexity; trialability; observability. For example, if a community perceives that a recommended dietary change has benefits for them by comparison with their existing diet; if the proposed change is compatible with lifestyle and culture; if it is not too complicated, e.g. to grow, collect and cook; if it is relatively easy to try out without making a full commitment; if the community can readily and rapidly observe the benefits – then the innovation stands a pretty good chance of being adopted!

CHANGE AGENT CHARACTERISTICS

The final facet of communication of innovations theory of interest to us has to do with the characteristics of the change agent, e.g. the health educator working with a community or group of people.

It is, of course, a matter of common sense to note that whether or not people are persuaded to modify their life-style may very well hinge on the repertoire of skills possessed by the health educator. However, Rogers and Shoemaker additionally remind us that the change agent must be acceptable to the community (or be sufficiently cunning to employ those who are acceptable). This notion is elaborated in the principle of homophily, to which further reference will be made in Chapter 8.

INDICATORS OF SUCCESS

Communication of innovations theory operates at a macro level and so we might expect that the insights which it provides for evaluation will also be at a macro level. To some extent this is true. In the last analysis the indicator of success for those whose goal is to produce a change in a social system will be the extent to which the innovation in question has been adopted. The theory should, however, also invite us to note the extent of the adoption process and the speed with which adoption has or is taking place. For instance, monitoring of, say, the adoption of a newly introduced vaccine will give an indication of the degree of steepness of the 'S-shaped' diffusion curve at any given point in a campaign. If it is relatively shallow, additional resources may be needed. On the other hand, a rapid move from early adopter into the early majority category would imply that the programme has gathered its own momentum.

Again, we have already noted the utility of the theoretical analysis in the process of standard setting, i.e. the establishment of realistic criteria for programme assessment: less ambitious standards must be set when a programme is seeking to influence that minority of the target group which has not yet had their children vaccinated. Alternatively, of course, and in accordance with the principles of herd immunity, it may be decided that an attempt to influence the remaining 5% or 10% of the populace is not a cost effective proposition.

Finally, Rogers and Shoemaker's theoretical formulations can help us with indirect indicators. For instance, if we know what constitutes the features of an innovation which maximize its chance of success, we can merely count the number of such features which any particular innovation possesses and we can, having made a similar assessment of change agent characteristics, etc., draw conclusions about the potential efficiency of the programme. The principle is, of course, similar to that embodied in pretesting, to which reference will be made later.

The possibility of monitoring the progress of a campaign was mentioned above. Process evaluation – a kind of micro level monitoring – might also be used to document potentially significant elements of any given programme. For instance, documenting the interaction between change agent and opinion leader in a neighbourhood, village or community group might illuminate, *ex post facto*, the reasons for the success or failure of the intervention. Of course, if the notion of formative evaluation is practised, appraisal of process can be used to maximize the chance of success by making successive modifications to the programme in response to the insights gained from observation and documentation, a point which was explained more completely in Chapter 2.

MICRO LEVEL THEORY: THE HEALTH ACTION MODEL

Having considered the usefulness of macro level theory in the form of Rogers and Shoemaker's formulation, we will now continue to argue that 'there is nothing so practical as a good theory'. This time we will be operating at the micro level and considering how an understanding of psychological, social and environmental factors may influence **individual** decision making and subsequent choices and behaviours. The health action model will be used to explicate the relationship between these psychosocial and environmental influences and to provide a framework for the prudent selection of indicators of performance. First, though, a few observations about the use of models may be opportune.

THE USE OF MODELS

As Green (1984) has pointed out, there are a wide range of theoretical models at the disposal of health educators and we might reasonably ask why one particular model should be selected at the expense of any other. Before addressing this issue, a brief explanation of model making would seem to be in order.

Models are derived from theory and thus seek to provide an explanation of some feature of our world. Models do not provide a detailed replica of reality but rather they offer a partial and simplified representation of whatever aspect of the real world is of interest to the theoretician or practitioner. The process of simplification is necessary because it allows us to concentrate on what is most important for particular needs while excluding irrelevancies and unnecessary detail. A good model will achieve this goal of simplification while including all key elements. For instance, a 'technical' (as opposed to 'ideological') model in health education should incorporate the various components which are essential to human decision making and explain their inter-relationships. A better model would quantify those relationships and facilitate predictions about the likelihood of an individual – or, more problematically, a group of individuals – adopting and sustaining a particular course of action under given circumstances.

Luck and Luckman (1974) provide a useful general definition of models.

A model is a representation of the significant features of the problem under study. It can be a simple verbal description or a three-dimensional design such as is produced by architects or engineers, or it can be an abstract logical or mathematical representation. Since it is usually too expensive and risky to experiment blindly with the problem in the real world we need a model to allow us to examine the effect of a range of possible changes, either initiated by the decision makers or coming spontaneously from the environment. The model builder always has to satisfy two conflicting needs: he wants his model to be a faithful representation of the problem; he also wants his model to be a powerful tool for examining a wide range of alternative courses of action, which implies that it must be simple to apply.

Some models offer no more than a useful but limited formula which may provide a rough guide for practice and the evaluation of practice. Although the authors would not consider it a model as such, it is useful to consider the '... framework of general goals and theoretical principles for health promotion ...' which was used in the successful North Karelia heart disease prevention programme (see Chapter 8). This framework included five programme elements which were considered the minimum necessary for coherent programme design.

1.   Improved preventive services;
2.   Information ('to educate people about their health');
3.   Persuasion ('to motivate people');
4.   Training ('to increase skills of self-control, environmental management and social action');
5.   Community organization ('to create social support').

(McAlister et al., 1982)

This scheme is clearly a much improved version of the simplistic 'K-A-P' model to which reference was made in Chapter 1 (i.e. the suggestion that the provision of knowledge together with the use of attitude change devices will routinely lead to a change in practice). The five point plan does

however, provide a guide for programme planning and offers clear indicators for evaluation: they include performance indicators, such as provision of services to detect and control hypertension, and various intermediate indicators, such as knowledge of CHD risk, positive attitudes to reducing risk and the acquisition of culinary skills for a healthy diet. It also offers examples of indicators which may be used as measures of social and environmental change, such as the establishment of networks of lay leaders and the development of healthy nutritional policy which among other innovations gave rise to the Karelian low-fat mushroom sausage!

THE HEALTH BELIEF MODEL

Rather more refined theoretical models provide a narrower and sharper focus. Probably the best known of these is the **health belief model** (HBM) (Becker, 1984). Although the HBM has undergone revision (Janz and Becker, 1984), its main contribution to programme planning has been the way it has highlighted the role of certain beliefs in stimulating preventive health actions. The HBM asserts that an individual must believe:

1.   That (s)he is susceptible to a given disease;
2.   That the disease or disorder is serious;
3.   That the proposed preventive action will be beneficial – i.e. will effectively protect the individual from the threatening disease;
4.   That these benefits will outweigh any costs or disadvantages that (s)he believes will be incurred as a result of the recommended preventive health action.

In addition the likelihood of action will be enhanced if the individual has a generally positive attitude to health (typically measured by totting up the number of preventive measures adopted by the individual in addition to the preventive action currently under consideration) and if some cue or trigger is provided. The most important indicators of success which are highlighted by the HBM are the four key beliefs (how many of these does the individual hold and how strongly are they held?), the number of preventive actions undertaken and the successful delivery of appropriate 'cues to action'.

THE THEORY OF REASONED ACTION

A second model merits comment in this context since it has frequently been used to good effect in the health field. This is Fishbein's **theory of reasoned action** (Fishbein and Ajzen, 1985; Ajzen and Fishbein, 1980). Fishbein and Ajzen complement and improve on aspects of an HBM analysis of health decision making by separating belief from attitude and emphasizing the paramount importance of the influence of 'significant others' on an individual's 'intention to act'. The often substantial gap between intention and practice is acknowledged and the relationship between beliefs, attitudes, normative factors, intention and practice is expressed in mathematical terms. The Fishbein model would typically generate the following indicators:

1. An often long list of different beliefs about a given specific health action;
2. The attitude which is created by these beliefs;
3. A series of beliefs about the likely reaction of various significant others to the proposed behaviour;
4. The individual's motivation to comply with the perceived wishes of the significant others;
5. The strength of the resulting behavioural intention;
6. The actual behavioural outcome itself.

REVISIONS AND DEVELOPMENTS

This chapter cannot provide a comprehensive review of the extensive literature on models and theories having relevance for health and illness behaviour. It would, however, not be appropriate to apparently question the value of models such as the HBM or TRA. This is certainly not the intention, especially since models such as the TRA were not specifically designed with health education in mind. It will, however, become apparent that we need to take account of a number of variables which do not figure in the two models which have been discussed so far. We must, though, acknowledge the fact that the models themselves have been extended or developed to meet criticisms about their lack of explanatory power in certain contexts. For example, one of the weaknesses of the HBM centres on its assertion that beliefs about susceptibility and seriousness give rise to perceived threat which, in turn, increases the likelihood of individuals adopting recommended preventive actions (along with beliefs about the costs and benefits of so doing). The effect of fear and arousal on decision making is, however, by no means simple and according to Prentice-Dunn and Rogers (1986), Rogers' formulation of a 'protection motivation theory' (1975) takes us 'beyond the health belief model' in its capacity to explain the effect of these important variables.

Again, one of the major criticisms of the theory of reasoned action has centred on its focus on volitional control. This limitation is of particular importance in health education since much health and illness related behaviour is profoundly influenced by emotional factors – and, of course, by environmental constraints. Acknowledging this limitation, Ajzen developed a 'theory of planned behaviour' (Ajzen, 1985; Schifter and Ajzen, 1985). This theory included a very important addition to the TRA: 'perceived behavioural control'. This concept of control is consonant with Bandura's notion of self-efficacy and the broader idea of reciprocal determinism (both discussed in Chapter 1). The revised model thus asserts that actions depend not only on beliefs and attitudes about behavioural outcomes and the reaction of significant others – they also depend on the extent to which people believe it is actually possible to translate intention into practice and, for example, adopt any given innovation.

THE WORK OF TRIANDIS

Before discussing the health action model, some reference must be made to a sophisticated model which lacks the popularity of HBM or TRA but which nonetheless has much greater relevance for health education. This model was developed by Triandis (1980). Two equations from Triandis model will be provided below so that readers may judge for themselves the relevance of the constructs used.

Equation 1

$$P_a = (wHH + wII)\ P.F.$$

where P_a is the probability of the act, indexed by a number between 0 and 1; wH and wI are weights; I is a behavioural intention or self-instruction to perform the act; H is the habit to perform the act that reflects automatic behaviour tendencies developed during the past history of the individual; and F describes the facilitating conditions.

Equation 2

$$I = w_S S + w_A A + w_C C$$

where I = behavioural intention; S = the individual's self-instruction to do what is viewed as correct from the point of view of the individual's moral code, and to do what has been previously agreed with others; A is the affect attached to the behaviour and C = the value of n perceived consequences of the behaviour. w = weights to be assigned to each factor.

In order to facilitate appraisal of the constructs which should be incorporated into an efficient explanatory model for health education practice, readers might care to compare and contrast the components within Triandis' system with the health action model. Before explaining the HAM, we would like to reiterate the point that although models should be judged on the basis of their sophistication and applicability, personal predilection should legitimately play a part in selection. Alternatively, practitioners may prefer to build their own model. Whatever the choice, a theoretical framework is a *sine qua non* for professional decision making.

THE HEALTH ACTION MODEL

The health action model was developed in an attempt to provide a comprehensive framework which would incorporate the major variables influencing health choices and actions (Tones, 1979; 1981). Although its original concern was with health education, it proved to be compatible with the formulation of health promotion described in Chapter 1. Figure 3.6 provides an overview of key system components.

It will be seen that there are two major sections to the HAM. The first of these contributes to an individual's intention to act, or behavioural intention (BI), and comprises an interacting system having three parts: cognitive, affective and normative. Central to the cognitive dimension is a belief system which interfaces with a kind of information processor. This includes a number of intellectual skills needed to handle incoming information and generally interpret environmental events.

The affective dimension, which has a reciprocal relationship with the belief system, is to all intents and purposes concerned with an individual's motivational state. The normative system signals the importance of different kinds of social pressure on people's intention to act.

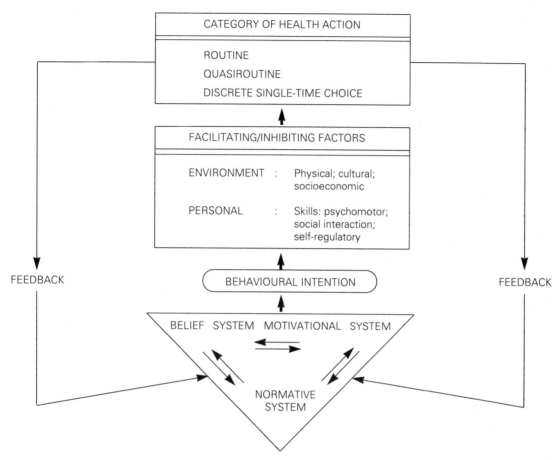

Figure 3.6 The health action model: an overview.

The second major section is concerned with all those factors which determine whether or not an intention is translated into practice; it is also concerned with whatever factors make it likely that an action will be sustained or become routinized or, on the other hand, lead to relapse or rejection of a previously made decision.

In terms of health promotion goals, the first section (belief system; motivation system; normative system) relates to the motivation of individuals to act; the second section is concerned with providing postdecisional support.

It is not, of course, assumed that behavioural intention is necessarily a conscious state; an individual will frequently make a decision in a choice situation without any conscious calculation of the costs and benefits and without weighing up alternatives. The decision is, however, influenced by a peculiar cluster of beliefs, motives and social pressures which have created a state of readiness for action when the appropriate circumstances arise. Clearly, efficient decision making will in fact require conscious calculations and many health education approaches will incorporate that goal into their rationale.

The term 'discrete single time choice' refers to a single specific decision. The goals of most educational programmes will include a large number of such decisions. Indeed, there may well be as many discrete choices to make as there are programme objectives.

Once the choice has been made there are two possibilities: the decision may be reversed or it may ultimately become routinized – for instance, purchase and preparation of a high fibre meal may result in a firm commitment never to try it again. Alternatively, the experience may prove enjoyable and subsequently may be incorporated into habitual dietary practice. Routines may be established in the way described above or may result from an often protracted process of socialization. Children do not routinely brush their teeth after meals as a result of a process of 'vigilant decision making' based on appraisal of costs and benefit. They do it as a result of Skinnerian conditioning in which parents shape their behaviour through the application of reward (and sometimes punishment). The whole procedure would typically be supported by the use of modelling' in accordance with the dictates of social learning theory.

Routine practices of any kind are not under direct conscious control and do not therefore require a conscious decision, except perhaps when they are becoming established, when they are disrupted or when attempts are made to change them. For example, drivers need to make a deliberate choice once they have formed an intention to wear seat belts; however, once the choice has become routine, it will recur automatically.

Figure 3.6 shows a feedback process. This indicates how the experience of performing a particular health action, a break in a routine or other related event can either consolidate action or, as it were, 'switch it off'. For instance, a negative experience at an antenatal clinic may cause a woman to modify her previous beliefs about the costs and benefits of attending. A woman who has been per-suaded to breastfeed her children may experience discomfort and pain from sore nipples and start to bottlefeed; a man who has succeeded in quitting smoking for several days may no longer be able to cope with the feelings of anxiety and irritability and relapses. On the other hand someone who has reluctantly decided to use a condom to assuage a sense of apprehension about risk of HIV infection may discover the experience is quite colourful and exciting!

The reference to 'quasi routine' in Figure 3.6 merits some explanation. It refers to the pervasive effect of normative pressure on the process of decision making. It describes a situation in which a particular practice (healthy or unhealthy) is so pervasive that the individual is unaware that a choice is really possible. A particular course of action may be so unusual or reprehensible that only the most reckless of deviants would ever contemplate the action in question. Note, for instance, Harfouche's (1965) description of the normative expectations of the maternal role regarding breast-feeding:

> Nursing is a duty; a mother who does not nurse denies her baby's right … she is stingy, lazy, negligent, lacks affection like a step-mother … no lactation, no affection.

In a case of this kind, although there would appear to be an alternative of artificial feeding, the only real choice is breastfeeding which is therefore described as a 'quasi routine'. The phenomenon is related to the process of 'inferior' decision making which Janis and Mann (1977) labelled 'quasi-satisficing'.

FACILITATING FACTORS AND THE PROVISION OF SUPPORT

Bearing in mind the importance attached by health promotion and the empowerment model to the provision of support to facilitate genuine decision making, it is essential to take account of those barriers or inhibiting factors which may be interposed between intention and action. Conversely, we might say that the identification of appropriate facilitating factors is a necessary prerequisite for effective health promotion. In Figure 3.6, two varieties of factor are depicted. The first and arguably the most important of these is the physical, cultural and socioeconomic environment, the significance of which has been fully debated in an earlier chapter.

The second set of factors are 'personal' in the sense that they refer to the knowledge and skills which the individual needs to ensure that the health action will materialize and be sustained. Skills may include psychomotor competences, such as the dexterity needed for the proper use of a condom or for the efficient practice of first aid techniques. They will also include social interaction skills – for instance, the capacity to communicate assertively with a partner about safer sex practices. Less obvious, perhaps, is a need for self-regulatory skills.

Sustaining behaviours which involve loss of gratification is one of the most difficult of the tasks which health education seeks to facilitate. The difficulties involved in controlling 'addictive behaviours' are well documented. Accordingly, a variety of techniques associated with behaviour modification have been evolved to help people monitor their behaviours and environmental circumstances, avoid temptation and discover substitute gratifications and rewards for successful maintenance of the healthy activities they have chosen to adopt. These various techniques are here referred to as 'self-regulatory skills' (Kanfer and Karoly, 1972).

While on the subject of gaining control over addictive behaviours, we might note how the popular and so-called 'revolving door' model developed by Prochaska and DiClemente might be incorporated in the HAM. The model in question describes how, for example, heavy smokers might move round a kind of cyclical trajectory before eventually succeeding in quitting their habit. They move through five stages of change: precontemplation, contemplation, action, maintenance and (quite probably) relapse before they re-enter the precontemplation stage. A less cursory description of the model may be examined elsewhere (DiClemente and Prochaska, 1982; Prochaska, 1992; Breteler *et al.*, 1990). However, in HAM terms, the stages of precontemplation and contemplation relate to the changing dynamic within the belief, motivation and normative systems following education and/or other influences leading to a behavioural intention which results in the action stage. Whether maintenance or relapse follows will be determined by the degree of support – including self-regulatory skills – available to the individual, the strength of behavioural intention and the degree of trauma associated with 'withdrawal'. In the case of 'relapse', the feedback loop cancels intention and the individual resumes the former unhealthy behaviour.

HAM: THE BELIEF SYSTEM

Some indication of the importance of health beliefs has already been provided in the earlier discussion of the health belief model. However, although the notions of susceptibility, seriousness and beliefs about costs and benefits are useful, they are not necessarily the beliefs which health education would seek to modify. As we will see, these HBM beliefs are the product of a series of subordinate beliefs.

It should be noted at this point that beliefs are defined in the HAM as cognitive rather than affective constructs. In this we follow Fishbein's (1976) formulation:

A belief is a probability judgement that links some object or concept to some attribute. (The terms 'object' and 'attribute' are used in a generic sense and both terms may refer to any discriminable aspect of an individual's world.) For example, I may believe that *PILL* (an object) is a *DEPRESSANT* (an attribute). The content of the belief is defined by the person's subjective probability that the object–attribute relationship exists (or is true).

The hierarchical nature of beliefs is illustrated in Figure 3.7 which considers the contribution of a number of beliefs to an individual's decision to seek early medical advice in relation to a skin lesion which might prove to be skin cancer.

Before seeking medical assistance, the individual in question must first recognize that (s)he has a skin lesion. She must then believe it might be skin cancer, i.e. she must form a level of subjective probability which justifies a visit to her doctor. For reasons to be stated below, it may indeed facilitate her medical consultation if she believes it is just possible that it is skin cancer but probably not.

The individual's belief about the likelihood of the sore on her hand being skin cancer will be influenced by her pre-existing belief about her susceptibility to that disease (which, in turn, will depend on her understanding and beliefs about the risk factors). Her intention to visit her doctor will also be influenced by her belief about the seriousness of the disease. Now, according to the HBM, the product of susceptibility and seriousness is a particular level of perceived threat. However, as we indicated earlier, this HBM formulation is a problematic since too high a level of fear generated by that perception of threat may give rise to defensive avoidance rather than 'rational' action. It is for that reason that it may be better if the individual discussed above should have only a moderate level of conviction about the likelihood of her particular lesion being cancer: a very high level of certainty may create too high a level of arousal and give rise to delay in service utilization.

The limitations of the HBM's notion of beliefs about seriousness as necessary precursors to preventive action are particularly well illustrated by cancer. Indeed, one of the major goals of cancer education is to reduce cancerophobia – an inappropriately high level of fear of the disease – and so rather than enhancing beliefs about seriousness it may be necessary to reduce their potency. Figure 3.7

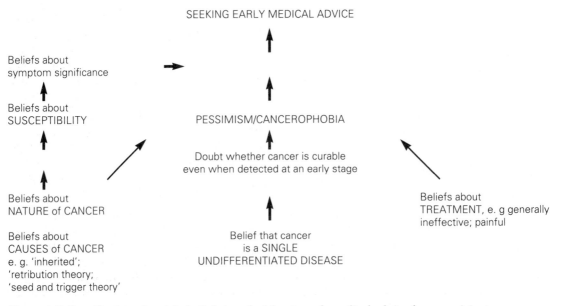

Figure 3.7 Contribution of certain beliefs to a decision to seek medical advice for a persistent sore.

shows cancerophobia (which derives from the general belief system which we label 'pessimism') as a significant barrier to action. It will also be apparent that this barrier derives from a number of subordinate beliefs, one of which is the belief that treatment for cancer is (i) generally ineffective and (ii) painful or distressing (in popular parlance, the treatment is worse than the disease).

Again, we need to probe further before structuring our education programme. We need to ask about the origin of these 'higher order' beliefs. If we do so, we realize that we must consider beliefs about the nature of cancer and its causes. For instance, it has been well documented that people may have a variety of 'theories' about the cause of cancer. A retribution theory considers that cancer has been visited on the individual as a punishment for past moral transgressions. The 'seed and trigger theory' posits that we all have cancer within us in a dormant form, like a kind of seed, which is merely waiting for some event (almost any event – a knock, death in the family, work stress) to trigger it.

More recently, according to audience research by the BBC (1983), it appears that many people consider that cancer is one single undifferentiated disease. This belief about its intrinsic nature will in turn affect the higher order belief that cancer may not be curable. After all, if people know that in many cases treatment fails and they believe that all cancers are the same, they may reasonably suspect that all treatment will be ineffective (and traumatic). Similarly, if you cannot prevent one cancer, you will not be able to prevent any.

Figure 3.8 provides a more detailed analysis of the systems which contribute to an individual's intention to act. The importance of beliefs about cause is acknowledged and they appear as 'attributional beliefs'. The theory of attribution in general provides valuable insights for health education although further discussion is not feasible here (Kelley, 1967).

A particular application of attribution theory centres on how people explain the various vicissitudes which they experience during their lives. More typically, this phenomenon will be discussed in terms of beliefs about control, such as self-efficacy, locus of control and the like. These notions were explored in Chapter 1 and we will merely reiterate their importance at this point. However, returning to Figure 3.7 it is worth observing that an 'empowered person' – i.e. one having internal locus of control, high self-esteem and the like – should be able to cope with a higher level of threat and be less likely to resort to defensive avoidance than an 'external'.

At all events, these various important beliefs about control appear in the HAM in the category, 'beliefs about self'. The sum total of these beliefs forms what is often defined as the self-concept. This includes the notion of 'body image', the importance of which for self-esteem needs no further elaboration.

We should perhaps draw attention to the fact that the HBM variable of susceptibility figures in the category of beliefs about self. Again, while it is not possible here to pursue the matter further, the question of susceptibility should be examined more critically than normally happens. We need in short to consider **why** people believe that they are susceptible. This takes us into the interesting area of risk perception and includes issues such as why people may not accept the level of risk to which their behaviour exposes them (Weinstein, 1982; 1984) and the tendency to overestimate the likelihood of the unlikely and underestimate the real frequency of relatively common threats (Lichtenstein *et al.*, 1978; Slovic *et al.*, 1982).

Before leaving the discussion of beliefs about self, a word of explanation may be needed about the appearance of 'existential beliefs' in the category associated with beliefs about health action. This is to acknowledge the significance of Lewis' (1987) conceptualization of 'existential control', to which

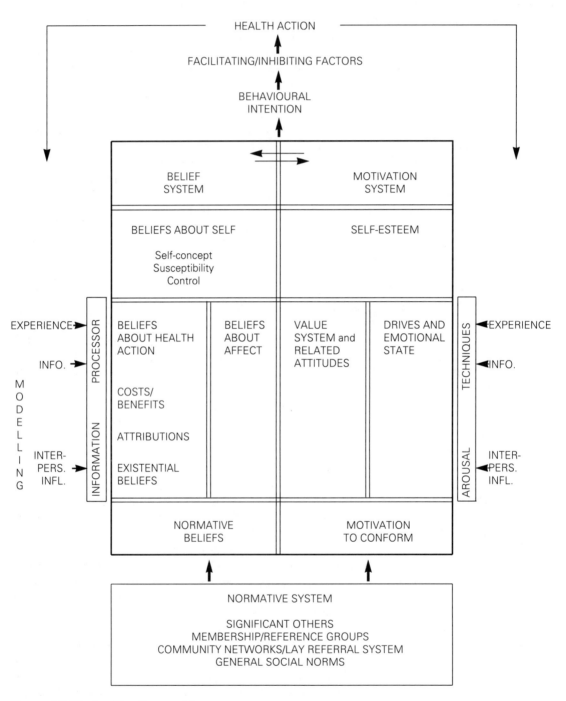

Figure. 3.8 The health action model.

reference was made in Chapter 1. This is viewed here as a set of beliefs not so much about self but rather about life. It is meant to indicate the importance of people's 'philosophy of life' or creed. It is paralleled in the motivation system by a set of associated values. In short, existential beliefs refer to the cognitive dimension, the nature of what a person believes to be true. The affective dimension describes the strength of the values associated with those beliefs.

It will also be evident from Figure 3.8 that a reciprocal relationship exists between all systems. Self-esteem, for instance, refers to the value attached to an individual's construction of self, which may or may not be a true construct. Again, beliefs in general influence feelings and the general level of motivation leading to intention to act. On the other hand, the motivation system influences personal beliefs. It is, for example, well known that we prefer to believe what it is comfortable to believe and often resolutely refuse to accept apparently rational argument due to this pressure from the motivation system. Freud, of course, talked about 'wish fulfilment'!

HAM: THE MOTIVATION SYSTEM

The **motivation system** describes a complex of affective elements which ultimately determines the individual's attitude to the specific action and his or her intention of adopting it. Part of this complex is the individual's value system. Values are acquired through socialization; they are affectively charged sets of beliefs referring to particular aspects of experience (see Rokeach (1973) and Horley (1991) for more detailed discussion). Religious and moral issues relate to all-embracing values; the feelings one has for a career or in relation to family or spouse may be important in underpinning many health related actions.

Attitudes, on the other hand, are more specific than values. They describe feelings

towards particular issues. Fishbein and Ajzen (1985) provide a definition which is both congruent with the HAM perspective and which shows how attitudes relate to beliefs:

> … an attitude (refers) solely to a person's location on a bipolar evaluative or affective dimension with respect to some object, action or event. An attitude represents a person's general feeling of favourableness or unfavourableness towards some stimulus object …
>
> Each belief links the object to some attribute; the person's attitude toward the object is a function of his evaluations of these attributes.

Each value will thus produce a large number of attitudes. For instance, the value associated with sex and gender roles will give rise to a series of attitudes towards, say, the employment of women, the nature of the marriage contract, the role of women in trade unions, the adequacy of medical care for female maladies and so on. The acquisition of new beliefs will, in turn, generate new attitudes energized by the value systems. For example, a belief that breastfeeding would militate against full sharing of the parental role might lead to a negative attitude to breastfeeding derived originally from the gender value mentioned above.

Obviously several values may conspire to produce one single attitude and this situation is illustrated in Figure 3.9. It is apparent from this analysis – indeed, it is a truism – that it will be much more difficult to change an attitude which derives its motivational force from several values, especially where such values are deepseated and salient. Almost by definition, then, one of the most powerful and influential values is that of self-esteem. As we noted, self-esteem refers to the extent to which the individual values the attributes which make up the self-concept. Just as we formulate attitudes to any aspect of our world in accordance with our value system, we

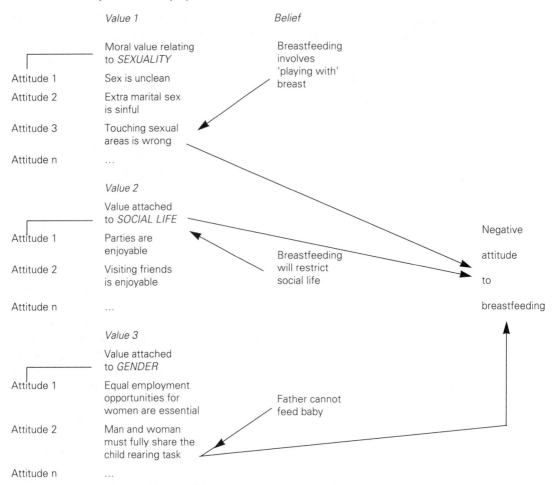

Figure 3.9 The contribution of values to attitude to breastfeeding.

develop attitudes to ourselves. The sum of these attitudes defines our self-esteem. The centrality of the notion to self-empowerment has already been mentioned.

Given our emphasis so far on the importance of recognizing the hierarchical nature of beliefs and the fact that belief strength may vary from doubt and uncertainty to absolute conviction, it is enlightening to note the possibility of a hierarchical categorization of values. Simon (1974) was a leading figure in the US 'values clarification movement' and he viewed values clarification as moving through a seven-stage process as follows:

1. Prizing and cherishing;
2. Publicly affirming;
3. Choosing from alternatives;
4. Choosing after consideration of consequences;
5. Choosing freely;
6. Acting;
7. Acting with pattern, consistency and repetition.

Arguably, those individuals who have clarified their values successfully and who have developed a fully integrated system, which is always consistently applied in their everyday life, will be much more resistant to change than those at an earlier stage of development. In relation to performance indicators, we are presented with a readymade 'scale' allowing us to measure the effectiveness of the values clarification (or values promotion) exercise.

In addition to values and attitudes, the motivation system incorporates 'drives'. The health action model differs from some of the approaches already mentioned in that it recognizes the fact that certain basic and powerful influences may override socially acquired values and attitudes. The term **drive** is therefore used to describe largely inherited, species specific motivational factors such as hunger, sex and pain. It is also used here to refer to those acquired motivators having drivelike qualities, such as addictions to drugs. The importance of drives is obvious at the commonsense level of explanation. For instance, a teenager might believe in the benefits of contraception and have acquired the appropriate techniques in using them; he or she may also have a well developed moral sense but congruent beliefs, values and attitudes may yield to the pressures of sexual passion! Similarly, the alcoholic may well know the damage(s) he is causing to his or her family life and may value children and spouse highly but it is the drivelike influence of the addiction which may determine behaviour.

Frequently, however, there may be no obvious drive influencing intention to act. Nonetheless the presence of certain emotional states may signify the existence of motivational factors derived from drives. For instance, guilt and anxiety may usefully be considered a fractionated or watered down version of pain or fear. Again at a commonsense level it is apparent that nagging feelings of anxiety at the prospect of a spouse's disapproval may prevent a person undertaking some otherwise valued healthy action.

According to the HAM, the classic notion of dissonance (Festinger, 1957) is best explained functionally in terms of derived drive rather than an all-embracing theory of attitude change. The state of dissonance is thus viewed as a feeling akin to that of guilt but created by perceptions of inconsistency between beliefs, attitudes and behaviours. As with other drivelike states, it is 'negatively reinforcing', i.e. it creates a state of discomfort which individuals are motivated to reduce by whatever means they have at their disposal. Dissonance reduction techniques may be 'rational', as for instance when a smoker who values his health stops smoking. Alternatively, dissonance may be reduced by denying the evidence that smoking causes disease and/or studiously avoiding any antismoking 'propaganda'.

Following our discussion of the most appropriate way of conceptualizing the HBM's notion of perceived susceptibility and our comments on risk taking, it would be remiss not to comment on the **positive** reinforcement which risk taking provides for many people. We have already suggested in the context of Jessor's propositions about 'problem behaviour' that risk taking can provide real functional benefits for adolescents struggling to cope with transition. Of equal interest is the argument that some individuals actively pursue risk for the sake of its physiological effects. To put it somewhat crudely, it would seem that they become 'addicted'. Lyng (1990) discusses a number of reasons why people indulge in high risk behaviour and cites Delk (1980) who describes high risk behaviour 'as a form of tension-reduction behavior with addictive qualities related to the build-up of intoxicating stress hormones'.

Lyng's own preferred explanation is in terms of 'edgework' which is seen as a way of handling 'the problem of negotiating the boundary between chaos and order'. Lyng's analysis could be said to have a certain authority since it was based on participant observation as a jump pilot! He asserts that all edgework involves:

> ... a clearly observable threat to one's physical or mental well-being or one's

sense of an ordered existence. The archetypical edgework experience is one in which the individual's failure to meet the challenge at hand will result in death or, at the very least, debilitating injury.

He also argues that many features of drug taking and even 'binge drinking' do not involve self-destructive behaviour as such but rather an attempt to demonstrate mastery and control.

Clearly, both categories of risk taking render the notion of susceptibility irrelevant in predicting likely behaviour. Indeed, in relation to edgework, an activity in which there is no susceptibility to danger would cease to be attractive. Whatever the explanation, it is the motivation system which incorporates the relevant constructs. In the first instance, we are dealing with the drivelike 'addictive' motives; in the case of Lyng's explanation, we are concerned with a mix of beliefs about control, the associated notion of self-esteem and, perhaps primarily, a particular value in relation to the meaning of life and living.

Needless to say, the various drivelike states described above may pose a substantial challenge to the metacognitive and self-referent processes involved in self-regulation – as is apparent in health educators' often desperate attempts to find competing but healthy alternative reinforcers!

A final point should be made about the motivation system and its reciprocal relationship with the belief system. It will be seen in Figure 3.8 that a potentially significant influence may be exerted on behavioural intention not only by any given drive or emotional state but also by **beliefs** about these. This is shown as 'beliefs about affect'. The point may be illustrated by the fact that many smokers may never form an intention to quit despite believing in the benefits of doing so and the costs of continuing smoking. The reason is perhaps obvious: they believe that they would be unable to cope with either the loss of gratification from smoking or/and the negative affect they would experience from withdrawal (Marsh and Matheson, 1983). In HAM terms, this belief about affect would contribute, *inter alia*, to a 'belief about self' in the form of a negative 'self-efficacy' belief.

The motivation system is, then, a composite of different drives, values and attitudes having different emotional charges and giving rise to a particular level of arousal – or a 'push' to take action. Drawing on the experience of those enthusiasts who observed the behavioural minutiae of the white rat's maze learning skills, we might reasonably expect that a 'goal gradient' effect will operate. In other words, whatever the initial level of arousal in relation to a given goal (for example, a sexual encounter), that level will increase proportionately as the individual approaches the desired stimulus object. The significance for the prevention of HIV and other STIs by avoiding unprotected sexual activity will doubtless be self-evident!

The normative system also contributes to the level of arousal mentioned above in the form of an individual's motivation to conform to pressures from other people. We will now consider this.

HAM: THE NORMATIVE SYSTEM

The term 'norm' describes cultural, subcultural and group behaviours together with the various values, beliefs and routines associated with such behaviours. The actual observable behaviours may be termed statistical norms while the beliefs held by the relevant population about such behaviours may be called social norms. Current figures on the prevalence of smoking in, for example, the UK and USA would indicate that the smoker is a deviant in higher social class groups. The notion of deviance underlines the importance of the coercive power of norms and their influence on behavioural intentions and decision making. The effect of the social norm is clearly most important here, for although it would often be correlated with the statistical norm, it is an individual's belief about other people's activities which is influential rather than the extent of the activities themselves.

Norms do not only operate within relatively large cultural units. The influence of norms within a small group on its individual members may be very powerful indeed and has been widely documented; the effect does of course depend on the extent to which the group member values membership of the group in question. Again the norms of a reference group, i.e. a group to which an individual does not belong but for which (s)he has membership aspirations, may also be influential in determining attitudes and behaviours. As indicated earlier, where norms exert a very high degree of coercive pressure, decisions may be reduced to the status of quasi routines.

The health action model describes the **normative system** from an individual and therefore psychological perspective (for a sociological point of view of normative influences, see Baric (1978). This individual perspective includes not only a person's belief about normal practices in the local or national community but also beliefs about the likely reaction of significant others, as described earlier in the discussion of Fishbein's model. It is, however, obvious – again as Fishbein indicated – that such beliefs will only influence behaviour where the individual is motivated to comply with the wishes of significant others or to conform to what (s)he perceives as acceptable norms.

It is apparent that the normative system generates further variables which might be used as diagnostic measures and indicators of success. These will include a description of the actual normative status quo (statistical norms), e.g. the prevalence of a particular practice in a given community; the 'norm sending' aspects of the environment, such as the advertising of unhealthy products or the availability of smoke-free places; the nature of the 'lay referral system' (Freidson, 1961); the nature of social support networks; group behaviours; the actions and attitudes of significant others. The catalogue of normative indicators would also incorporate individual perceptions and beliefs about all of the aforementioned measures, such as people's interpretations of the significance of the presence or absence of healthy foods in works canteens; their awareness of prevalent lay constructions of illness; their beliefs about the level of peer smoking and the likely reaction of their friends to their proposed membership of a health and fitness club. These indicators, incidentally, might be used in an evaluation of a health promotion programme having as its main goal either a change in the normative status quo or a change in people's beliefs about the normative situation.

Before moving on to provide a more detailed discussion of indicators, we will comment on how HAM might provide guidance for the construction of health promotion programmes.

HAM: IMPLICATIONS FOR HEALTH PROMOTION

As already argued, health promotion is viewed as a synergistic combination of education and 'healthy public policy'. Any consideration of HAM would suggest that there might be two policy 'inputs'. First and most important, policy measures would be essential if environmental barriers to choice are to be removed and/or healthy choices are to be encouraged. These measures might range from substantial financial and legislative effects to handle disadvantage, unemployment and more general 'social pathogens'. More particularly, specific measures such as food labelling and ready access to condoms would be needed to facilitate healthy dietary choice and safer sex practices respectively.

Less obviously perhaps, policy measures may be needed to counter 'norm sending' features of the environment (which therefore influence individual intentions to act via the normative system). For instance, the most cogent argument against government's continued refusal to ban direct and indirect promotions of tobacco products is its norm sending effect which signals a degree of approval of smoking and legitimizes individuals' doubts about the health damaging properties of smoking tobacco.

In relation to health education, it is important to make a distinction between 'supportive' health education, which seeks to facilitate people's intentions to act, and education which operates at an earlier stage and facilitates the intention itself. Supportive health education would provide the knowledge and skills needed to achieve the health action: for instance, knowing where to apply for benefits; having the psychomotor skills needed to use a condom in the approved manner and the social interaction skills assertively to negotiate its use with a partner. In relation to indicators of performance and standards of achievement, it is clearly much easier to demonstrate success in, for example, providing people with knowledge and skills for which they acknowledge they have a need than in influencing the beliefs and intentions of individuals who are firmly opposed to a recommended health action.

If we consider the ways in which health education might influence behavioural intention, we can identify from Figure 3.8 two possible sources of input. One of these influences the belief system while the other, as it were, feeds into the motivation system.

The most common and most ethical way in which health education operates is via the belief system. The belief system is in turn influenced by three major processes: experience, the provision of information and interpersonal persuasion. It is well recognized that experience is the most powerful of these: in a real sense, we are likely to believe what

we experience, whether this is at first hand or vicariously. For instance, the relatives of a patient who has died from cancer are less likely to be convinced by health education messages seeking to reduce cancerophobia than those who have had neither first nor secondhand experiences of this kind. The provision of information is undoubtedly the stock in trade of health educators and clearly takes many forms. These will include interpersonal 'teaching' and the use of a wide variety of written media.

A third situation must also be recognized. As traditional attitude theory tells us, people may be influenced not so much by the message but by the person delivering it. We have, in fact, already mentioned the importance of communicator credibility in our discussion of communication of innovations theory. And so, this category of 'input' into the belief system will refer to any instance where people's beliefs are influenced by the characteristics of the health educator: their perceived expertise, trustworthiness, homophily, attractiveness or charisma.

It will be noted that a reference is made to one of the central tenets of social learning theory – that modelling is the most common form of promoting learning. Clearly, modelling usefully describes deliberate attempts to persuade by using prestigious or otherwise attractive personalities. However, modelling also has a strictly informational function: we learn many things merely by observing what happens to other people.

In Figure 3.8, a kind of information processing function provides an interface with the belief system. The purpose of this is to acknowledge that existing knowledge, concepts and principles and various cognitive skills such as decision making competences will provide interpretation and analysis of incoming data from all sources and subsequently reinforce, challenge and even change old beliefs and create new ones.

Three similar inputs – experience, information and interpersonal – are also shown as having a kind of direct access to the motivation system (rather than influencing it less directly via the belief system). This indicates deliberate attempts to arouse emotions – of which perhaps the most controversial and notorious is the use of fear appeal. The distinction between the persuasive modelling effect of using an attractive or credible communicator may be slight in practice and would depend on whether the effect on the client resulted from merely believing the communicator's message or was, alternatively, due primarily to the direct emotional impact arising from, say, sexual attraction or identification with the model's perceived power. Both situations, of course, rely essentially on non-rational techniques.

In relation to the use of information to create a direct emotional impact, the message would be deliberately designed to create either positive or negative affect. Typically pictures would be used – for example, to arouse disgust or anxiety or, alternatively, to trigger nostalgia or feelings of parental warmth.

Experience again is likely to have the most powerful impact although on this occasion it would exert its effects directly on the emotions. For example, the deliberate use of role play in which smokers underwent the unpleasant experience of having lung cancer diagnosed from X-rays provides a prime example of such a technique. Incidentally, according to Janis and Mann (1965), such techniques 'had a marked influence on smoking habits and attitudes'.

Hopefully, our fairly extensive discussion of HAM will substantiate our assertion that an understanding of the dynamics of health related decision making provides a large number of potential indicators for signalling the success of health promotion. More importantly, we have argued that an understanding of theory is essential before we can choose appropriate sets of indicators – and justify our claims of success when challenged by our managers!

INDIRECT INDICATORS AND THE IMPORTANCE OF PRETESTING

At the beginning of this chapter we identified three major kinds of indicator: indicators of outcome, intermediate indicators and indirect indicators. As discussed earlier, intermediate indicators are frequently more appropriate or practicable measures of success than outcome indicators. However, even intermediate indicators may prove to be impracticable in certain instances and planners must resort to indirect measures of success.

As we have seen from Figure 3.8, educational inputs are designed to influence one or more of the various psychosocial or environmental factors affecting health related decision making. If the measurement of these factors should prove problematical – perhaps because of lack of time or resources – or if it should be considered unnecessary because the effectiveness of a given educational input had already been demonstrated, then an evaluation may be concerned only with verifying that the educational programme in question had been properly delivered.

For instance, let us consider an educational programme in which family doctors routinely provide their patients with advice about smoking cessation as part of opportunistic health promotion during the consultation. As Russel *et al.* (1979) have demonstrated, the provision of such advice can produce a smoking cessation rate of 5.1% after one year when supportive leaflets are given to patients. This compares with a rate of 0.3% in a control group. If all 20 000 general practitioners were to adopt this approach as a matter of course, then the researchers argued there would be half a million fewer smokers in the first year. This level of success could only be matched by increasing the number of special smoking cessation clinics to 10 000! Having demonstrated this cost effective result – and in the absence of unlimited resources – it would make sense to assume that a programme of this sort would be at least as effective in future and would continue to reduce smoking in a practice population. An indirect measure of effectiveness might then legitimately be used to monitor the extent to which doctors delivered the service – for instance, by recording the number of practitioners who requested dispensers of leaflets designed to be used as a support for the interpersonal advice on smoking cessation.

Other examples of commonly used indirect indicators of anticipated success would include the following: (i) adoption by schools of a new curriculum package, (ii) teacher attendance at courses designed to familiarize them with the package and, most indirect of all, (iii) the pretesting of the package during construction to determine reading ease and consumer acceptability. In other words, it is often possible to describe a chain of indicators starting with an indirect measure and leading on through other indirect measures via various intermediate indicators until finally some indication of a successful outcome is reached. A record of the successful completion of the early links in the chain may be all that is needed or all that is possible in the case of many evaluation enterprises. This chain of possible indicators is illustrated in Figure 3.10.

McGuire's discussion (1981) of this chain of indicators might usefully be noted at this point. He refers to the 'distal measure fallacy' involved in evaluating a campaign solely on the basis of the early indicators and describes

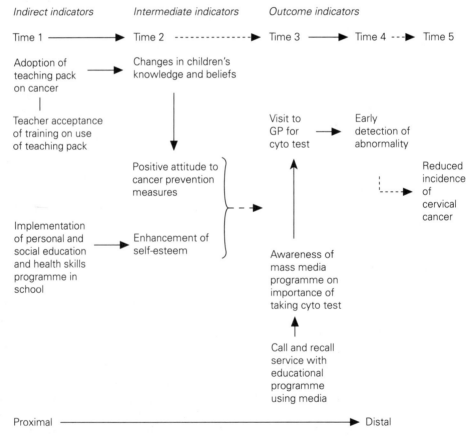

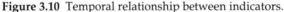

Figure 3.10 Temporal relationship between indicators.

also an 'attenuated effects fallacy' where the evaluator fails to take account of the 12 or so links in the chain and recognize that the probability of achieving all of them is a function of the probability of achieving step 1 multiplied by the probability of achieving step 2 and so on until step 12 is reached. In other words, the chances of success are relatively small!

PRETESTING THE PROGRAMME

Pretesting must form part of any well de-signed health education programme. It is also an integral part of the process of evaluation. Two main pretesting goals may be distin-guished: the first is to pretest relevant charac-teristics of the target population, the second is to pretest the programme and its com-ponent parts.

The first form of pretesting has to do with audience segmentation. Its purpose is two-fold. Relevant population or target group measures indicate those group and individual characteristics which the programme de-signers must take into consideration if they are to meet consumer needs and foster effective learning. They also serve as a baseline or yardstick against which the programme's success may be judged through the application of post-tests as part of the normal function of summative evaluation. The data provided can then be fed back into the system to enhance future similar activ-ities. Formative process evaluation is, as indicated in Chapter 2, an integral part of effective programme development and such formative research is also central to the pretesting of messages and general pro-gramme content.

Palmer (1981) provides an excellent ex-ample of audience pretesting in formative research in his description of the develop-ment of the Children's Television Workshop Health Minutes programme – a series of minute-long presentations on health topics. Pretesting focused on ten measures:

1. Individual needs and values (to which programmes could appeal as part of the 'canalization' process);
2. Barriers to health behaviours;
3. Family members' involvement in health decisions;
4. Prior improvements in lifestyle (seeking to associate new health behaviours with prior health promoting decisions);
5. Subject matter explorations (previous relevant knowledge or ignorance);
6. Knowledge of symptoms;
7. Health lexicon (in order to devise an appropriate vocabulary for hispanic speakers);
8. Prior influence of television and radio (impact of earlier programmes on health behaviours);
9. Inventory of household medications;
10. Parents' perceptions of themselves as child trainers.

Clearly the measures of individual charac-teristics and their immediate socioenviron-mental situations will depend on programme purposes and may be defined in various ways, technical or non-technical. Romano (1985) describes research into smoker charac-teristics using focus group interviews which resulted in the development of four psycho-graphic profiles. These were 'the Fatalists; the Diligent; the Avoiders; and the Oblivious'! Subsequently programme materials were developed to take account of these different personality types.

Turning now to the pretesting of pro-grammes rather than potential audiences, Romano (1984a), in one of the most useful guides available on the subject, has identified two major stages: concept development and message execution. The first of these is concerned with the evolution of potential messages and associated rough artwork – often in the form of animatics. These are devised initially as a result of *a priori* decisions about their likelihood of achieving programme goals. The tentative messages are then pretested on a representative sample of the target group (Romano, 1984b). Leathar (1980) provides a classic example of the way in which a message had to be modified in response to evidence of misperception after pretesting. He describes the reactions to an antismoking poster developed to remind people of the link between smoking and ill health. The setting was a graveyard; the cigarette was represented symbolically as a tombstone. A line of copy at the bottom of the picture asked the rhetorical question 'Why do you think every packet carries a government health warning?'. Although the original version received several awards from professional advertisers, it was misperceived by the primary target group, smokers. This example of selective perception and defensive avoidance is described by Leathar as follows:

Smokers, on the other hand, saw things somewhat differently. In general, they showed a high level of psychological defensiveness towards the entire advert. Initially, they claimed to see the cigarette as a variety of unrelated objects: a stick of rock, lipstick, even a telegraph pole. Furthermore, they superficially assumed the bottom line simply to be the conventional government health warning itself, thus failing to see it as a statement relating the visual material to the warning. They thus not only misperceived the symbolic visual presentation of the cigarette tombstone, but saw little, if any, relationship between this and the factual copy line which was intended to be the main theme of the advertisement. This confusion was further compounded by the image presented. Like non-smokers, smokers attributed a certain 'lightness' to the impression created, but this was attractive and pleasant and in no way symbolic of ill health. It reminded them of pleasant and rather idyllic country scenes, of bluebells and daffodils and pretty girls; of sunshine and ploughmen's lunches in 'nice' country pubs.

The scene was subsequently restructured as a result of the pretesting in order to provide a rather more funereal impression and the line 'Ashes to ashes' was introduced as a symbolic link.

One of pretesting's major functions is to develop messages and programmes tailored to a given market segment. In commenting on the irrelevance of many messages for lower social class groups, Player and Leather (1981) underlined the importance of providing socially sensitive advertising. They challenged the advice given to those requiring support in coping with the withdrawal symptoms following attempts to give up smoking – advice such as 'suck a clove', 'doodle with a paper clip' or 'start a new social activity'! In order to avoid such middle class bias at the concept development stage, Leathar (1980) used a projective technique to determine target group reactions to the packaging of two alternative forms of booklet offering advice on how to stop smoking. Working class respondents showed a clear preference for one of the two covers when asked to describe the 'personality' which each of the covers conveyed to them. The preferred cover was associated with a person who drank in typical pubs, was open and friendly and could be relied upon to lend money and help you out. In the words of communication of innovations theory, the most attractive cover was more homophilous. In advertising parlance the preferred booklet had a better brand image.

The techniques and instruments used in pretesting are, of course, not fundamentally different from those used in evaluating health education programmes generally. The various indicators of success listed later in Table 3.4 could equally be applied to pretesting and it is not difficult, for instance, to relate these to the standard pretesting questions developed by the US Office of Cancer Communications Health Message Testing Service (Romano, 1984b). Table 3.2 is particularly interesting because it not only provides a

Table 3.2 Guidelines for interpreting responses to standard pretesting questions (from Romano, 1984b)

	High score range (%)	Average score range (%)	Low score range (%)
Attention/recall (Per cent remembering seeing message after one exposure)	41 or higher	30–40	29 or lower
Main idea (Per cent remembering main idea of message after one exposure)	36 or higher	25–35	24 or lower
Worth remembering (Per cent indicating 'yes')	76 or higher	60–75	59 or lower
Personally relevant (Per cent indicating message is talking to someone like themselves)	66 or higher	50–65	49 or lower
Anything confusing (Per cent indicating 'yes')	9 or lower	10–20	21 or higher
Believable	91 or higher	75–90	74 or lower
Well done	66 or higher	50–65	49 or lower
Convincing	71 or higher	55–70	54 or lower
Informative	76 or higher	60–75	59 or lower
Made its point	91 or higher	75–90	74 or lower
Interesting	66 or higher	50–65	49 or lower
Pleasant	66 or higher	50–65	49 or lower

pragmatic list of measures related to the pretesting of television public service advertisements (PSAs) but also provides guidelines for interpreting the results. It will be recalled that establishing meaningful and realistic standards of success is a fundamentally important task for health education programming.

Standard pretesting techniques comprise: individual indepth interviews, central location intercept interviews, self-administered questionnaires, focus group interviews, gatekeeper review and readability testing. As may be imagined, these are based on standard quantitative and qualitative research approaches as discussed in Chapter 2. One or two further comments will serve to illustrate the particular flavour of pretesting approaches.

The focus group interview or panel testing seeks to gain insight into the characteristics of given communications and programmes by recording the discussion of a panel consisting of representatives of the target group and noting their reactions to the pilot materials. Conversation, questioning or more specialized tactics – such as the projective technique mentioned above – may be used in this context.

The central location intercept interview may also be called a 'hall test' since interviewees, typically identified by quota sampling, will be invited to a hall or other convenient central location for panel testing – or indeed any other kind of research into audience reactions. Romano (1984a) also describes a more expensive version of the hall test – 'theatre testing' – which allows larger numbers to respond to visual and electronic communications.

The technique of gatekeeper review acknowledges the importance of researching the reaction of key individuals who will control the target audience's access to given health education programmes.

One of the more important and specialist applications of pretesting involves the analysis of written materials. A detailed discussion of this area is beyond the scope of this chapter but requires some brief review. Since the majority of communication and learning materials in health education are in written form, it is clearly important that the target group responses are properly tested. It is of course possible to use any of the techniques discussed above to judge the suitability of written materials. For instance, a 'copy editing' technique could be used in conjunction with individual or group interviews. This involves the respondents actually writing on, say, a pamphlet or leaflet and scoring out offensive items, underlining confusing phrases and writing in alterations or additions. However, the testing of written materials normally comprises three broad approaches: content analysis, typographical analysis and measuring readability. Content analysis has its own technology but in its simpler form consists of systematically sampling written passages or books and categorizing content in whatever way is most likely to illuminate the particular research and its goals. For instance, Davison (1983) analysed the questions asked at a series of public cancer education sessions and examined their implications for the content of cancer education. The study of mass media programming by Best *et al.* (1977) was based on a content analysis of news reporting just as Hansen's (1986) observations on the incidental portrayal of alcohol on mass media documented references to and depiction of alcohol in advertising, documentaries and entertainment programmes such as soap opera. Redman (1984), in a useful chapter on printed and non-print materials in patient education, reports a content analysis of 27 mental health pamphlets which demonstrated that:

> ... approximately 60% of the content was in the middle-class cultural mould and that another 30% consisted of ambiguous

platitudes ... The conclusion of this analysis was that the mental health movement was unwittingly propagating a middle-class ethic under the guise of science ...

Research into the design of print has received rather less attention in health education and tends to focus on the relative legibility of different typefaces, use of upper case compared with lower case letters and the general aesthetic presentation (see, for instance Hartley (1980)). On the other hand the assessment of readability is or should be part of the routine process of developing written communications.

Three main strategies tend to be used in measuring reading ease. The first of these uses a frequency count principle arguing that people will be more likely to comprehend commonly used words. And so vocabulary is checked to see if it forms part of an agreed core of basic, i.e. frequently used, language. Perhaps the best known of these approaches is the Dale–Chall list which includes the 3000 most commonly occurring words in the American language (Dale and Chall, 1948). A second procedure is based on calculations of the redundancy inherent in particular written passages, i.e. the amount of repetition, overt or covert. The Cloze procedure (Holcomb and Ellis, 1978) removes every fifth word from a passage and invites respondents to estimate the meaning of the missing word. The higher the success rate, the greater the comprehensibility of the passage.

However, the most commonly used approach to assessing readability is based on the empirical finding that the comprehensibility of written material is correlated with sentence length and number of polysyllabic words within the sentence. Short sentences containing words having few syllables tend to be easier to read than long sentences containing a high proportion of long words. Although the most popular of these various formulae internationally is undoubtedly the Flesch formula (Flesch, 1948), a simpler version is the FOG (Frequency of Gobbledegook) formula (Harrison, 1980). The Office of Cancer Communications, on the other hand, uses the SMOG (Subjective Measures of Gobbledegook) formula (McLaughlin, 1969).

It is important to be aware that all of the reading ease measures referred to above do not pretest a representative sample of the actual target group and are thus not as reliable nor as valid as genuine pretesting. For instance, the popular Dale–Chall, Flesch, FOG and SMOG formulae were all indirectly derived from results of the McCall–Crabbs Standard Test Lessons in Reading and thus relate to average developmental stages of reading competence in American children. As Pichert and Elam (1985) point out, 'Readability formulas may mislead you'! Nonetheless there are real correlations between these formulae and the intelligibility of written data and they provide valuable pretesting tools when used with caution. In any case, once we move beyond the realm of checking comprehension and recall into the realm of attitudes and intentions, we would be advised to take the results of all pretesting with the proverbial pinch of salt. Attempts to discover how people will actually react to communications and programmes on the basis of their comments about acceptability, interest, personal preference or stated intention should always be guided by a degree of scepticism. This of course applies even more so when observations are made about other people's likely responses!

AIMS AND OBJECTIVES

There is some degree of terminological confusion between various statements of educational intent. Reference is made to aims, goals, targets and objectives almost interchangeably and indiscriminately. While there may be no universal agreement about the meaning of all of the above terms, there is general agreement about the difference between two of them: aims and objectives. An

aim would normally describe a general statement of intent; it would usually provide an indication of the value underpinning a given health education programme – but little else. For instance, an aim for a nutrition education programme might be to improve the nutritional status of the nation. The implicit assumption is that this is worth doing, but because of the generality of the aim and the value position embodied within it, it is difficult to challenge its appropriateness (as opposed, say, to its practicability). On the other hand, **objectives** are much more specific and precise. Any one aim might generate a large number of objectives. The nutritional aim referred to above might be translated into dozens of objectives including, for example, that a target group should reduce '...average saturated fatty acids (SFA) intake from 59 g (18% of total energy) to 50 g (15% of total); i.e. a 15% reduction' (NACNE, 1983).

Two observations may be made about the term objective: first, an objective is likely to generate more controversy than an aim – because it provides specific details of what is intended; and second, it is considerably easier to measure (for the same reason). Objectives have an especially important part to play in evaluation. On the one hand it has been argued that evaluation designs derived from objectives may well corrupt the educational programme while, on the other hand, it has been stated with equal vigour that the attainment of properly constructed objectives provides the best of all possible indicators of programme success. For the present, however, we will merely consider the objective as an indicator of performance. Before doing so, we need to give some further thought to the question of specificity.

It is possible to envisage a spectrum of specificity ranging from the delightfully vague to the almost pedantically precise. The aim would be located at the general end of this spectrum while the other pole would be occupied by a particularly specific variety of goal statement generally known as a behavioural objective. This highly refined statement describes the behaviours which a learner (as opposed to a teacher, educator or instructor) will produce in order to demonstrate that the desired terminal outcome has been achieved. The behavioural objective will, moreover, specify the conditions under which the learned outcome will emerge and criteria (or standards of acceptable performance) which will be used to signal success. Figure 3.11 illustrates this specificity spectrum as a goal continuum. In accordance with standard practice, an aim is positioned at the general end of the continuum while a behavioural objective is located at the other end in acknowledgement of its high degree of specificity. While a properly constructed behavioural objective could hardly be rendered more specific – being, as it were, at a pinnacle of precision – other educational goals could be placed at virtually any point on the continuum. Their location would depend entirely on how general or specific they were. The example of alcohol education has been used to illustrate the potential variation in specificity and it can immediately be seen that the general aim of promoting moderate drinking could be translated into literally hundreds of more specific goals. The intermediate goal of helping young people to resist social pressure represents one of these and, in turn, could be translated into a much more limited number of more detailed, precise objectives.

It is not the purpose of this book to explore the merits and demerits of using behavioural objectives – although earlier discussion of quantitative and qualitative research methods has an important bearing on this. However, the interested reader should consult an amusing article by Popham (1978) in which he describes the rise and fall of the 'behavioural objectives movement'. The zenith of this quest for precision and specificity in his own personal position is symbolized by a 1962 bumper sticker which read 'Help stamp out non-behavioural objectives' and which indicates the degree of emotional involvement which curriculum design can inspire in its devotees. Since that highpoint, there has been a move away from what Parlett and Hamilton (1978) have called the 'agricultural-botany paradigm' of educational evaluation and this has been accompanied by a demise in the popularity of the behavioural objective – certainly among educationalists (Popham modified his position to the point at which his bumper sticker read 'Help stamp out *some* non-behavioural objectives!).

However, whatever the fashion, the advantages of the behavioural objective are very real. Once the objective has been constructed, the success of the related educational programme can be determined in an objective, reliable and observable way by merely noting whether or not the objective has been attained – in other words, by means of a simple yes/no decision. It is worth adding here the observation made by a doyen of the behavioural objective movement, R.F. Mager (1962): '... if you give each learner a copy of your objectives, you may not have to do much

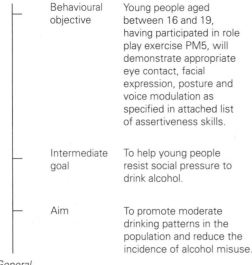

Specific

	Behavioural objective	Young people aged between 16 and 19, having participated in role play exercise PM5, will demonstrate appropriate eye contact, facial expression, posture and voice modulation as specified in attached list of assertiveness skills.
	Intermediate goal	To help young people resist social pressure to drink alcohol.
	Aim	To promote moderate drinking patterns in the population and reduce the incidence of alcohol misuse.

General

Figure 3.11 A goal continuum. An example from alcohol education.

else'. This somewhat cryptic statement makes the entirely justifiable assertion that in many instances the specificity and clarity of the goal statement embodied in behavioural objectives are sufficient to generate learning. Unfortunately, one of the main difficulties in constructing this kind of goal statement stems from the fact that many educators are insufficiently clear about their goals! Without such clarity a behavioural objective cannot be produced.

It would, at first glance, appear that a behavioural objective might be inappropriate for programmes which measure their effectiveness by means of intermediate indicators of success. This would, however, be a misconception since the behaviour in question may refer not only to an 'action' outcome – such as attending a clinic for immunization – but may equally well apply to such cognitive or affective indicators as the acquisition of knowledge or attitude change. Behaviour therefore refers to any observable act: for instance a behavioural indication of successful learning about the involvement of fats in coronary heart disease might include producing a list (verbally or in writing) of various cooking oils and fats which correctly indicated which of these were saturated and which were polyunsaturated.

Apart from the advantages of specificity, behavioural objectives have two further benefits to offer evaluators. These derive from their emphasis on the importance of including the conditions under which a given learned outcome is to be demonstrated and the standards which have to be met if the learning is to be adjudged successful. The former requirement serves as a useful reminder that a given learning outcome will only be achieved if the conditions necessary for any learning situation are fulfilled (for instance, the acquisition of social interaction skill requires repeated practice and feedback, perhaps using a role play technique; attitude change, on the other hand, might require the use of 'group discussion–decision' (Bond,

1958) or some other appropriate methodological tactic). The matter of standards merits rather more detailed consideration since it has an important bearing on the politics of evaluation.

STANDARDS

Green and Lewis (1986) identify four kinds of standard which might be used to determine the relative success of any given intervention. The results of a health education programme might simply be compared with the degree of success achieved in previous ventures of a similar kind (historical standards) or, alternatively, a comparison might be made with the level of performance produced by other workers in programmes of a similar nature designed for similar target groups (normative standards). A third kind of yardstick is provided by 'theoretical standards' in which the criteria of success are derived from a knowledge of relevant theory – which indicates what one might reasonably expect on the basis of a conceptual analysis which is ultimately derived from all previous research in a given area. Green and Lewis contrast these with a fourth level of expectation based on 'absolute standards' which demands nothing less than perfection, i.e. 100% success!

The reference to absolute standards should remind us of the important political dimension to evaluation – a dimension which we ignore at our peril. While our political paymasters may not really be so naive as to expect complete success, they frequently appear to have entirely unrealistic expectations of what health education might achieve, both in general and in relation to particular programmes. It is an interesting paradox that these same politicians – whose whole experience in politics will typically have led them to redefine the ambitious and idealistic goals of their youth so that their expectations have come to be more consistent with the 'art of the possible' – may expect health education to achieve substantial switches in public opinion and the deepseated values which frequently underpin these attitudes. For instance, a mass media campaign might be expected significantly to shift lifestyles in a way which is largely inconsistent with existing social norms. If such a change were to happen in the political arena, it would be akin to achieving a dramatic reversal of political allegiance in large sectors of the population as a result of a series of party political broadcasts. It would rightly be viewed as little short of miraculous!

More commonly, perhaps, political goals for a programme may differ, consciously or unconsciously, from overt health education goals. On the surface a hypothetical media based drug education programme might be seeking to harden attitudes against heroin use or even to reduce the proportion of the population misusing that substance. However, the hidden agenda may well be to demonstrate governmental concern to an irrationally anxious public and to placate vocal and influential party supporters who have been outraged at what they perceive to be a major social and moral problem. In such cases it is essential that this hidden agenda be explored with the paymasters so that false expectations are not established and the subsequent and often inevitable failure of the programme is not used as evidence of the ineffectual nature of health education. Logically, the purpose of evaluation in these circumstances should be to provide a kind of performance indicator which will record activity, energy and perhaps enthusiasm! It should not seek to measure changes in the stated target population, i.e. drug abusers or those at high risk of misusing drugs; only minimal change would be set as a theoretical standard in a programme of this sort.

While it may not be possible precisely to specify standards of success, a sound understanding of existing theory in health education should allow us to establish criteria for programme evaluation and to indicate what we might expect from any given intervention. Clearly, past experience and specific ad hoc research will sharpen our predictions but even where such prior knowledge is limited, our understanding of health related behaviour and educational theory should enable us to make realistic estimations of likely success. For example, we should be able to comment on the very best standard we could hope to achieve (a theory-based 'absolute standard'). The so-called 90/90 rule, which was used as a rough guide in developing linear teaching programmes in the heyday of programmed learning, would attempt to achieve a success rate of 90% in 90% of a relatively homogeneous target group. This is sometimes expressed as a 90/90/90 criterion (Davies, 1981), i.e. 90% of students will achieve 90% of the objectives 90% of the time. Further attempts at refining programmes would be subject to a law of diminishing returns and not be cost effective. One might therefore say that a properly structured and essentially cognitive programme which has been pretested on a homogeneous target group might hope to achieve a comparable 90% success rate but no more.

Let us consider a second hypothetical example, this time in the affective area. Let us assume that a vaccine has been developed to immunize against AIDS. The vaccine can be administered in a one-shot, once-for-all form on a lump of sugar at any doctor's surgery, outpatient department, health centre or chemist. There are no side effects and effectiveness has been proven. Little knowledge of attitude change theory is required to predict the success rate of a properly pretested mass media based programme which utilizes all appropriate channels to deliver the message and which provides specific information about where to obtain the vaccine – and, of course, uses minimal fear appeal! The 90/90/90 criterion mentioned above might even be surpassed in certain high risk groups!

SOME REFLECTIONS ON COST EFFECTIVENESS

Before closing the discussion on standards of success, it is important to give some consideration to the measurement of effectiveness in economic terms. In other words we must confront some of the thorny issues raised by cost effectiveness and cost–benefit analysis. In a very real sense economics is the ultimate arbiter of programme implementation even if, on occasions, it is not the primary concern. All programmes must take account of cost since all programmes consume resources and resources are finite. The most obvious situation where economic analysis is viewed as an essential part of programme planning and evaluation is where health education's raison d'etre is considered to be one of saving on expensive health care costs so that money may be spent on other and presumably better things. However, even where the health education model of choice is, say, to create a sense of wonder at the marvellous workings of the human body, resources are necessary. Even where society values knowledge for its own sake (currently a somewhat eccentric view), it is manifestly better to create such knowledge efficiently, i.e. with minimal rather than profligate use of resources.

We can therefore argue that whatever the precision of the objectives set or the sophistication of the criteria of success adopted by a programme, some measure of efficiency should be considered. The term **effectiveness** is commonly used to denote the extent to which programme objectives have been achieved. The term **efficiency** normally refers to relative effectiveness, i.e. how well a programme has done by comparison with actual or potential competing programmes and strategies – or specific methods within programmes. Behavioural objectives have, of course, an inbuilt measure of efficiency in the form of conditions and standards. Health economics seeks to quantify efficiency by expressing it in monetary terms.

Three common analytical tools are employed in health economics:

1. Cost analysis – which merely indicates the financial cost of competing programmes or other initiatives;
2. Cost effectiveness analysis – which compares the efficiency of competing interventions in achieving a given goal by stating the relative financial costs involved;
3. Cost–benefit analysis – which, unlike cost effectiveness analysis (CEA), not only states the costs in monetary terms but also seeks to fix a price tag on the benefits accruing from the programme. A calculation of the cost per given benefit is then possible (typically expressed as a cost–benefit ratio).

It is important to note the difference between cost–benefit analysis (CBA) and CEA. Cost effectiveness analysis seeks only to state the cost involved in, say, using smoking cessation clinics compared with family doctors providing routine advice on giving up smoking (as illustrated earlier in this chapter). On the basis of the quoted study, GP involvement is clearly more cost effective.

Cost–benefit analysis, on the other hand, would not necessarily assume that smoking cessation was a worthwhile goal under any circumstances and would compare the financial costs of delivering the programme with the financial costs of the benefits resulting from smoking cessation. It is therefore controversial insofar as many people will fundamentally question the morality of attaching a financial label to human life and health; others will merely question the feasibility of doing so. The arguments used here are somewhat similar to those involved in the debate about behavioural objectives. The objection on grounds of ethical principle suggests that cherished human values are somehow demeaned by the process of subjecting them to critical analysis. The second category of objection is manifestly different:

its criticism is based on accusations of incompleteness or naïvety.

The fact is, however, that just as behavioural objectives clarify goals through their precision and specificity, CBA and CEA may provide useful information to help decision making under conditions of resource limitation. They may also be politically useful for health educators who, in the face of criticism of the costs of proposed programmes and demands for proof of efficiency, may be able to point out the relative cost of routinely accepted medical practices and non-educational preventive procedures. It is clear that the amount of money spent on different life-saving interventions varies enormously in relation the pay-off in terms of lives saved, as may be seen in Table 3.3.

An important health economics concept is that of opportunity cost. Any service expenditure involves not only the cost of delivering that service but also the loss of some other facility which might have been financed by the money spent on that service provision. Thus while it might be argued that the money spent on prevention and health education could have been spent on curative services, it would seem equally reasonable to stand the argument on its head and assert that the resources used in high technology acute

Table 3.3 Cost per life saved for various preventive measures

Preventive measure	Cost per life saved (£)
Screening for stillbirth	50
Childproof containers	1 000
Department of Environment (road safety)	39 300
Screening for cancer of the cervix	10 000– 41 700
Trawler safety	1 000 000
Alterations to high rise flats after Ronan Point disaster	20 000 000

Derived from Mooney, G.H. (1977)

medicine might be better spent on health education and preventive services. Cochrane's (1972) classic 'random reflections on the health service' showed how many routinely practised medical procedures had never been evaluated. Townsend (1986), in discussing cost effectiveness, cites Bodmer (1985) who commented on the escalating cost of chemotherapies in the treatment of cancers and asserted that despite '... very serious side effects...' these had '... no more than a marginal effect at the present time on increased survival'. Again, if we were to take account of evaluations of coronary care units (Mather *et al.*, 1971; Colling *et al.*, 1976) we would conclude that the prospect of surviving an acute myocardial infarction would be enhanced by being nursed at home or in a general hospital ward rather than in a coronary care unit.

It is certainly not the intention of this book even to begin to explore the intricacies of CEA and CBA and interested readers are referred to authoritative discussions (Green and Lewis, 1986; Windsor *et al.*, 1984). Two points are worth making, however. First there is evidence that health education has been both effective and efficient, even when judged by the rigorous criteria of CBA. Second, despite such evidence of success, we should be very careful before allowing ourselves to be seduced into making such analyses routinely. Prevention in general and health education in particular may prove to be eminently worthwhile but intrinsically expensive!

Let us, nonetheless, consider an example where on the basis of existing theory a health education intervention could be expected to be cost effective. Townsend (1986) considered how a hypothetical mass media antismoking campaign costing £250 000 might be judged in a cost effectiveness analysis. Assuming that 1000 people gave up smoking permanently, 10 000 gave up temporarily, 2000 cut down temporarily and 15 000 seriously considered giving up, then 2991 life years would be saved at a cost of £84 per life. The cost would appear to be reasonable by comparison with Table 3.3. The reader will be better able to judge whether, on the basis of historical, normative and theoretical standards, such a campaign could be expected to deliver these results after referring to Chapter 6 which discusses the effectiveness and efficiency of mass media.

Terris (1981) has enthusiastically argued the cost effectiveness case for prevention, estimating that a moderately effective programme in the USA might save each year at least 400 000 lives, six million person-years of life and five billion dollars' worth of medical costs. Green has provided several much more closely argued examples of favourable cost – benefit ratios for specific health education programmes (1974). One of these demonstrates a saving of $7.81 per dollar invested in a hypertension screening and education programme; the other, which analysed the impact of using group discussion techniques to modify unnecessary use of emergency rooms for asthma patients, notched up a cost–benefit ratio of 1:5.

A British study by the Policy Studies Institute (Laing, 1982) on the benefits and costs of family planning identified conservative benefit to cost ratios of 1.3:1 for the typical prevented unplanned pregnancy; a ratio of 4.5:1 for prevented pregnancies among mothers of three or more children; and a 5.3:1 ratio for unplanned, premarital conceptions. In other words, '... for every £100 spent on family planning services, the public sector can expect a benefit of £130, £450 and £530 respectively'. Although this illustration does not refer to a health education programme per se, it is clear that family planning, like other health promotion initiatives, cannot be achieved without an educational component.

There is, then, clear evidence that health education may not only be effective but its benefits can outweigh programme costs. However, as indicated above, we must strike a cautionary note. Just as health education

should resist attempts to cajole it into using medical or epidemiological indicators of success, it should also be wary of adopting CBA too enthusiastically. While a favourable cost–benefit ratio is possible, there will be many instances where health education may in the long run prove expensive. For example, the cost of successful alcohol and smoking programmes in terms of lost employment in those industries and lost government revenues is well known and although many if not all of these costs can be offset by savings on health service treatment costs, the balance sheet is still complex. The longer people live, the more demands they make on the welfare state. As Smith (1977) elegantly reminds us:

'Various kinds of false optimism are invoked by many doctors... First, they argue that preventive and curative medicine may one day be as successful with diseases that are currently chronic and incurable as it has been in the past with those acute diseases that relatively speaking no longer trouble us. But unless we succeed in abolishing death we shall always have to treat the dying. The optimists sometimes seem to look forward to a time when most people will make their exit from this world without causing inconvenience to doctors. The evidence provides little ground for any such hope. In general, the older we are when we die the longer the period of alleviative care we require before death. Since it seems reasonable to suppose that the older we are when we die the more likely it is that we have died of old age, it follows that when most people die of old age rather than intercurrent disease, the demands they make on medical care are greater. When we all die of old age, after a lifetime of health, the main task of the health service will be with the alleviative care of terminal illness. If we should succeed in abolishing death the main preoccupation of the health service will be with contraception.

Although health economists may offset some of the costs of future health care by the process of 'discounting' – so that future costs are rated as less important than current costs – or by resorting to the somewhat casuistic notion of 'merit good' (Cohen, 1981) which appears to acknowledge that some social benefits are so intrinsically meritorious that financial costs are deemed irrelevant, nonetheless and in the last analysis, we have to be prepared to pay for health.

If the entire focus of our evaluation is, however, to be on achieving favourable cost–benefit ratios, presumably the ideal intervention is one which ensures that individuals achieve a level of health which is just sufficient to enable them to carry out an approved social role while indulging themselves in unhealthy activities to the extent that they avoid sickness absence, are productive but manage to damage their constitution to the extent that they die quickly on the day after they achieve pensionable age. In reality, though, Draper's observations are nearer the mark: health promotion, he argues, is inherently inconsistent with the goal of economic productivity. In which case we are more likely to have to choose health or wealth (Draper, Bert and Dennis, 1977).

INDICATORS: A REVIEW

Throughout this chapter we have explored in some detail the range and variety of indicators of successful health promotion and education programmes. An attempt was made to demonstrate the theoretical elements contributing to various outcomes via individual decision making and showing how these might be assessed by means of a 'chain' of indicators ranging from indirect through intermediate to outcome. It was also, hopefully, apparent that intermediate indicators might be considered outcome indicators of success for certain models of health education. For instance, in Figure 3.10, a measure of self-esteem might be an intermediate

indicator for a preventively oriented cancer education programme but an outcome indicator for a personal/social education programme having as its goal self-empowerment. These points should be borne in mind when considering Table 3.4 which lists and exemplifies various indicators in roughly ascending order of their approximation to 'distal' outcome indicators. It will be noted that the term 'personality measure' has been used as one variety of intermediate indicator and this, perhaps, requires some explanation. It is clearly inappropriate here to venture into the field of personality theory, nor is it particularly profitable since classic measures of personality type have little relevance to the evaluation of health promotion programmes.

It is difficult to draw a fine line between measures of personality and measures of other individual characteristics such as knowledge and beliefs. For the purpose of the present discussion, only those variables which define a relatively enduring personal attribute will be described as measures of personality (or which describe a cluster of characteristics more or less peculiar to the individual). Both self-esteem and perceived locus of control could be viewed as personality measures or as an example of a value and a belief respectively. Similarly the notion of ego strength would legitimately be seen as a personality trait which would be part of mainstream personality theory (see Cattell's 16 PF Test (Cattell, 1965)) and also have relevance for health related behaviour. For instance an increase in both self-esteem and ego strength would be expected to help individuals resist social pressure to engage in unhealthy behaviours.

Again, while not a recognized and standardized test of personality, profiles of smoking type would also qualify (although this might be a useful indicator for research in health education, it would have no value as an indicator of evaluation since it is presumably not desirable to change type of smoker –

Table 3.4 Taxonomy of indicators which may be used in evaluating health promotion/health education programmes

Types of measure	Examples
Clinical/epidemiological measure	Measures of mortality and morbidity (incidence and prevalence rates); sickness absence rates; bed occupancy, etc.; disability indices; plaque index; serum cholesterol level; control of diabetes; blood pressure
Subjective indicators/ measures of 'quality of life'/well-being	Level of reported satisfaction; Nottingham Health Profile; Bradburn Affect Balance Scale; Personal Competence Scale; level of assertiveness; level of self-esteem
Behavioural indicators	
Routines	Dietary behaviours; exercise; routine use of stress management skills
Single time choices	Visit to doctor for cyto test; writing letter to MP about sports sponsorship by tobacco industry
Skills (psychomotor)	Breast self-examination; cardiopulmonary resuscitation
Skills (social interaction)	Assertiveness; resisting social pressure to smoke
Intermediate indicators	
Awareness/attention	Paying attention to poster; awareness of TV public service advertisement about coronary heart disease
Perception/interpretation	Correct interpretation of doctor's advice
Recall of information	Remembering that saturated fats are unhealthy (but not necessarily understanding why)
Understanding	Understanding that cancer is not a single undifferentiated disease
Decision making skill	Making appropriate choice of heart healthy food in a supermarket
Values	Valuing deferred gratification when superior pay-off to immediate gratification
Beliefs	Belief in susceptibility to accident; belief that life after retirement may be productive and enjoyable
Attitudes	Positive attitude to breastfeeding baby; feeling it is important to lose weight; satisfaction with doctor's communication
Drives	'Addiction' to alcohol; dependence on tobacco
Personality measures	Self-esteem; health locus of control; ego strength
Indirect indicators	Number of leaflets distributed; teacher's attendance at course on new approaches to drug education; schools buy new health education teaching package; schools use teaching package correctly

even if it were possible – but rather to achieve smoking cessation).

The various personality measures discussed above serve to illustrate nicely the point made earlier that an indicator might be either intermediate or outcome depending on the health education model adopted. For instance, enhanced self-esteem and increased internality might be an entirely self-sufficient goal for a mental health programme or alternatively it could be only an intermediate point in a programme which considers these attributes as necessary precursors to a more distal goal of resisting social pressure to smoke or drink immoderately.

The present chapter has examined indicators of success and the theoretical framework which should help evaluators make appropriate choices. The remaining chapters will consider evaluative aspects of major strategies for delivering health education – in schools, health care contexts, via mass media, in the workplace and by means of various community interventions, including community development.

REFERENCES

Ajzen, I. (1985) From intention to actions: a theory of planned behaviour, in *Action Control: From Cognition to Behaviour*, (eds J. Kuhl and J. Beckman), Prentice-Hall, New Jersey.

Ajzen, I. and Fishbein, M. (1980) *Understanding Attitudes and Predicting Social Behavior*, Prentice-Hall, New Jersey.

Allen, D., Harley, M. and Makinson, G.T. (1987) Performance indicators in the National Health Service. *Social Policy and Administration*, **21**(1), 70–84.

Barić, L. (1978) Health education and the smoking habit. *Health Education Journal*, **37**, 132–7.

Becker, M.H. (ed.) (1984) *The Health Belief Model and Personal Health Behavior*, Charles B. Slack, Thorofare, New Jersey.

Best, G., Dennis, J. and Draper, P. (1977) *Health, The Mass Media and The National Health Service*, Unit for the Study of Health Policy, London.

Black, N. (1992) The relationships between evaluative research and audit. *Journal of Public Health Medicine*, **14**(14), 361–6.

Bodmer, W.F. (1985) Understanding statistics. *Journal of Royal Statistical Society*, **148**, 69–81.

Bond, B.W. (1958) A study in health education methods. *International Journal of Health Education*, **1**, 41–6.

Bradburn, N. (1969) *The Structure of Psychological Well-being*, Aldine, New York.

Breteler, R.H., Mertens, N.H.M. and Rombouts, R. (1990) Motivation to change smoking behaviour: determinants in the contemplation stage, in *Theoretical and Applied Aspects of Health Psychology*, (eds L.R. Schmidt *et al.*), Harwood Academic Publishers, London.

Briscoe, M.E. (1982) Subjective measures of well-being; differences in the perception of health and social problems. *British Journal of Social Work*, **12**, 137–47.

British Broadcasting Corporation (1983) *Understanding Cancer*, BBC Broadcasting Research Special Report, BBC Research Information Desk, London.

Cattell, R.B. (1965) *The Scientific Analysis of Personality*, Penguin, Harmondsworth.

Catford, J. (1993) Editorial. Auditing health promotion: what are the vital signs of quality? *Health Promotion International*, **8**(2), 67–8.

Cochrane, A.C.L. (1972) *Effectiveness and Efficiency: Random Reflections on the Heath Service*, Rock Carling Lecture 1971, Nuffield Provincial Hospitals Trust, London.

Cohen, D. (1981) *Prevention as an Economic Good*, Health Economics Research Unit, University of Aberdeen.

Colling A., Dellipiani A.W., Donaldson, R.J. and McCormack, R. (1976) Teesside coronary survey: an epidemiological study of acute attacks of myocardial infarction. *British Medical Journal*, **2**, 1169–72.

Dale, E. and Chall, J.A. (1948) A formula for predicting readability: instructions. *Education Research Bulletin*, **27**(37), 11–20.

Davies, I.K. (1981) *Instructional Technique*, McGraw-Hill, New York, p. 22.

Davison, R.L. (1983) Questions about cancer: the public's demand for information. *Journal of the Institute of Health Education*, **21**, 5–16.

Delk, J.L. (1980) High-risk sports as indirect self-destructive behavior, in *The Many Faces of Suicide*, (ed. N.L. Farberow), McGraw-Hill, New York.

Department of Health (1992) *Health of the Nation*, HMSO, London.

DiClemente, C.C. and Prochaska, J.O. (1982) Self change and therapy change of smoking behaviour: a comparison of processes of change in cessation and maintenance. *Addictive Behaviours*, **7**, 133–42.

Draper, P., Bert, G. and Dennis, J. (1977) Health and wealth. *Royal Society of Health Journal*, **97**, 121–7.

Festinger, L. (1957) *A Theory of Cognitive Dissonance*, Row Peterson, Evanston, Ill.

Fishbein, M. (1976) Persuasive communication, in *Communication Between Doctors and Patients* (ed. A.E. Bennet), Oxford University Press, Oxford.

Fishbein, M. and Ajzen, I. (1985) *Belief Attitude, Intention and Behavior: An Introduction to Theory and Research*, Addison-Wesley, Reading, Mass.

Flesch, R. (1948) A new readability yardstick. *Journal of Applied Psychology*, **32**, 221.

Forsberg, B.C., Barros, F.C. and Victora, C.G. (1992) Developing countries need more quality assurance: how health facility surveys can contribute. *Health Policy and Planning,* **7**(2), 193–6.

Freidson, E. (1961) *Patients' Views of Medical Practice,* Russell Sage, New York, pp. 146–7.

Green, L.W. (1974) Toward cost–benefit evaluations of health education: some concepts, methods, and examples. *Health Education Monographs,* **2**, 34–64.

Green, L.W. (1984) Health education models, in *Behavioural Health: A Handbook of Health Enhancement and Disease Prevention,* (eds J.D. Matarazzo *et al.*), John Wiley, New York.

Green, L.W. and Lewis, F.M. (1986) *Measurement and Evaluation in Health Education and Health Promotion,* Mayfield Publishing Co., Palo Alto, CA, pp. 174–6.

Hall, J. (1976) Subjective measures of quality of life in Britain: 1971 to 1975: some developments and trends. *Social Trends,* **7**, 47–60.

Hansen, A. (1986) The portrayal of alcohol on television, *Health Education Journal,* **45**(3), 127–31.

Harfouche, J.K. (1965) *Infant Health in Lebanon: Customs and Taboos,* Khayats, Beirut.

Harrison, C. (1980) *Readability in Classrooms,* Cambridge University Press, Cambridge.

Hartley, J. (ed.) (1980) *The Psychology of Written Communication* (Part 3), Kogan Page, London.

Holcomb, C. and Ellis, J. (1978) Measuring the readability of selected patient education materials: the Cloze Procedure. *Health Education,* **9**, 8.

Horley, J. (1991) Values and beliefs as personal constructs. *International Journal of Personal Construct Psychology,* **4**, 1–14.

Hovland, C., Lumsdaine, A. and Sheffield, F. (1949) *Experiments on Mass Communication,* University Press, Princeton.

Hunt, S.M. and McEwen, J. (1980) The development of a subjective health indicator. *Sociology of Health and Illness,* **2**, 231–46.

Janis, I.L. and Mann, L. (1965) Effectiveness of emotional role playing in modifying smoking habits and attitudes. *Journal of Experimental Research in Personality,* **1**, 84–90.

Janis, I.L. and Mann, L. (1977) *Decision Making,* Free Press, New York.

Janz, N.K. and Becker, M.H. (1984) The Health Belief Model: a decade later. *Health Education Quarterly,* **11**, 1–47.

Jessor, R. and Jessor, S.L. (1977) *Problem Behavior and Psychosocial Development: A Longitudinal Study of Youth,* Academic Press, New York.

Kanfer, F.H. and Karoly, P. (1972) Self-control: a behavioristic excursion into the lion's den. *Behavior Therapy,* **3**, 398–416.

Kelley, H.H. (1967) Attribution theory in social psychology, in *Nebraska Symposium on Motivation, 1967* (ed. D. Levine), University of Nebraska Press, Lincoln.

Laing, W.A. (1982) *Family Planning: The Benefits and Costs,* No. 607, Policy Studies Institute, London.

Leathar, D.S. (1980) Defence inducing advertising, in *Taking Stock: What Have We Learned and Where Are We Going?* Proceedings of the ESOMAR Conference, Monte Carlo, September, pp. 153–73.

Lichtenstein, S., Slovic, P., Fischoff, B., Layman, M. and Combs, B. (1978) Judged frequency of lethal events. *Journal of Experimental Psychology: Human Learning and Memory,* **4**(6), 551–78.

Luck, G.M. and Luckman, J. (1974) *Patients, Hospitals and Operational Research,* Tavistock, London.

Lyng, S. (1990) Edgework: a social psychological analysis of voluntary risk taking. *American Journal of Sociology,* **95**(4), 851–86.

Mager, R.F. (1962) *Preparing Instructional Objectives,* Fearon Publishers, Belmont, CA.

Marsh, A. and Matheson, J. (1983) *Smoking Attitudes and Behaviour,* HMSO, London.

Mather, H.G., Morgan, D.C., Pearson, N.G. *et al.* (1971) Acute myocardial infarction: home and hospital treatment. *British Medical Journal,* 334–8.

Maxwell, R.J. (1984) Quality assessment in health. *British Medical Journal,* **288**, 1470–1.

McAlister, A., Puska, P., Salonene, J.T. *et al.* (1982) Theory and action for health promotion: illustrations from the North Karelia Project. *American Journal of Public Health,* **72**, 43–53.

McGuire, W.J. (1981) Theoretical foundations of campaigns, in *Public Communication Campaigns,* (eds R.E. Rice and W.J. Paisley), Sage, Beverly Hills.

McLaughlin, G. (1969) SMOG grading: a new readability formula. *Journal of Reading,* **12**, 639.

Moon, B. (1990) Patterns of control: school reform in Western Europe, in *New Curriculum – National Curriculum,* (ed. B. Moon), Hodder and Stoughton, London.

Mooney, G.H. (1977) *The Valuation of Human Life* (Appendix C), Macmillan, London.

NACNE (1983) *A Discussion Paper on Proposals for Nutritional Guidelines for Health Education in Britain,* Health Education Council, London.

Pack, B.E., Hendrick, R.M., Murdock, R.B. and Palma, L.M. (1983) Factors affecting criteria met by hospital based patient education programmes. *Patient Education and Counselling,* **5**, 76–84.

Palmer, E. (1981) Shaping persuasive messages with formative research, in *Public Communications Campaigns*, (eds R.E. Rice and W.J. Paisley), Sage Publications, Beverly Hills.

Parlett, M. and Hamilton, D. (1978) Evaluation as illumination: a new approach to the study of innovatory programmes, in *Beyond the Numbers Game* (eds D. Hamilton *et al.*), Macmillan, London.

Pichert, J.W. and Elam, P. (1985) Readability formulas may mislead you. *Patient Education and Counselling*, **7**, 181–91.

Player, D.A. and Leathar, D.S. (1981) Developing socially sensitive advertising, in *Health Education and the Media*, (eds D.S. Leathar, G.B. Hastings and J.K. Davies), Pergamon, London.

Popham, W.J. (1978) Must all objectives be behavioural? in *Beyond the Number Game*, (eds D. Hamilton *et al.*), Macmillan, London.

Prentice-Dunn, S. and Rogers, R.W. (1986) Protection motivation theory and preventive health: beyond the Health Belief Model. *Health Education Research*, **1**(3), 153–62.

Prochaska, J.O. (1992) What causes people to change from unhealthy to health enhancing behaviour? in *Preventing Cancers*, (eds T. Heller, L. Bailey and S. Pattison), Open University Press, Milton Keynes.

Redman, B.K. (1984) *The Psychology of Written Communication* (Part 3), Kogan Page, London.

Rogers, E.M. and Shoemaker, F.F. (1971) *Communication of Innovations*, Free Press, New York.

Rogers, R.W. (1975) A protection motivation theory of fear appeals and attitude change. *Journal of Psychology*, **91**, 93–114.

Rokeach, M. (1973) *The Nature of Human Values*, Free Press, New York.

Romano, R. (1984a) *Pre-testing in Health Communications*, National Cancer Institute, Bethesda, MD.

Romano, R. (1984b) *Making PSAs Work*, National Cancer Institute, Bethesda, MD.

Romano, R. (1985) Pre-testing smoking messages, in *Smoking Control*, (eds J. Crofton and M. Wood), Health Education Council, London.

Rosenman, R.H. (1977) History and definition of the type A coronary-prone behavior pattern, in *Proceedings of the Forum on Coronary-Prone Behavior*, (ed. T. Dembroski), Dept of Health, Education and Welfare, Pub. No. (NIH) 78-1451, Washington DC, pp. 13–18.

Russell, M.A.H., Wilson, C., Taylor, C. and Baker, C.D. (1979) Effect of general practitioners' advice against smoking. *British Medical Journal*, **2**, 231–5.

Schifter, D.B. and Ajzen, I. (1985) Intention, perceived control and weight loss: an application of the theory of planned behavior. *Journal of Personality and Social Psychology*, **49**, 843–51.

Simon, S.B. (1974) *Meeting Yourself Halfway*, Argos, Niles, Ill.

Slovic, P., Fischoff, B. and Lichtenstein, S. (1982) Why study risk perception? *Risk Analysis*, **2**(2), 83–93.

Small, N. (1989) *Politics and Planning in the National Health Service*, Open University Press, Milton Keynes.

Smith, A. (1977) The unfaced facts. *New Universities Quarterly*, **Spring**, 133–45.

St Leger, A.S., Schnieden, H. and Walsworth-Bell, J.P. (1992) *Evaluating Health Services' Effectiveness*, Open University Press, Milton Keynes.

Terris, M. (1981) The primacy of prevention. *Preventive Medicine*, **10**, 689–99.

Tones, B.K. (1979) Past achievement, future success, in *Health Education Perspectives and Choices*, (ed. I. Sutherland), Allen and Unwin, London.

Tones, B.K. (1981) Affective education and health, in *Health Education in Schools*, (eds J. Cowley, K. David and T. Williams), Harper and Row, London.

Tones, B.K. (1986) Preventing drug misuse: the case for breadth, balance and coherence. *Health Education Journal*, **45**, 197–203.

Tones, B.K. (1987) Devising strategies for preventing drug misuse: the role of the health action model. *Health Education Research*, **2**, 305–18.

Townsend, J. (1986) Cost effectiveness, in *Smoking Control: Strategies and Evaluation in Community and Mass Media Programmes*, (eds J. Crofton and M. Wood), report of a workshop, Health Education Council, London.

Triandis, H.C. (1980) Values, attitudes, and interpersonal behavior, in *Nebraska Symposium on Motivation*, 1980, (ed. H.E. Howe), University of Nebraska Press, Lincoln.

Warner, K.E. (1981) Cigarette smoking in the 1970s: the impact of the anti-smoking campaign on consumption. *Science*, **211**, 729–31.

Weinstein, N.D. (1982) Unrealistic optimism about susceptibility to health problems. *Journal of Behavioral Medicine*, **5**(4), 441–60.

Weinstein, N.D. (1984) Why it won't happen to me: perceptions of risk factors and susceptibility. *Health Psychology*, **3**(5), 431–57.

Windsor, R.A., Baranowski, T., Clark, N. and Cutler, G. (1984) *Evaluation of Health Promotion and Education Programs* (Appendix C), Mayfield Publishing Co., Palo Alto, CA.

HEALTH EDUCATION IN SCHOOLS

4

Schools have long been promoted as a major setting for the provision of health education and a number of justifications offered. First, in recognition of the significance of early learning of health related knowledge, attitudes and behaviours for future health, the schools offer a convenient way of reaching a significant proportion of children and young people over extended periods of time. Second, if schools are concerned to promote complete development, of which health would be an integral part, specific health related activities including education need to be provided. Third, children have been accorded the right to knowledge about health, recently formalized in the Universal Declaration of Children's Rights (United Nations, 1989). Schools have a major role to play in providing for this right.

The link between health and education is not, however, associated solely with participation in health education. Access to education in general has positive impacts on individual and community health. A number of health indicators are correlated with population literacy levels and consequently one of the Health for All by the year 2000 goals is the number of countries where literacy levels for both men and women exceed 70%.

The importance of the education of girls in relation to health has been particularly emphasized in official statements. A child born to a mother with no education is twice as likely to die in infancy as a child born to a mother with four years schooling. Educated women (Dhillon and Philip, 1992) act more decisively in family health matters, take appropriate steps to improve nutrition and prevent illness and seek care in times of illness. It should be noted that education as

an empowering process for girls does not always emerge as clearly from the literature as education for preparing girls for lives as wives, mothers and for key roles in the production and maintenance of health.

Given the widespread support for the view that education for health should occur during childhood it becomes important to reach not only children in schools but also those who are unable to attend school or whose attendance is shortlived. UNESCO estimates in 1985 suggested that 105 million children in the world between six and 11 years did not receive formal education, of which 70% were in the least developed countries and 60% were girls. By 1990 the estimate rose to 130 million out of school (Dhillon and Philip, 1992). Many of these children will be living in families and stable communities which have traditionally provided some education for health but there is also a large and growing number of children who lack these traditional networks of support. There are, for example, estimates of 30 million street children (Dhillon and Philip, 1992) in the world with approximately half of these in Latin America. In response to the recognition of the importance of health education in childhood and youth, there are a growing number of initiatives designed to reach those who are not in the schools. While this chapter is focusing on health education in schools we will be exercising latitude and commenting briefly on initiatives with out of school children and young people.

One of the emerging themes of the 1980s was the attention to the school as a health promoting environment and this provides the context within which school health education will be discussed. In addition, however, schools are set within communities and the potential of the school to have an influence on the health of this community has increasingly been addressed. For example, the Alma Ata Declaration on Primary Health Care (WHO, 1978) gave the education sector a major role:

> Schools could provide the efficient means to attain all of the eight components of primary health care and could ensure that young people can be educated to have a good understanding of what health means, how to achieve it, and how it contributes to social and economic development.

This chapter will begin by providing a brief discussion of the development of school health education and of the philosophical approaches within it, prior to posing some general questions on its evaluation. The remainder of the chapter will consider the evaluation of health education in schools at a number of levels.

HISTORICAL BACKGROUND AND APPROACHES TO SCHOOL HEALTH EDUCATION

While schools in most countries will have included, for differing periods of time, some health teaching, however minimal, planned efforts to develop comprehensive programmes of health education are relatively recent. In the UK, for example, particular energy has been devoted since the late 1960s to the development of school health education but a slow development, focusing particularly on physical health, had been taking place since at least the beginning of the century.

While the stimuli to development have varied over time and between countries, the WHO, alone or in association with other agencies, has had a background international influence. Beginning in 1950 a number of documents have been published offering discussion of school health education together with recommendations. The 1950 Expert Committee on School Health Services (WHO, 1951) emphasized the importance of developing satisfactory health education programmes, supportive teacher training and the use of innovative teaching methods. Endorsement of the emphasis on health education in schools was provided by a subsequent Expert Committee on Health Education of the Public (WHO, 1954). Although this document did not use the current language of 'health promoting schools', many of the criteria now specified for such schools are mentioned in this early document. It also recommended that as part of teacher training, students should experience co-operative relationships between school and community public health workers and collaborative working. The committee recommended that the WHO, in collaboration with UNESCO, should convene a conference or study group to explore the fostering of teacher training for health education. A joint committee was convened in 1959 and a source book, *Planning For Health Education in Schools*, was published in 1966. The emphasis on the schools in the Alma Ata document has already been noted and a further Expert Committee on New Approaches to Health Education in Primary Health Care (WHO, 1983) noted the special position of teachers because of their potential to affect the health of students and, in turn, of the community.

Throughout the 1970s and 1980s, WHO produced a number of reports and technical discussions which addressed features of health of children and young people and included observations on school health education (WHO, 1977, 1979, 1986, 1989). A number of similar principles and recommendations can be seen running through the documents: the need to recognize the two-way relationship between health and education; the matching of health education programmes to local needs and problems; enhancement of the role of schools in local communities by establishing closer relationships between children, teachers, parents and community members; greater co-operation between health, education and social authorities and increasing interdisciplinary collaborative research; basic and in-service interdisciplinary health education training for teachers; and the use of innovative teaching methods including the participation of children in community health projects. When discussing the health of 'adolescents' or, more recently, of 'youth' the documents of the 1980s give emphasis to the participation of young people themselves in assessment of their needs and the planning, implementation and evaluation of programmes.

A global review of the status of school health education in 1990 was prepared by WHO for presentation at the World Conference of Education for All in Thailand. It documented the nature and range of successful initiatives, stressed the importance of health education for all children whether or not they are able to attend schools and set out challenges and issues for action, including:

1. Linkage of health education with the Education For All initiative;
2. Need for policies on school health education and for joint education and health sector implementation strategies;
3. Curriculum development based on health needs of different age groups and taking the sociocultural context into account. Inclusion of parents and community leaders on curriculum development committees;
4. The need to give due weight in schools to personal and social development;
5. Teacher training and other curricula support for health education;
6. High priority to the pivotal role of teachers in the promotion of health in schools and communities;
7. Schools must be health promoting institutions;
8. School health education must be planned and implemented in the context of the pupils' families and the wider community.

(WHO, 1990)

In 1991 WHO, UNESCO and UNICEF convened health and education experts from 16 countries to form a joint Consultation on Strategies for Implementing Comprehensive School Health Education/Promotion programmes. The Consultation arrived at a consensus and issued guiding principles for action which will be referred to in the course of the chapter. In its conclusions this report stated that:

We have a growing understanding of which programmes work and under which circumstances. Much of what we still need to know will be learned through designing, implementing and evaluating school health education programmes.

(WHO/UNESCO/UNICEF, 1992)

Chapter 1 discussed alternative ideologies of health education and the outcomes associated with each of them. First thoughts might lead to the conclusion that schools, with their requirement to be educational, would confine themselves to the use of educational and empowerment approaches to health education. On closer consideration, however, acknowledgement of the constraints imposed by the developmental stage on achieving key competencies such as informed decision making which are central to these models leads us to expect to find, in addition, some adoption of preventive medical models. Furthermore, since schools have a role in socialization ranging, according to viewpoint, from relatively benign socialization through to active social control, preventive approaches are likely to have a part in fulfilling such activities. In all countries we can find interplay between educational/empowerment approaches and preventive medical ones. The balance varies according to time, place and age of pupils. The support of aims associated with both approaches was reported in a study by Charlton (1980) of students and tutors in initial teacher training. Asked to rate each of a list of aims, the provision of information was consistently listed first, followed closely by influencing pupils' attitudes and behaviours. Increasing decision making skills was rated first by only a very small percentage of students but by a higher percentage of tutors.

The last 15 years have seen the development of more sophisticated thinking about educational models in health education and a broadening out to become what this text labels as an empowerment approach. Influences came from child centred progressive educational ideology, the personal growth movement, the writings of Freire and ideas from postindustrial theorizing. Concepts associated with child centred educational ideology – e.g. self-esteem, developmental organization, decision making – have more strongly influenced primary education and many of the early health education projects informed fully by educational and partly by empowerment approaches were for younger children (Schools Council/HEC, 1977; HEC, 1983a).

In very general terms it is the radical–political model which has been less evident in school health education. While the raising of awareness about social and environmental causes of ill health has not been ignored, it has not seemed to rank highly in importance as an aim with teachers. In a survey in Welsh secondary schools (Nutbeam *et al.*, 1987) teachers rated topics in order of perceived importance. The environment and health were rated as very important by only 28% of respondents. There are relatively few health education projects for schools which have embodied some commitment to a radical approach. A good example in the UK was the Health Careers Project (Dorn and Nortoft, 1982) although it was very little used in schools. While incorporating consciousness raising and consideration of health promotion policy strategies, its approach was predominantly educational:

> The aim of the course is that young people develop a conception of health relating to the broader social and economic conditions

that together with their responses to these conditions affect their health and that they actively explore some of the practical possibilities of changing these circumstances and their responses, with the object of enhancing health.

It is possible that the development of thinking and practice around the health promoting school in alliance with other health promoting settings will act as a stimulus to the adoption of more radical approaches in school health education.

In conclusion, it should be stressed that teachers themselves may not articulate categorizations of health education approaches and their practice is likely to be informed by concepts associated with more than one approach. Most of the major statements of aims for health education from a range of countries clearly incorporate outcomes which derive from more than one philosophical approach.

EVALUATING SCHOOL HEALTH EDUCATION – GENERAL DISCUSSION

While it has been a commonplace to note the overall paucity of evaluation in health education, it can be suggested that schools in most countries have been particularly slow to evaluate fully their activities. Williams (1986) commented on this:

> Evaluation and assessment are words we need to hear more of. We must help teachers to evaluate and assess the gains they make with pupils in terms of knowledge, attitudes, and of course the influence on their decision making skills and health behaviour.

A whole variety of reasons can be offered for past shortcomings as far as evaluation is concerned.

1. The general policy on evaluation in education as a whole. While the formal assessment of pupil attainment, especially in

the cognitive domain, and the informal appraisal of all features of the curriculum have always been school activities, comprehensive formal evaluation of a wide range of processes and outcomes has been slower to emerge;

2. The failure to recognize the importance of evaluating a subject which has generally had low status within the curriculum;

3. The lack of skills for evaluating the range of objectives addressed in health education. Teachers are generally skilled in the assessment of cognitive and some skills areas but less so when assessing attitudes or the complex social interaction and decision making skills;

4. The general shortage of time and other resources to support evaluation;

5. In the absence of agreed aims for school health, the specification of outcomes to be addressed in evaluation can generate conflict and consequent inaction.

The changes in education which have occurred in many countries over the last ten years have contributed to a reduction in some of the above barriers. These changes have been a result of both external pressures and ongoing professional development. Some governments, of which that of the UK is a good example, are making schools more accountable through, for example, the regular testing of performance. Although major reservations exist in education about such government policy it is likely that this climate of accountability will lead to an increase in evaluation skills. At the same time a number of developments, such as the production of records of achievement, profiling and the assessment of a wider range of competencies at school leaving level have broadened evaluation skills. More specifically, courses disseminating health education projects have emphasized and tried to develop evaluation skills and the inclusion of evaluation sheets in associated pupil materials has served as a reminder to teachers.

There are probably no aspects of evaluation which are unique to schools but there are features which may be more of an issue in this context than others.

1. Delineating what should be evaluated as health education. The broader its definition the more difficult it becomes to differentiate health education from education in general.

2. Health education can be organized in a number of ways in schools. In the secondary sector, for example, it may be provided through co-ordinated inputs across a number of curriculum subjects such as biology, home economics and physical education; as a constituent strand of personal, social and health education (PSHE) courses; in the context of tutorial time; as a timetabled subject in its own right; or through varying combinations of these and other arrangements. If attempting, for example, to evaluate sex education in schools, identifying all the contributions from the formal curriculum can be difficult. If, in addition, those contributions from the other elements of the total school curriculum are also to be considered, evaluation becomes even more complex.

3. Where health behaviours are a focus for evaluation there are two particular issues. First, many of the behaviours which are a focus for attention typically occur outside the school environment and evaluators must rely on reported measures. Second, some activities will be oriented towards behaviours that do not occur for variable periods after leaving school. Because of the difficulties in carrying out long term evaluations there may need to be a heavy reliance on intermediate indicators.

4. With the expectation that schools will be strongly committed to the goals of educational and empowerment approaches there may be a greater need than in some contexts to engage with the difficulties of operationalizing and measuring the more

complex outcomes of empowerment, decision making, etc.

5. Decisions about who should plan and carry out evaluations have particular significance. Where there is a commitment to empowerment approaches pupils ought to be participating in, rather than merely co-operating with, the evaluation process.

In evaluating school health education there are a number of points of focus. An obvious starting point could be the learning outcomes of pupils achieved within the formal curriculum. This learning could be directed both to present and to future health. As can be seen in Fig. 4.1, the other elements of the school curriculum also contribute to the health education of pupils – they may reinforce the classroom work but equally could work in opposition to it. If we wish to see health education happening within an institution which as a whole promotes health, a second focus of evaluation is on the school as

a health promoting institution. Children and young people can take their learning into their families and communities. There is increasing attention to developing and evaluating this role.

While it may be possible to demonstrate considerable success in small scale health education activities in some schools, it is also important to assess the extent to which the schools system as a whole provides effective health education. Finally, in order for schools to be effective in their health education, facilitating policies are needed. In the following sections we shall be discussing examples of successful activities at each of these levels.

EVALUATING SCHOOL HEALTH EDUCATION – LEVELS OF ANALYSIS

PUPIL ACHIEVEMENTS

Much of the evaluation of school health education, taken as a whole, has addressed

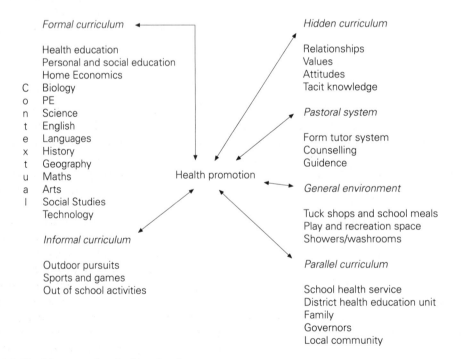

Figure 4.1 Health promotion in the school.

classroom activities offered within the formal curriculum. Studies may address single indicators but more usually there is attention to various combinations of the intermediate and outcome indicators discussed in Chapter 3. Earlier evaluations tended to focus on knowledge and beliefs, attitudes and relatively simple health behaviours. There is a growing optimism that school health education can be effective in addressing these variables. Back in 1981 Bartlett concluded that the best developed programmes were successful in increasing knowledge, somewhat successful in improving attitudes and infrequently successful in achieving lifestyle change. Only four years later Mason and McGinnis (1985), reporting on the School Health Evaluation study in the USA which involved 30 000 children, said:

> The study unequivocally demonstrates that school health education is an effective means of helping children to improve their health knowledge and develop healthy attitudes. It also shows that school health education can decrease the likelihood that children will adopt behaviours that are hazardous to health, such as cigarette smoking.

Others around the same time concurred with this view (Kolbe, 1985; Reid and Massey, 1986) although the latter authors saw progress as somewhat uneven and thought it desirable to consider results for different health topics individually. They concluded from their review:

> ... given suitable methods used in appropriate contexts, schools can favourably affect teenage health related behaviour in relation to smoking, oral hygiene, rubella and immunization and teenage fertility. There is also some evidence for potential success in the field of diet and exercise.

Although an exhaustive review would probably now lead to a modification in the topics listed, the general tenor of their conclusion would probably still hold. The extent and sophistication of evaluation activities varies according to health topic and approach. Where programmes have been oriented to the goals associated with the preventive model there has been growing attention, particularly in the area of smoking, to varying combinations of intermediate indicators associated with specified behaviour outcomes. These have included developing resistance to smoking pressures with the use of peer educators, decision making skills and values clarification (Hansen, 1992).

The variations in effectiveness between health areas continues to be significant. As we will discuss later, the psychosocial approaches adopted in the case of smoking have not been as successful where alcohol is concerned and a recent reviewer has expressed strong reservations about the potential impact of individualized alcohol education in the schools setting (May, 1993). Currently throughout the world considerable resources are being put into HIV/AIDS education and it is hoped that schools can play a significant role in prevention. However, when it has been so difficult to introduce sex education, even in quite limited forms, in many countries of the world, the barriers to success are considerable for this major health concern. In developing countries of the world the long-standing problems of infectious diseases such as malaria and diarrhoeal disease are ones where it is expected that schools can play a significant role in prevention. Because relatively few published evaluations exist it is more difficult to comment on progress for these health areas.

While there has been a widespread tendency to organize health education around health topics – whether these be the major concerns of countries of the 'north', those of the 'south' or shared concerns – this is not the only approach. An alternative is to identify the personal attributes and competencies needed to achieve health – of the individual and of the community – and to develop a curriculum around their development.

Although specific health topics will be drawn on in the process it will be as vehicles in developing what are hoped to be transferable skills. Emphasis would be on such things as self-esteem, self-efficacy, locus of control, empowerment, decision making, assertiveness, advocacy and so on. The Healthskills project in the UK provides a good example of such an approach (Anderson, 1988). Clearly the variables listed may be developed in the course of projects oriented towards behavioural goals but within the empowerment approach they move from being intermediate to outcome indicators.

In addition to addressing questions of the effectiveness of school health education, we also need to ask about efficiency and equity. There can be interest in the efficiency of alternative methods and resources in achieving desired outcomes, on identifying both the most appropriate timings for health education and the extent and timing of reinforcement in order to maintain achievements. We have earlier noted the problems of ensuring that children outside the school system have access to health education. Within the system we also need to monitor the extent to which education is planned taking into consideration the needs of all children and that provision addresses equal opportunities.

In making observations about health education at the pupil level we are interested in examining not only what has been published in the evaluation literature but also in commenting on the omissions. Across the world health education happens in very different contexts, in many of which it is difficult to organize evaluation and bring findings to a wider audience. The literature on school health education and evaluation is not, therefore, fully representative of activity and achievements. The remainder of this section will provide discussion of a selection of indicators followed by some discussion of efficiency and some conclusions.

KNOWLEDGE AND BELIEFS

Health education activities oriented towards knowledge can be undertaken for different purposes; as a first stage in what is hoped to be a progression towards attitude development or change and ultimately behavioural outcomes; or with the objective of developing transferable knowledge skills. It is difficult to generalize about the extent of continuing belief in the K-A-P progression. In an extensive review of drug prevention health education activities Hansen (1992) recorded that they almost invariably included knowledge components but with little conviction that, alone, they would achieve anything.

Given the amount of health education activity which is solely concerned with transmission of information there must still be widespread beliefs that this is to some degree an effective way of generating desired attitudes and behaviours. For maximal impact on specific health behaviours any such knowledge may need to be very specifically focused, as for example in specifying frequency of sugar intake as a preventive measure in dental caries.

We need also to ask, however, if pupils develop knowledge in ways which leave them open to reassessing it in the light of later developments in epidemiological knowledge or using it in situations where social and other pressures exist. Health education can offer many examples of adherence to educational messages effectively communicated in the past but now superseded. If this is to be prevented it might be better if school health educators emphasized the general skills of acquiring and appraising knowledge rather than efficient delivery of current wisdom.

While it would be unrealistic to expect children to 'discover' all the health knowledge appropriate for them it is important to give sufficient attention to the use of active approaches in knowledge oriented work. This point was recognized in the UK document

Health Education from 5–16 (DES, 1985) which proposed as one of the objectives of health education that people should know how to distinguish between fact, promotion and polemic and how to weigh and interpret information about health from a variety of sources. Brierley (1983) had earlier observed that the experience of weighing evidence on diet, smoking, immunization, fluoridation and other health issues was rather thin in health education.

Clearly active enquiry approaches are central to much educational thinking – although under attack from the 'back to basics' movement – but the opportunities and means of achieving them will vary. It can be relatively easy in contexts where classes are small, schools well resourced and the educational culture accepts the ideas associated with child centred, progressive philosophy. It is more difficult when classes are very large, resources are minimal and the culture of education expects learners to be relatively passive. Nonetheless the success of the 'Child to Child' project has demonstrated the power of active learning approaches in very varied school settings (Aarons, 1979). In assessing knowledge oriented activities we are looking for a recognition of the need for some emphasis on active enquiry as a contribution to development of transferable knowledge skills. For example, an evaluation of peer teaching in the Netherlands (de Vries *et al.*, 1992) included some information seeking activities as part of the programme. More generally health education in primary schools in some countries is often built around projects incorporating active knowledge seeking.

There is abundant evidence that schools can increase health knowledge – it would be surprising if they didn't. This knowledge gain may, however, range from the increase in facts to development of concepts and principles that can be used in problem solving. It is the more complicated cognitive goals that are the more difficult to achieve. With simpler cognitive goals as its target, Natural Nashers (HEC/Dental Health Study, 1984), a dental health education programme for the lower secondary years (11–13), demonstrated significant differences in knowledge between study and control groups after teaching the programme. Of the three knowledge measures assessed (Table 4.1), correct responses were more likely from girls, from pupils from non-manual backgrounds and regular attenders at a dental practice. While the project was successful in developing a new belief in the study group in the role of sugar in dental caries, it was not so successful in changing the already held belief about the preventive action of toothbrushing on dental caries.

An interesting discussion of developing knowledge so that it provides an adequate

Table 4.1 Changes in knowledge

	Eruption, first permanent		Frequency of sugar intake		Reasons for teeth	
	Study	*Control*	*Study*	*Control*	*Study*	*Control*
Pre(%)	13	13	18	19	53	51
Base	1399	1453	1401	1419	1613	1636
Post (%)	29	17	46	25	82	57
Base	1373	1319	1364	1275	1460	1435
	$z = 4, p < 0.05$		$z = 6.33, p < 0.05$		$z = 8.33, p < 0.05$	

basis for future health activity is provided by Eisemon and Patel (1990) in a study of diarrhoea education in Kenyan schools. In community research they had found that mothers who had attended school understood that diarrhoea could lead to severe dehydration and might routinely give oral rehydration solution (ORS) to their children. However, even mothers who had completed the full stage of primary education could not always explain why ORS was necessary and effective and the treatment was sometimes combined with other, harmful treatments. Health is a compulsory paper in the primary school leaving examination in Kenya so Eisemon and Patel set out to show how the test items which assessed knowledge about ORS, immunization, control of communicable diseases and child nutrition could be changed so that teachers were encouraged to explain disease processes and enhance understanding of preventive measures and treatments. In a small scale demonstration project they reported success in developing understanding in addition to facts.

BEHAVIOURS

Health related behaviours are a main goal of much health education – ranging from sensible drinking, adoption of safe sex practices, hygiene behaviours, reductions in smoking recruitment, behaviours associated with prevention of a range of infectious diseases such as malaria, guinea worm, diarrhoeal disease and accident prevention, to name but a few. As noted earlier the successes in relation to health behaviours are variable – in part reflecting the levels of time and other resources directed towards specific issues (not necessarily highly correlated with the importance of these issues in mortality or morbidity terms or for young people themselves) but also the different challenges that they offer to the educator.

Smoking education, for example, has been a major component of school health educa-

tion in developed countries and has been subjected to consistent evaluation. A typical finding was offered by the School Health Curriculum Project (Owen *et al.*, 1985). Using a self-reported measure of smoking with 7th grade pupils, it was found that 12.7% of control students smoked compared with 7.7% who had participated in the programme. It was estimated that if the results were extrapolated nationwide 146 000 7th graders would delay the onset of smoking. The related My Body project in the UK (Health Education Council, 1983a) reported a probable halving of the rate of experimental smoking associated with participation in the programme. Smoking behaviour was discussed comprehensively by Reid (1985) who observed that:

There has been a remarkable reversal of fortune since Thompson concluded in an earlier review of smoking that most methods had shown little success. One can almost claim that most methods have been highly successful in the short term. Even approaches based largely on information have been successful.

Some of the reasons suggested to account for the successes were the fall in prevalence of smoking in the adult population and consequent changes in the social environment in which smoking choices are made; the use of non-didactic approaches with an emphasis on discussion and active finding out from films and books and an emphasis on the immediate effects of cigarette smoke as opposed to long term hazards.

An issue which received relatively little attention until recently was the differential impact on boys and girls of smoking education. Murray *et al.* (1984) reported that boys who were taught the My Body project were less likely than boys in the control groups to smoke subsequently while, in contrast, girls who were taught the programme were more likely than controls to adopt smoking. When allowance was made for the effects of parental and siblings smoking the differential effect persisted. The purpose of the My Body project is to provide children with a thorough understanding of personal health and to 'inoculate' them against pressures to smoke after entering secondary school. This appeared to have been successful with the boys; with them the intentions in relation to smoking at 11–12 years were a good predictor of behaviour two years later. It was concluded that the My Body project had been taught at an age which would have maximum impact on smoking incidence among boys. In the case of girls, whose smoking careers lagged behind those of boys, the intervention had come too early.

Of particular interest in smoking has been the use of methods which address the social influences on this behaviour. Evans *et al.* (1978) identified peers, parents and the media as major sources of pressure in relation to smoking and in response, attempted to familiarize children with these pressures and ways of dealing with them. Others (McAlister *et al.*, 1979; Botvin, Eng and Williams, 1980) developed the ideas further and added the use of peer leaders as educators, activities to increase the social commitment not to smoke and the role playing of situations that needed resistance to social pressure. A variety of studies have reported significant results using these approaches (Hansen, 1992) although there have also been negative findings. Comparisons between studies are not easy because the precise elements and their organization vary. It is also difficult to deduce which elements are of particular significance, as noted by Flay (1986) in a review of this literature.

As commented earlier the successes in smoking education have not been equally matched in the case of alcohol. In a critical review of the literature May (1991) noted that methodologically sound project evaluations were rarely encountered in this body of literature. He reported that the commonest educational approach has been the provision of facts which might be an effective response

to any perceived knowledge needs but evaluated programmes had generally failed to demonstrate positive effects on attitudes or alcohol use. He notes the modest positive effects achieved by Bagnall (1987) in an experimental study in which student participation was an important component. As in the case of smoking, alcohol education has developed the use of various combinations of approaches which draw on psychological theory and incorporate social skills development, resistance to peer pressure using role play, enhancing self-esteem and attention to locus of control.

Although skills based approaches may be marginally more effective than knowledge based ones, May concludes that reviews and meta-analyses have drawn negative conclusions. For example, he cites the study of Mauss *et al.* (1988) which evaluated a programme designed to 'enhance students' knowledge of alcohol and its effects, to improve self-esteem and decision making skills and impart appropriate attitudes regarding the responsible use of alcohol'. They were unable to demonstrate any appreciable effect. May goes further to question the assumptions underpinning skills based approaches and contends that there is little by way of empirical research to support the view that the young use or misuse alcohol because of lack of competence, inability to resist peer pressure or lack of decision making skills. The emphasis on psychological models of behaviour, he argues, has tended to over determine the individual as the source of behaviour change with a consequent neglect of the social context.

In comparing the modest successes in smoking related education with the apparent lack of success in alcohol education, May suggests possible reasons. First, there is the relative ease in the case of smoking of conveying the message of total abstinence in comparison with the more ambiguous message of 'sensible drinking'. Second, as noted earlier, smoking related education has achieved greater success because of the changing social climate of growing opposition to tobacco use. The apparent success of some tobacco education interventions may be only partly related, therefore, to their technical efficiency. To have prospects of greater success alcohol education must, May claims, attend to the complex social contexts in which alcohol use takes place; to the meanings which young drinkers attribute to these situations; and to their drinking behaviours within them.

A thoroughgoing review of 'substance use prevention' studies carried out between 1980 and 1990 has recently been completed by Hansen (1992). His review excluded programmes that targeted tobacco alone but included those where it was addressed in conjunction with other substances. He notes that previous reviews had placed emphasis on type 1 errors but that type 2 errors (Chapter 2) had been relatively ignored. He stresses that in assessing the state of the art both type 1 and type 2 methodological critiques are essential. He drew up a classification of the projects reviewed around what he describes as the 'building block theoretical concepts' used by researchers in describing their programmes. For each of these concepts theoretical or quasi-theoretical assumptions have been claimed about the link of the component with behaviour. Hansen identified 12 components: information, decision making, pledge (encouragement of personal commitment not to use substances), values clarification, goal setting, stress management, self-esteem, resistance skills training (identification and assertive resistance of pressures from peers, parents, siblings, adults and the media), life skills training, norm setting, assistance (intervention and counselling) and use of alternatives (experience of activities incompatible with substance use). Most of the programmes reviewed included at least two of the foregoing components while seven out of the 41 studies focused on a single component. Hansen was not able to document the relative effort given to separate components, the time spent on

specific tasks and quality measures of components. While such factors are important much of the literature had provided insufficient information to permit classification.

The most frequent programme component was information giving (90.2% of programmes reviewed) although Hansen notes that few of the researchers of multicomponent programmes expected information to change important mediating variables. The commonest educational approach to knowledge work was the use of the socratic method in which knowledge and beliefs of students are elicited through structured discussion. Resistance skills (44% of programmes) and decision making skills (42%) were the two next most common components.

The programmes were subsequently grouped into six categories to facilitate analysis. Some programmes from five of the six groups were effective at preventing the onset of substance abuse while at the same time all groups included programmes with neutral or negative outcomes. The most promising strategies appeared to be 'comprehensive' ones and 'social influences'. Programmes in the comprehensive group included multiple components – on average seven strategies (range 5–9). All included information, decision making and resistance skills training; four included pledge and norm setting components and the only component absent from all of these programmes was the teaching of students to assist each other with problems. The social influences group included programmes with a major objective of teaching students about peer and other social pressures and the development of skills to resist them and nearly all included information activities. Hansen comments that as both these categories of programmes contained multiple components he was unable to deduce from studies whether it was the addition of components or inclusion of one or more key components that was the key to success. He did suggest that many researchers drew unjustified conclusions about the causes of programme effectiveness.

Some themes emerged from his analysis. The most promising component appeared to be social influences but he cautioned against emphasizing too strongly the identification and resisting of peer pressures as the major reason for success of these programmes since several studies which specifically tested these variables failed to produce positive effects. In the studies he had reviewed, the knowledge component had been pervasive and while noting that it was not sufficient by itself to achieve prevention, its ancillary benefits were not known. While social influence and comprehensive programmes were most consistently effective, success cannot be guaranteed. Intervening characteristics needed further consideration including the training and background of teachers, fidelity of presentation and the target population. Hansen concludes by pointing to the weakness of much of the research conducted on programmes and the need for 'the adoption of a systematic approach that tests basic approaches to prevention, which in part may require more conceptual specification and tighter experimental control'.

In the foregoing discussion there has been mention of the development of social skills, of decision making and of other personal attributes identified earlier as goals of the empowerment model. They were, however, being addressed as intermediate variables in the pursuit of behavioural goals. Quite clearly, in many of the projects reported there may have been secondary objectives that the skills developed would be transferable ones but in most cases the goals of the preventive model, whether or not clearly explicated, appeared to be dominant. Botvin, however, in his evaluation of a life skills approach to smoking, noted the wider benefits. He included a number of variables in his programme (locus of control, anxiety, self-image, susceptibility to social influence, need for acceptance and peer identification) and commented:

The emphasis on self-empowerment and acquisition of basic coping skills not only makes the program intrinsically interesting to students but indirectly addresses other important areas of health. Such a program may serve as a core around which an entire health education curriculum might be developed.

In 1981 Bartlett, in his assessment of school health education, said that its effects on such pupil outcomes as decision making and social interaction abilities have seldom, if ever, been measured. In the intervening period these outcomes have been emphasized in all statements on health education and, as discussed in the previous section, have been included and evaluated as components of preventively oriented programmes. They are integral to much thinking about school health education, as emphasized by Anderson (1986).

... the need for personal growth and skill enhancement leading to the development of responsible, autonomous and assertive young people capable of making rational and informed decisions about their health is the foundation of successful health education.

It is probably fair to say that there is still less reported evaluation of empowerment related attributes as project outcomes in themselves in comparison with their evaluation as part of preventive model projects. This need not be a criticism if we are seeking to identify the successful ways of achieving decision making, social interaction skills, etc. There can be a problem if the skills of interest are embedded in multistrategy programmes and are not separately evaluated. As an illustrative example of empowerment model outcomes, we can comment on successes in developing decision making skills.

DECISION MAKING

Decision making is a skill which has been rated highly in statements of aims of health education and it has been addressed in one way or another in the majority of specially produced health education projects. How successfully decision making skills have been developed is still difficult to assess from the literature available. Developing measures for assessing these skills is more complex than for knowledge or attitudes.

It is necessary in the first place to define an act of decision making. People do not make decisions in the same way on all occasions – strategies vary according to the choice in question, situational factors and characteristics and competencies of the actual decision maker(s). Much decision making education is directed towards the development of a rational or what is described by Janis and Mann (1977) as a 'vigilant' decision making strategy although in real life this may not be the most useful or the most appropriate one in many health choice situations. For example Hansen, in the review discussed above, noted that decision making skills components focused extensively on teaching a method for evaluating information and drawing a conclusion using a rational process. Briefly, a rational 'vigilant' approach requires the decision maker to be able to recognize a choice situation, generate the alternatives available, collect and appraise information on each alternative, clarify values related to each alternative, order alternatives and make a choice.

A number of personal and social skills are often needed to implement a decision. Teaching activities may address either individual elements of the whole skill or the complete decision making act. Skills may be taught in a general sense or be related to specific health decision making situations and there may be varying emphases on the cognitive act of decision making and the personal competencies to use skills when required. Both objective and subjective measures can be included in evaluations and the degree of importance attached to each may relate, in part, to the philosophical approach of the evaluator. Feelings of self-empowerment can result from active involvement in decision making and this development may be seen as more important than objective measures of skill. Clearly in many cases there is likely to be a correlation between objective and subjective assessments. On the whole the literature includes more evaluations of elements of decision making than of complete acts.

Lammers *et al.* (1984) assessed the effects of the School Health Curriculum Project (SHCP) on health knowledge and selected cognitive dimensions of decision making skills with reference to smoking. Using the Health Decision Making Index, the focus was on the generation of reasons for and against smoking, identifying the three most important and developing a behavioural intention. At the post-test there was a significant difference between experimental and control group pupils with the former producing a higher total number of reasons. This study endorsed the earlier findings by Duryea (1983) and concluded that the SHCP had the potential to affect the cognitive dimension of the decision making process. Duryea considered that the more alternatives considered for a given decision, the greater the possibility that the decision would be a rational one.

Botvin *et al.*'s (1980) life skills training approach discussed earlier included two sessions related to the decision making process. In the first, students discussed how they made important decisions and a strategy for making decisions was suggested. The second session dealt with techniques used by advertisers to influence consumer decisions. Evaluation of the approach indicated a reduction of new smoking by 50% in junior high school students.

In conclusion it should be noted that the evaluated studies of decision making are oriented particularly towards rational models. An increase in studies focusing on the range of strategies used in decision making would be welcomed.

EFFICIENCY

It is important to identify the most efficient way of reaching planned objectives even though these may not always be the preferred strategies to adopt. In the school contexts in which health education is provided, resources may be scarce and competition for them acute. Whatever one's political stance on the decisions taken at national or international levels which leave schools in such difficult positions, it would be naive to think that educators can avoid developing justifications for the use of expensive strategies.

The use of multicomponent strategies in the drugs prevention area demonstrates successes but there is need, as stated above, to understand the separate contributions of individual components. Not all might be important to include and attention to efficiency demands the identification of not only what is necessary but also sufficient. In addition, if we are to sustain the learning gains from specific activities, a more detailed knowledge is needed about the needs for, and the timing of, reinforcing activities. Some evidence on the cumulative impact of repeated instruction was included in the evaluation of the School Health Curriculum Project (Cooke and Walberg, 1985). Student performance was tracked over two years to provide an estimate of the benefits of cumulative exposure. For all three classes of variables examined, groups with two units of exposure performed better than those with one, regardless of grade levels.

Some approaches to health education are popular with pupils and while this is clearly an important justification for their use, in cost conscious times it may also be very necessary to spell out the educational gains from their use. A particularly good example is the use of drama and in particular the use of theatre in education (TIE) groups specializing in health related productions. An evaluation by McEwan *et al.* (1991) examined the costs of using TIE in HIV AIDS education and concluded that:

> The costs of Theatre in Education may be too high in cases where the programme objectives are to impart information, but may be justified in programmes which seek to empower young people or to change their attitudes.

In all countries of the world the educational process has, at one time or another, been dominated by formal, highly structured and teacher controlled approaches to learning. In some countries participatory learning methods are widely established in school health education but still have to be adopted in others. The Geneva Consultation document (WHO/ UNESCO/UNICEF, 1992) recommended that health education be based on participatory learning and engage children in community action projects. In any context it is helpful to consider how active methods can be effectively and efficiently developed. Quite simple and relatively cheap techniques can often be used. In classrooms the use of the flannelgraph, for example, can stimulate greater active participation in the achievement of knowledge goals than use of a chalkboard. Drawing on active methods which are well known in specific cultures also makes teacher training an easier prospect. The use of puppets and other folk media spring to mind as examples. Currently there is little to report on rigorous evaluations of such techniques.

PARTICIPATION

In this section we have said little if anything about participation of young people themselves in defining their health education needs, their preferred methods for learning and their involvement in deciding on the focus and process of evaluation. This is not to underplay the importance of participation but while it may be seen as important in the planning and implementation of many school health education activities, it does not as yet command a high profile in published evaluations.

Bremberg (1991), for example, in a review of health education studies published between 1976 and 1989 in which authors claimed an effect on health related behaviours using quasiexperimental designs identified only one in which students identified their own health needs and set up goals accordingly (Bremberg and Arborelius, 1991). This was a Swedish programme entitled 'It's Your Decision' which involved the identification with 15–16 year olds of personally relevant issues, followed up by self-initiated activities directed towards personally relevant goals. The programme was facilitated by health counsellors from outside the schools. In the post-test, participating students reported more health enhancing activities than controls during the previous term – about half of which were oriented to physical health and the remainder to psychological and social health. The experimental group also gained in self-esteem and internal locus of control in comparison with the control group. Many would prefer to see participation evaluated by qualitative research methods.

Finally, a comment on an indicator that does not emerge as strongly from evaluative studies as perhaps it might – the satisfaction of young people themselves with the health education programmes in which they participate. Undoubtedly much informal and formal evaluation does take place and many of the health education projects contain good suggestions for monitoring pupil views – the 'field of words' in the *Taught Not Caught* materials (Clarity Collective, 1985) is an example that can be particularly recommended. The nature and degree of participation of young people themselves in planning, implementing and evaluating health education should, it is suggested, be one indicator used in monitoring the health promoting status of schools.

CONCLUSION

In this section we have commented, albeit briefly, on a selection of indicators that may be used in evaluating the success of health education with individual pupils. Some aspects of health have been subjected to much closer attention than others, typically where specific behaviours have been associated with immediate or future physical health. The most sophisticated evaluations have taken place for some of these areas, smoking education being a main example. While some of the apparent successes in the smoking area have not been replicated in others it has also been stressed that the complex psychosocial approaches to smoking education are, in essence, special programmes rather than typical of ongoing educational processes in schools.

If school health education is to be effective it has been suggested that educational methods developed by behavioural scientists will need to be adopted (Bremberg, 1991). Some people would wish to challenge the emphasis on behavioural changes associated with health outcomes especially where these are professionally or adult defined rather than the concerns of young people themselves. The literature is still rather short on separate evaluation of some of the indicators associated with the empowerment model. While some, such as decision making skills and self-efficacy, are frequently embedded in some of the comprehensive psychosocial programmes they may not be individually or comprehensively evaluated.

THE SCHOOL AS A HEALTH PROMOTING COMMUNITY

The school promotes the health of its pupils in a variety of ways: through education in both the formal and informal curriculum; through the hidden curriculum – the values and relationships within the school; through the general school environment; and through health and other caring services.

While there has always been a recognition of the fact that features of the school environment can be antagonistic to the health education in the curriculum and early WHO documents on school health education noted this importance of the school environment as a support to classroom work, it wasn't until the 1980s that there was a concerted focus on the school as a health promoting environment. One of the significant early health education projects in England, the Schools Health Education Project 13–18, encouraged teachers in its training workshops to consider the nature of the health promoting school (Schools Council/HEC, 1982). Trefor Williams and Christine de Panafieu, in a review of health education in European countries (1985), concluded that the major emphasis in Europe was still placed upon the development of health education curricula with their attendant materials and methods and that more needed to be placed on a consideration of the ways in which what is taught in the classroom might be supported and reinforced through the values and attitudes implicit in the organization, structure and staffing of the school. For successful curriculum development in health education, Williams had earlier proposed three criteria:

1. An understanding of the content and process of health promotion;
2. An understanding of curriculum development and school organization;
3. An understanding of the potential of the school as a health promoting community and also of the school's place in the setting of the wider community.

Since this was written there has been a major initiative within the European Region developed jointly by WHO, the European Community and the Council of Europe on Healthy Schools (WHO, 1991). *The Health of the Nation* document has stated that Britain should play its full part in this initiative and

its development and will seek to establish, in co-operation with European partners, a pilot network of health promoting schools.

Definitions of a health promoting school vary as do the specifications of the separate but interacting elements which contribute to the whole. For example, Young (1992) identifies three main elements:

1. Health education in the formal curriculum and through pastoral care;
2. The hidden curriculum – including the caring relationships, the examples set by teachers, the relationships developed between home and the school, and the physical environment and facilities of the school;
3. The health and caring services providing health screening, immunization, first aid and psychological services.

Young's use of 'hidden curriculum' is a wider one than is usual in the educational literature and it would probably be better to use a more general heading.

Conceptualizations of the specific criteria of a health promoting school can yet again be related to the ideological position of commentators. Some may be looking for criteria which are related to the achievement of empowered young people who are enabled to reach their full potential and develop health as a resource for living within health promoting communities. *The Health of the Nation*, however, seems to have rather more restricted ideas in stating that the pilot network of health promoting schools in England will develop, and assess, the effectiveness of strategies for changing and shaping pupils' patterns of behaviour, with the aim of safeguarding their long term health. These criteria for assessing the health promoting nature of schools will be debated and different conclusions drawn from place to place – as will the emphasis on specific ones. The core elements of the health promoting school – the formal curriculum, the school environment and school health services – are related to and informed by school policies on health promotion and by wider education policies. The health promoting school in turn is ideally set within and interacts with a health promoting community with which it forms coalitions.

Although there is now a strong impetus to focus on the whole school as a health promoting setting earlier evaluations recorded that schools had tended to focus on specific elements rather than the whole. In particular there was the development of specific policies on smoking and nutrition and, as required in England and Wales, on sex education. In the case of nutrition this can be seen as a response to the growing interest in many countries in the links between diet and health and to a longstanding recognition that school meals and tuckshops can counteract classroom education. Where smoking is concerned the groundswell of support for the abolition of smoking and a recognition of teachers as role models in the smoking career acted as triggers. In both cases the existence of district smoking and nutrition policies in some countries may have provided facilitative environments.

In a 1987 survey of one third (n = 74) of Welsh secondary schools, Nutbeam (1987) reported that 71 (83%) had a policy on smoking directed towards pupils but only 25 had one regarding smoking by staff in the school. However, 55 did have a restriction on smoking outside the staffroom with 43 specifying that no teacher should smoke in the presence of children. The basis for the smoking policies generally seemed to be narrower than would be expected from a fully fledged health promotion policy with many schools regarding smoking as mainly a disciplinary issue.

Teachers' attitudes and behaviours are important in ensuring that smoking education in the classroom is supported in the environment as a whole. Another study by Nutbeam *et al.* (1987) in 29 primary and secondary schools in the south of England addressed teachers' attitudes and behaviours. Twenty two per cent (n = 192) of the men and 15% (n = 196) of the women were smokers which compared favourably with the norm for smoking in the socioeconomic group to which teachers belonged (29% in 1984). It was found that 70% of teachers in the sample accepted their exemplary role in relation to smoking and over 80% agreed that they had an active role in influencing children's health behaviour as it related to smoking. There was general consensus on the need to provide a smokefree environment for non-smokers but less agreement on efforts to restrict smoking by teachers.

In the Welsh study (Nutbeam, 1987) only a minority of schools had nutrition policies. More than half of the respondents reported the existence of such policies in their local education authorities although at the time of the survey none in fact existed. In a more recent survey of a random sample of 87 Welsh secondary schools (Smith *et al.*, 1992) three fifths of schools reported written policies or rules about smoking but less than a third mentioned policies about alcohol and illegal drugs. As in the earlier survey, policies which addressed teachers' smoking were still rare – one in seven schools – although restrictions on smoking had increased a little since the earlier survey. In this more recent survey most of the health education co-ordinators in the schools were unfamiliar with the 'health promoting school' term. Smith *et al.* note:

> Many of those who thought their school was a health promoting one or close to becoming one were incorrect in their belief, judged by criteria concerning curriculum organization, supportive policy developments and community involvement.

The writers conclude that these findings were disappointing and illustrated a gap between the concept of health promoting schools and current practice.

Integral to much of the discussion of health promoting schools has been the recognition that such schools should address the health of all their members – pupils, teachers and support staff. In the past it was not usual to include schools in workplace education. However, the Carolina Healthstyle Program (Maysey *et al.*, 1988), which was established in 1982 for 20 000 state employees, was broadened to include school employees in one pilot district in 1985 and a further four districts in 1987. The programme has a formal structure with a programme co-ordinator at district level, a steering committee at school district level and a smaller Healthstyle committee in each school building. This last committee plans and implements a health promotion programme for its school building which:

1. determines employees' needs and interests in health promotion programmes;
2. determines what facilities, health services and other resources are available within the worksite;
3. develops plans and commitments to conduct specific activities over the year;
4. implements and evaluates plans and modifies them for the next year.

In the pilot district employees paid a small sum to join the programme and 75% participation occurred.

Clearly in seeking comprehensive evaluations of the health promoting nature of schools and most particularly when there is some commitment to empowerment approaches, there is little in the school environment which does not have some bearing on its health promotion standing and to which attention needs to be given. As Anderson (1979) has said:

> To have an effect it is essential that self-empowerment is part of an approach and a philosophy applied throughout the whole school – not just something that happens on Friday afternoons in personal, social and health education lessons.

The Healthskills project has made the examination of the ways in which schools empower or depower their members and the discussion of possible changes an important component of its staff development workshops. Without this attention on the whole school, Anderson proposes, 'the notion of informed decision making, so important to health education, but requiring a degree of personal autonomy and self belief, is likely to remain nothing but a notion'. This project has also recognized the need for teachers to address their own health in the context of the social setting of the school as a prelude to the curriculum development of health education.

It is too early to review evaluations which comprehensively assess schools as health promoting settings. It will be interesting to note the criteria which are used as well as the successes which are achieved. It is to be hoped that, in addition to very obvious health criteria, there will be efforts to review more diffuse and difficult to assess criteria such as contribution to the reduction of health inequalities. Schools routinely make a commitment to equal opportunities but can fall far short of fulfilling this aim in practice. Very many factors can be considered in evaluating a school's success in this respect: the appropriateness of the curriculum as a whole and of health education in particular in the context of multiracial societies; respect for cultural diversity; proper integration of young people with special needs; avoidance of racism and sexism; and appropriateness of teaching methods and resources. The Schools Council in the UK produced a number of documents to assist schools in carrying out appraisal of the curriculum in a multiracial society and for tracking sex stereotyping in teaching materials and some schools have developed 'user friendly' statements (ALTARF, 1984) of their policies on equalities which are given to all newcomers.

SCHOOL HEALTH EDUCATION AND THE HEALTH OF FAMILIES AND COMMUNITIES

One of the objectives of health education is the development of young people who, as adults, will contribute to the development and maintenance of health in their families and communities. Increasingly, however, attention has been directed both to the immediate impact of school health education on family and community health and also to the potential contribution of families and communities to the health education curriculum.

The 1991 Geneva Consultation Conference (WHO/UNESCO/UNICEF, 1992) proposed that schools and communities are natural partners in health promotion and disease prevention. It encouraged the development of school–community projects which could provide learning opportunities for the children but could also be designed to 'involve, inform, and facilitate education of parents, family members and others in the community'. As we have seen above, the school interactions with the home and the wider community are factors to consider in assessing its health promoting status. Major importance has also been given to the school–community nexus by Hewett (1992) of UNICEF who has suggested placing the school at the centre of the development process. He says:

> The school and its immediate physical environment would be seen and treated as a first priority of health related development. It would be, for example, the location of a community's first safe water source, sanitary latrine and fuel efficient stove, a dependable source of nutrition and home garden knowledge and advice, a place for parents to meet and discuss practical improvements in various aspects of community life and wellbeing ... in general, the centre of social development in every community where a school existed.

Depending on the country in question different examples might need to be substituted in the above statement but the sentiment expressed is widely relevant. Schools could, for example, act as the centre of community recycling initiatives, as bases for food co-operatives, centres for monitoring environmental health, community education centres and so on.

When he reviewed the development of school health education in 1986, Williams said that remarkably little attention had been paid to its effects on families. In the interim more attention has been given to this matter. In an earlier study Wilcox *et al.* (1981) in evaluating the My Body project reported considerable discussion between parents and children following lessons in primary schools. Murray *et al.* (1984), in a long term evaluation of the same project, examined the smoking practices of children's parents as reported by the children. They found that the overall prevalence of parents' smoking was slightly lower in the intervention group. Charlton (1986) reported differential effects on the two sexes when using a two-lesson smoking topic directed at children and their parents. Significant impact on boys and their fathers occurred but there were less positive results on girls and their mothers.

In the USA the 3 Rs High Blood Pressure Program was developed in Georgia in response to high blood pressure as a major health problem in the state. The project was based on the proposition that 6th grade students could be taught practical information about high blood pressure. They could then facilitate the health education of families and peers and help effect blood pressure control within the community (Davis *et al.*, 1985).

The very important Child to Child project, which addresses a wide range of health issues, has a somewhat similar rationale. It is an international programme designed to teach and encourage children to concern themselves with the health of their younger brothers and sisters. Adopted initially in developing countries, it is now in use in more than 70 countries. It teaches children simple prevention and curative activities which they pass on to other children and their families.

Activity sheets and teachers' guides are available in a range of languages. In some countries very attractively produced readers are available, incorporating good story lines and health themes and an excellent means of developing health education through the language part of the curriculum. A Child to Child project in Bolivia using interactive radio as the initial teaching method was reported by Fryer (1991).

A radio Health curriculum on diarrhoea prevention and oral rehydration was developed for use with the 8–13 age group who often act as carers of their younger siblings and are also involved in household activities relating to food preparation and sanitation. Because of these responsibilities it was felt to be critical that these children had the ability to make informed decisions. Interactive radio requires participants to react quickly to a series of questions and the broadcast is then reinforced immediately afterwards by teachers. This project included five broadcasts transmitted weekly followed by teacher led instruction. Teachers' guides and also take home exercises were produced. Both formative and summative evaluation were used. From a pretest/post-test comparison, significant knowledge gains were recorded. The ability of children to adopt the prescribed behaviours and to teach them to family members was reported from interviews with parents. Parents were open to children acting as 'educators' and collaborated in the production of home water filters. Parents subsequently requested that the programmes be broadcast in the evenings so that they could also participate.

There is a history in some countries of bringing members of the community in to contribute in various ways to health education in the curriculum. African countries report the involvement of parents in school water and sanitation projects. In the Welsh study discussed earlier (Nutbeam, 1987), schools were asked about the involvement of parents and outside agencies in the planning

and teaching of health education. A wide variety of people and agencies were listed, headed by the health education service and other community health services. Fifty-seven schools (78%) reported involving parents and half of the schools consulted parents in the development of health education programmes, although in relatively passive ways. One quarter of the schools teaching health education neither consulted nor informed parents.

THE OVERALL IMPACT OF SCHOOL HEALTH EDUCATION

As we discussed at the beginning of the chapter, much hope has been invested in the capacity of schools to make significant contribution to health and/or health related outcomes. Evaluative studies, many small scale, some large scale, have provided evidence of the capacity of health education in the school setting to achieve outcomes associated with the various health education approaches. We may wish to assess the total impact of school health education at national or international levels using a variety of appropriate indicators. In addition we can evaluate the range of policy and other activities which contribute to the initiation and ongoing support of school health education. These could include, for example: international as well as national and local education policies which relate to health education; specific national curriculum statements; patterns of organization of school health education; initial teacher and inservice teacher training, and intersectoral collaboration. We will consider these factors before commenting on the overall outcomes of classroom activities.

Over the years there has been a series of international policy statements on school health education. These have emerged from international conferences and various representative bodies. While it is difficult to assess the impact of such statements on policy making and implementation in individual countries, it is a level of influence that needs to be addressed. We may wish to evaluate the changing emphases over time in the content of such documents and also to study their impact. A useful example for ongoing evaluation will be the national responses within Europe to this Region's Healthy School Initiative. On a global scale evaluations of primary health care developments in the period since Alma Ata, given the importance attached to the role of the school in PHC, could have reported on this contribution. Since this document did not operationalize in detail the roles of schools in PHC, potential for evaluation was reduced.

At the national level we need to consider policies on education and the curriculum, health sector policy as it relates to schools, teacher training policy and policies in other sectors related to school health education. While concerned to examine policies which focus on the provision of health education in the curriculum, it is important to recall the earlier observation that it may be, globally, that health is improved first and foremost through the effective provision of a number of years of basic education. Within national education policies the curriculum for schools can be prescribed, either in total or for specific core areas. When this is the case health education can be specified. Where no national curriculum is laid down, as was the case in England and Wales prior to 1988, what is provided in schools results from a network of influences and constraints: examinations; governors; parents; policy documents, etc.

Taking England and Wales as the example, schools were exhorted to develop and change the curriculum by competing interests, amongst which was the lobby for health education. Most of the educational reports from the 1970s onwards encouraged the development of health education and the Department of Education produced discussion documents (DES, 1977a, b, 1985). Despite this support neither health education nor personal and social education were listed as core or foundation subjects within the new National Curriculum. Although expected to appear as a cross-curricular theme, and guidance was later provided on the knowledge, attitudes and skills to be achieved at stages of education, this area of the curriculum is not subject to statutory control.

In examining national curriculum statements it is necessary to check for the inclusion of health education, to examine the detail in which objectives might be set and also to examine whether the subject is required or advised and if required, whether or not achievements are monitored. Such documents can be variously detailed in the specification of time for health education, its organization and objectives to be set. At the same time obligations to meet national curricula will be differentially enforced – between countries and within any one country in respect to specific subjects. For example, not all countries have national monitoring of progress and where it does exist it may not apply to all named subjects within the formal curriculum. English, maths and science have been selected, for example, for testing at seven, 11 and 14 years of age in England and Wales within the National Curriculum. It may be that national curriculum documents specify some subjects as compulsory, others as voluntary. Health education may well appear in the latter category.

Although we can gain some impression of health education provision from national documents where these exhort rather than set out specific goals to which schools will be accountable, a better impression of existing provision comes from national surveys. In England and Wales a survey in 1981–2 (Williams and Roberts, 1985) reported that 85% of secondary schools and 87% of primary schools provided some formal health education although this amounted to a planned programme in less than one third of the primary and two thirds of the secondary schools. In a later Welsh survey (Nutbeam, 1987) 72 out of 76 schools reported the teaching of health education and 59 (78%) had a planned programme. Fifty-nine also reported having a person designated as responsible for co-ordinating health education and in 43 of these schools the co-ordinator had undertaken specific inservice training. Increases in the number of schools having a co-ordinator was also recorded by the Health Education Authority in England. A 1983 survey recorded 18% of primary schools and 49% of secondary schools with a health education co-ordinator. By 1989 a further survey recorded increases to 55% and 80% respectively. Nutbeam *et al.* (1987) pointed out that where planned programmes existed coverage fell short of the ideal. Relatively few schools offered health education to all pupils in all years and a higher proportion timed inputs for the later years rather than the arguably more important early ones.

With the development of health promotion there has been increased attention to the role of intersectoral collaboration in achieving goals although, as we noted at the beginning of the chapter, reference has been made to it in WHO school oriented documents for the last 30 years. The 1989 Technical Discussion on the Health of Youth said:

> Promoting health in and through schools is a major challenge. It is a challenge that can only be met through collaboration between the education sector and the health sector and with assistance from related local, national and international organizations, policy makers, funding sources and non-governmental organizations.

This was emphasized in a recent speech by Nakajima (1992) who said that such collaboration was essential for the proper management and planning of school health education programmes. Successful activity designed to improve collaboration with reference to family life education was reported by Campbell (1984) and the history of intersectoral collaboration by the education sector has been reviewed (Tilford, 1991).

Some sense of the current provision of school health education internationally emerged from a series of country reports in the *Journal of School Health* (1990) and from the Geneva Conference (WHO/UNESCO/UNICEF, 1992) in which 16 countries participated and reports from each included comment on national responsibilities, policies, training, organization, objectives and evaluation. While there is currently considerable activity directed towards developing school health education, including the development of national policies, there are wide variations in the extent and type of provision and in the importance attached to health education within the school curriculum. In some countries it continues to be a heavily medically oriented activity. Ways of organizing health education within school curricula are diverse although cross-curriculum provision is a common pattern. The importance of co-ordination is recognized but is not necessarily fully developed.

Where teacher training for health education is concerned it is apparent that there is still a long way to go. Most countries report that some health education occurs in teacher training but does not necessarily form a statutory component. While it may exist as a separately provided subject it is more often provided as part of the curriculum of other subject areas. It is probably accurate to conclude that comprehensive core courses of health education in initial teacher training are still relatively uncommon. On the basis of surveys in a number of regions in the world, Dhillon and Philip (1992) commented that teacher preparation and motivation for health education were not as they should be.

MEASURED SUCCESSES

The difficulties in providing evidence for the success of school health education at national levels is well recognized. In 1985 Newman commented that schools are organized to facilitate learning, not to conduct evaluative research. In the interim period the growing pressures on schools in many countries to be more accountable in respect of pupil achievements has, as previously noted, changed the educational climate. While there are growing expectations that evaluation will happen these do not necessarily apply equally to all subjects, with the lower status health education less open to pressures.

Pessimistic comments have been made about the general successes of school health education. The USA contributor to the Geneva Conference reported progress over the previous ten years but felt that there was evidence that the 'gap between the state-of-the-art and actual practice was larger than in any other area of the curriculum'.

Some of the better evidence which can be offered as illustrative came from national level surveys in the USA in the 1980s. The School Health Education Evaluation (SHEE) (Gunn *et al.*, 1985) was a study of four different health education programmes in 20 states and involved 30 000 children. As an evaluation it addressed the issue of the need for experimental studies of teaching carried out in exemplary fashion and also the need for representative studies of the curriculum in natural surroundings. The total evaluation included studies of the four curricula in normal classroom situations and an experimental study of the School Health Curriculum Project (referred to earlier). Reviewing the SHEE, Cooke and Walberg (1985) described it as of the highest quality with respect to inferences about causal connections and the generalizations that it promoted. Health educators now had, they said, a large scale credible study to support their advocacy for school provision. The evaluation was made using a pretest/post-test questionnaire which addressed the learning objectives that experts and parents stated to be the most important in grades 4–7. These objectives included ten knowledge areas, four attitude areas and three practice areas.

The evaluation reported significant increases in knowledge for study classrooms compared with controls. Smaller but still significant increases were also found for attitudes and self-reported practices. The effectiveness of programmes was linked, not surprisingly, to the extent to which the projects in question were fully implemented. The impact of full implementation was, however, considerably less on knowledge items than on attitude and practice ones. In other words, teachers appeared to be quite effective in meeting the specific knowledge related objectives while only partially implementing programmes involving attitudes and practices. The amount of inservice training received by the teachers was also related to programme implementation measures: the fully trained completed a greater percentage of the programmes with greater fidelity than the partly trained, who were in turn better than the untrained. The overall results of the study have been summarized.

> The study shows, in general, that health education does make a difference, that it works better when there is more of it, and that it works best when it is implemented with broad scale administrative support for teacher training, integrated material and continuity across school years.

Although received with some enthusiasm the School Evaluation Study does have its limitations. On its own admission the study sample was mainly white and middle class although the reasons for this are not clear. The follow-up period was not as long as would have been liked and the study was addressed only to younger children. Although it did focus on some outcomes associated with the empowerment approach no comprehensive assessment of these outcomes was offered. Most importantly, it needs to be stressed that the gains identified in this evaluation were recorded when the programmes concerned were in the early active stages of implementation. As very many curriculum evaluations have demonstrated, maintaining long term implementation is very difficult. A 1992 study (Smith *et al.*, 1992) followed up the original eight sites selected for support in implementing the School Health Curriculum Project. Most districts had not continued to implement the programme, giving as reasons the loss of the 'programme champion' and insufficient administrative leadership. Those districts continuing were the smaller ones who also employed a part time co-ordinator for the project.

In time, sufficient evidence may be available to make detailed comparisons of successes across countries. One of the simplest ways of monitoring achievement of some health education objectives could be through incorporation of questions and tasks in national assessment of curriculum subjects. For example, as we noted earlier the biology curriculum in Kenya includes questions on oral rehydration therapy as part of the primary school leaving examinations. Decision making skills are also an objective within the curricula of some subject areas in the England and Wales National Curriculum and could, therefore, also be examined in the examinations taken at 16.

While it might seem to be rational to identify, at a very general level, global learning objectives for school health, van den Vynckt (1992) has questioned this. She acknowledges that health education is globally relevant but that implementation is likely to be slow in many developing countries. Although there is currently much emphasis on 'comprehensive' programmes she is not clear what this means in situations where social and economic conditions limit actions. She cautions against universalizing parameters of school health. Issues and concerns will be different, she argues, depending whether you are in the 'north' or the 'south'. Transferability of some goals may not be possible where training and resources are not avail-

able. She recommends the planning of phased actions with the initiation of programmes to solve immediate and pressing needs which can serve as relevant entry points on which to build other aspects.

CONCLUSIONS

Schools are widely seen as having a key role in health education whether the desired outcomes are changing behaviours or the personal and social skills associated with empowerment. In a large number of countries there have been gradual developments of health education in the curriculum although sophisticated co-ordination of the contributory elements and appropriate back-up from teacher and inservice teacher training are slower to develop. There is a growing recognition of the contributions of all aspects of the school to health education whether or not 'health promoting school' initiatives have been set up. The potential of the school to make an ongoing contribution to primary health care has also been acknowledged, particularly in developing countries. There is now a substantial literature which has evaluated certain outcomes of school health education; individual knowledge, attitudes and health related behaviours. There is still rather less evaluation of empowerment related indicators aside from incorporation within comprehensive programmes of preventive oriented education.

It is difficult to decide on the limits of what should be evaluated as health education – the broader the aims of health education become, the more evaluation could be addressing the education process as a whole. Reviewers have all noted successes in achieving certain outcomes. Kolbe (1985) reviewed 15 meta-evaluations published between 1980 and 1985 which together synthesized the findings of several hundred studies related to nine specific areas. The most important generalization from these was that school based health education programmes consistently improve targeted health knowledge, attitudes and skills and inconsistently improve target health behaviours. We have noted, for example, the inconsistencies between smoking and alcohol education. The successes noted have been welcomed, both as achievements in their own right and as potentially useful when seeking resources for health education. Newman (1985) stressed that:

> At a time when the efficacy and efficiency of all education is under scrutiny and the public is encouraging schools to 'return to basics', supporters of subjects like health education, thought by some not to be basic, need to show the effectiveness of health instruction.

At the beginning of this chapter we noted the large number of children in the world who do not have access to school and stressed the importance of developing strategies for providing these children with effective health education. The Geneva Conference (HYGIE, 1991) gave due consideration to this issue. It said that countries need to identify the population groups involved, determine why they are not in school and design or adapt appropriate educational programmes to meet specific conditions and needs. A variety of initiatives have been set up in countries across the world. If schools increasingly see themselves as health promoting units within a wider health promoting community with which alliances are built we may expect the development of outreach activities which could make a substantial contribution to the health of 'out of school' children.

We have noted as a weakness of school health education its relative slowness to consider the social and environmental causes of health and to debate collective as opposed to individually focused solutions to the problems of ill health. Some evaluators have stressed the need to give greater emphasis to the social contexts of young people when designing health education activities. The evidence of the participation of young people in planning, implementing and evaluating health education activities still does not emerge particularly strongly from the literature, although high levels of participation may take place in some contexts of practice.

Finally, if the range of expectations which are held for health education are to be achieved schools need to offer comprehensive, co-ordinated programmes, backed up by adequate resources, teacher training and continuity through the school years. Last, but perhaps most important of all, health education should be responsive to young people's expressed needs and they should also be able to play a participatory role in the evaluation which takes place.

REFERENCES

Aarons, A. (ed.) (1979) *Child to Child*, Macmillan, London.

ALTARF (1984) *Challenging Racism*, ALTARF, London.

Anderson, J. (1986), Health skills: the power to choose. *Health Education Journal*, **45**(1), 19–24.

Anderson, J. (1988) *HEA Health Skills Project: Training Manual*, Counselling and Career Development Unit, University of Leeds, Leeds.

Bagnall, G. (1987) Alcohol education and its evaluation: some key issues. *Health Education Journal*, **46**, 162–5.

Bartlett, E.E. (1981) The contribution of school health education to community health promotion: what can we reasonably expect? *American Journal of Public Health*, **17**, 1384–91.

Botvin, G.J., Eng, A. and Williams, C.L. (1980) A comprehensive school based smoking prevention program. *Journal of School Health*, **50**, 209–13.

Bremberg, S. (1991) Does school health education affect the health of students, in: *Youth Health Promotion: From Theory to Practice in School and Community* (eds Nutbeam, D., Haglund, B., Farley, P., and Tillgren, P.) Forbes Publications

Bremberg, S. and Arborelius, S. (1991) A student centred health education model at school for adolescents in Sweden: it's your decision – evaluation and implementation, in *Youth Health Promotion: From Theory to Practice in School and Community*, (eds D. Nutbeam, B. Haglund,

P. Farley and P. Tillgren), Forbes Publications, London.

Brierley, J. (1983) Health education in secondary schools, *Health Education Journal*, **42**, 48–52.

Campbell, G. 1984 Interprofessional cooperation in school health education, in *Health Education and Youth*, (ed. G. Campbell), The Falmer Press, London.

Charlton, A. (1980) An experimental methodology for HE in teacher training: a baseline survey with reference to cancer. *International Journal of Health Education*, **XXIII**, 25–34.

Charlton, A. (1986) Accuracy in the measurement of the prevalence of smoking in young people. *Health Education Journal*, **45**, 140–4.

Clarity Collective (1985) *Taught not Caught: Strategies for Sex Education*, LDA, Cambs.

Cooke, T.D. and Walberg, H.J. (1985) Methodological and substantive significance. *Journal of School Health*, **55**, 340–2.

Davis, R.L., Gonser, H.L., Kirkpatrick, M.A., Lavery, S.W. and Owen, S.L. (1985) Comprehensive school health education: a practical definition. *Journal of School Health*, **55**, 335–9.

Department of Education and Science (1977a) *Education in Schools: a Consultative Document*, HMSO, London.

Department of Education and Science (1977b) *Curriculum 11–16*, HMSO, London.

Department of Education and Science (1985) *Health Education from 5–16*, HMSO, London.

De Vries, H., Djikstra, M. and Kok, G. (1992) A Dutch smoking prevention project: an overview. *HYGIE*, **XI**(2), 14–18.

Dhillon, H.S. and Philip, L. (1992) Health in education for all: enabling school age children and adults for healthy living. *HYGIE*, **XI**(3), 17–27.

Dorn, N. and Nortoft, B. (1982) *Health Careers*, Institute for the Study of Drug Dependence, London.

Duryea, E. (1983) Decision making and health education. *Journal of School Health*, **53**, 29–32.

Eisemon, T.O. and Patel, V.L. (1990) Strengthening the effects of schooling on health practices in Kenya. *HYGIE*, **IX**(3), 24–9.

Evans, R.I., Rozelle, R.M., Mittelmark, M.B. *et al.* (1978) Deterring the onset of smoking in children: knowledge of immediate physiological effects and coping with peer pressure, media pressure and parental modeling. *Journal of Applied Social Psychology*, **78**, 126–35.

Flay, B.R. (1986) Psychosocial approaches to smoking prevention: a review of findings. *Health Psychology*, **4**, 449–88.

Fryer, M.L. (1991) Health education through interactive radio: a child-to child project in Bolivia. *Health Education Quarterly*, **18**(1), 65–77.

Hansen, W.B. (1992) School based substance abuse prevention: a review of the state of the art in curriculum 1980–90. *Health Education Research*, **7**(3), 403–31.

Health Education Council (1983a) *My Body*, Heinemann Education, London.

HEC/Dental Health Study (1984) *Natural Nashers*, HEC, London.

Hewett, A. (1992) Life, health and the community. *HYGIE*, **XI**(3), 33–6.

Janis, I. and Mann, L. (1977) *Decision Making*, Free Press, New York.

Journal of School Health (1990) (whole issue) International Perspectives on School Health, **60**(7).

Kolbe, L. (1985) Why school health education? An empirical point of view. *Health Education*, **16**, 115–20.

Lammers, J.W., Kreuter, M.W. and Smith, B.C. (1984) The effects of the SHCP on selected aspects of decision making among 5th graders. *Health Education*, **15**, 14–18.

Mason, J.O. and McGinnis, J.M. (1985) The role of school health. *Journal of School Health*, **55**, 299.

Mauss, A.L., Hopkins, R.H., Weisheit, R.A. and Kearney, K.A. (1988) The problematic aspects of prevention in the classroom: should alcohol education programmes be expected to reduce drinking by youth? *Journal of Studies in Alcohol*, **49**, 51–61.

May, C. (1991) Research on alcohol education for young people: a critical review of the literature. *Health Education Journal*, **50**, 195–9.

May, C. (1993) Resistance to peer group pressure: an inadequate basis for alcohol education. *Health Education Research*, **8**(2), 159–65.

Maysey, D.L., Gimarc, J.D. and Kronenfeld, J.J. (1988) School worksite wellness programs: a strategy for achieving the 1990 goals for a healthier America. *Health Education Quarterly*, **15**, 53–62.

McAlister, A., Perry, C. and Maccoby, N. (1979) Adolescent smoking: onset and prevention. *Paediatrics*, **63**, 650–8.

McEwan, R.T., Bhopal, R. and Patton, W. (1991) Drama on HIV and AIDS: an evaluation of a theatre-in-education programme. *Health Education Journal*, **50**(4), 155–60.

Murray, M., Swan, A.N. and Clarke, G. (1984) Long term effects of a school based anti-smoking programme. *Journal of Epidemiology and Community Health*, **38**, 247–52.

Newman, I. (1985) Comments from the field. *Journal of School Health*, **55**, 343–5.

Nakajima, H. (1992) Health, united efforts. *HYGIE*, **XI**(2), 5–7.

Nutbeam, D. (1987) Smoking among primary and secondary teachers. *Health Education Journal*, **46**, 14–21.

Nutbeam, D., Clarkson, J., Phillips, K. *et al.* (1987) The health-promoting school: organization and policy development in Welsh secondary schools. *Health Education Journal*, **46**, 109–15.

Owen, S.L., Kirkpatrick, M.A., Lavery, S.W. *et al.* (1985) Selecting and recruiting health programs for the school health education evaluation. *Journal of School Health*, **55**, 305–8.

Reid, D. and Massey, D. (1986) Can school health education be more effective? *Health Education Journal*, **45**, 7–13.

Schools Council/HEC Project (1977) *Health Education 5–13*, T. Nelson and Sons, London.

Schools Council/HEC Project (1982) *Health Education 13–18*, Forbes Publications, London.

Smith, C., Nutbeam, D., Roberts, G. and Macdonald, G. (1992) The health promoting school: progress and future challenges in Welsh secondary schools. *Health Promotion International*, **7**(3), 171–80.

Tilford, S. (1991) *Intersectoral Collaboration and the Education Sector*. Background paper, Intersectoral Collaboration and Health For All Project, Leeds Metropolitan University.

United Nations (1989) Draft convention on the rights of the child, in *The Next Generation: Lives of Third World Children*, (eds J. Ennew and B. Milne), Zed Books, London.

Van den Vynckt, S. (1992) Primary school health: where are we and where are we going? *HYGIE*, **XI**(3), 45–9.

Wilcox, B., Gillies, P., Wilcox, J. and Reid, D.J. (1981) Do children influence their parents' smoking? *Health Education Journal*, **40**, 5–10.

Williams, T. (1986) School health education 15 years on. *Health Education Journal*, **45**, 3–7.

Williams, T. and de Panafieu, C.W. (1985) *School Health Education in Europe*, Health Education Unit, University of Southampton.

Williams, T. and Roberts, J. (1985) *Health Education in Schools and Teacher Training Institutions*, Health Education Unit, Department of Education, Southampton University.

World Health Organization (1951) *Technical Report Series 30*, Expert Committee on School Health Services, WHO, Geneva.

World Health Organization (1954) *Technical Report Series 89*, Expert Committee on Health Education of the Public, WHO, Geneva.

World Health Organization (1966) *Planning for Health Education in Schools*, WHO, Geneva.

World Health Organization (1977) *The Health Needs of Adolescents*, Report of a WHO Expert Committee, Technical Report Series 308, WHO, Geneva.

World Health Organization (1978) *Primary Health Care: Report of the Conference on Primary Health Care*, WHO, Geneva.

World Health Organization (1979) *The Child and Adolescent in Society*, Report on a WHO Conference, Copenhagen, WHO European Regional Office, Copenhagen.

World Health Organization (1983) *Expert Committee on New Approaches to Health Education in Primary Health Care*, WHO, Geneva.

World Health Organization (1986) *Young People's Health: A Challenge for Society*, Report of a WHO Study Group on Young People and 'Health For All by the year 2000', Technical Report Series 731, WHO, Geneva.

World Health Organization (1989) *The Health of Youth*, WHO, Geneva.

World Health Organization (1990) *Enabling School-Age Children and Adults for Healthy Living*, Report prepared for the World Conference on Education for All, Jontien, Thailand, WHO, Geneva.

World Health Organization (1991) *Promoting the Health of Young People in Europe: A Training Manual*, Scottish Health Education Group, Edinburgh.

WHO/UNESCO/UNICEF (1992) Comprehensive school health education: suggested guidelines for education. *HYGIE*, **X1**(3), 8–15.

Young, I.M. 1992 The health promoting school encouraging parental involvement. *HYGIE*, **XI**(3), 40–44.

INTRODUCTION

In 1974 the President's Committee on Health Education in the USA described it as an integral part of high quality health care. Hospitals and other health care institutions had obligations to promote, organize, implement and evaluate health education programmes. Four years later the Alma Ata Declaration on Primary Health Care (WHO, 1978) located health education as the focal activity in the development of acceptable and accessible primary health care. In the interim period official statements in many countries have made recommendations on education in health care settings, of which *The Health of the Nation* in Britain is a recent example (DOH, 1992).

This chapter will examine health education in primary care and hospital settings around themes addressed in previous chapters: the conceptions of health education held in these contexts, debates on philosophical approaches, the organization and delivery of health education and the nature and outcomes of evaluation activities. As in the previous chapter it is not intended to provide comprehensive reviews of evaluative studies of which a growing number exist (Mullen *et al.*, 1985, 1992; Haynes *et al.*, 1987; Simons-Morton *et al.*, 1992).

TERMINOLOGY

Some initial comment is called for on terminology. The literature includes a variety of terms to cover educational activities in hospitals and primary care: health education, patient education, client education, patient counselling, health promotion, patient teaching and so on. While there is some consistency in the use of terms there is also confusion. A particular difficulty is associated with the varying usage of 'health promotion' – at times describing a total package of education, health care and policy, at other times specific health education activities. The differential use may not always matter but it can be significant if it leads to failures in communicating about and developing effective practice.

In examining health promotion in health care settings as a totality, different strands of activity can be identified. In addition to preventive and curative health care we can identify three strands of activity as shown in Table 5.1.

The distinction between patient education and general health education may seem an artificial and inappropriate one to make if we are taking a holistic approach to people but it does reflect much of the existing literature. Early work in health care contexts, especially in hospital settings, was oriented towards education specific to the immediate condition and only later was general health education given more attention. The use of 'patient' rather than 'client' is also open to criticism. The former term is said to carry connotations of the passive recipient of whatever aspect of health care is under consideration and 'client' is preferred. The term 'client', notwithstanding the growing consumerism in many health services, may also be challenged as not fully reflecting the relationship between users and providers of health services. Since the term

Table 5.1 Health promotion in health care

Patient education	General health education	Health promotion policy
Condition specific education with patients. Frequently focused on tertiary levels of prevention but includes activities directed to primary and secondary prevention	Aimed at primary prevention and promotion of positive health. For hospital patients and hospital workers. For patients in GP consultation in primary care. For all people on GP practice lists	General or specific health promotion policies. Focused on health care institutions or local communities

'patient education' remains widely used in the literature it will be used in this chapter to describe education that takes place with people who are participating in health care but does not imply a particular relationship between them and health care workers.

APPROACHES TO EDUCATION IN HEALTH CARE SETTINGS

As in other contexts, a diversity of approaches to education exists in health care contexts. Until comparatively recently education in hospitals was largely a condition specific activity with patients and strongly influenced by a preventive medical model. Much of the health education in primary care was also oriented to achieving lifestyle change. With the development of conceptions of the patient as an active rather than as a passive participant in health care, elements of educational and empowerment approaches have been more apparent. Much of the debate about approaches has centred on the activity of 'patient education' and Fahrenfort (1987) commented:

> In sum the call for patient education or information comes from two different directions – a patient centred one in which autonomy is the key word and a medico-centred one in which compliance still reigns.

These two calls for patient education have generated what can be seen as two literatures using two rather different languages, different arguments for providing education and different criteria for assessing outcomes. The language of the two approaches is illustrated in Table 5.2.

Actual practice does not fall neatly into one or other of these polarized positions and it may be more helpful to see them as points on a continuum. Individuals or specific occupational groups may adhere consistently to one position or the approach may vary according to client group, health condition and the preferences expressed by patients. The differences of approach can give rise to conflicts: between professional groups; within professional groups; between health professionals and patients and between patients themselves. In some circumstances people may be seeking an active involvement in the specification of their educational needs and be denied it; at other times there may be reluctance to respond to opportunities for active involvement and a preference for a passive role.

There have been advocates of both preventive and educational approaches throughout the history of patient education. Early demands for education were a response to the acknowledged lack of compliance with prescribed medical regimens and to the perceived need to secure behavioural change in the prevention of contemporary chronic diseases.

Table 5.2 Language and meaning associated with approaches to patient education

Medico-centred	Patient-centred
Compliance	Autonomy
Adherence	Patient participation
Planning for patients	Planning with patients
Behaviour change	Decision making/empowerment
Passive patient	Active ('activated') patient
Dependence	Independence
Professionally determined needs	Patient defined needs
Patient	Client

The term 'compliance' fitted in with the classic Parsonian model of the patient role – passive, dependent, co-operating with the doctor and an unequal partner in the relationship.

With the recognition that in many chronic conditions the individual needed to be more fully involved in the working out of lifestyle changes and in planning adherence to complex regimens, a development from the guidance/co-operation model to a mutual participation model was proposed (Szasz and Hollender, 1956). Although this model may appear to use more patient centred language its underlying implication is that patients will comply with rational behaviour as defined by the professional. Health services were first persuaded of the value of patient education because of its reported successes in improving compliance, increasing patient satisfaction and contributing to reducing costs of care. From the 1960s onwards a number of social movements led to a challenge to compliance oriented patient education. These included the women's, consumer, primary health care (WHO, 1978) and self-care movements. Although the focus of their concerns with health issues varied they shared a commitment to self-determination and active participation in health care. Rights to information and to an active role in health decision making were central concerns and the language of compliance was rejected.

There can be little surprise at the long term dominance and continuing prominence of preventive approaches to education in health care contexts, given their commitment to the medical model. It is rather more useful to consider the extent to which it is possible to move towards a wider acceptance and adoption of empowerment models. This issue was discussed by Fahrenfort (1987) who identified a gap between the promotion of patient emancipation and self-empowerment in theory and the possibilities of achieving these goals in practice. She found examples of humanistic patient centredness, more often in nurses than in doctors, but saw this as a long way from incorporating what Freire described as dialogue. This would imply not simply two-way communication in which doctors took notice of patients and their needs but would require a conviction on the part of doctors that the patient's own knowledge was as relevant to the situation as medical knowledge.

In actual practice, Fahrenfort contends, medical knowledge remains the norm in the hospital situation and is consolidated in two ways: through the assumption that it is medical knowledge that is to be disseminated to patients and through patients' own efforts to gain power in the situation by appropriating medical knowledge. In the process patients become 'lesser' doctors but the real doctors remain the guardians of the knowledge that is imparted in efforts to educate.

Considerable practical barriers also exist to the establishment of true dialogue: sufficient time, for example, may be difficult to secure in the relatively short periods of time people are typically in contact with health care institutions. Were success to occur, Fahrenfort suggests, it could not survive sanctions from medical practitioners towards truly autonomous patients. She concluded that patient education is not the royal road to emancipation.

Roter (1987), in a further examination of models for patient education, offers a 2 × 2 model which addresses, in particular, decision making and responsibility in client–provider relations (Figure 5.1). Of the four possible models, she sees the 'active participation' one as meeting ethical and philosophical concerns and meeting the realities of therapeutic encounters. This model assumes that the interaction should at minimum provide a client with a basis for effective participation in sound decision making.

It has to be asked if there is a general wish of patients for an active participatory role in health care. Steele, in reviewing the active patient concept, notes that patients in general want to be informed about their illnesses and the treatment options open to them. He argues, however, that while there is evidence that some patients do desire an active role in decision making and may benefit from such a role, there is little evidence that this is sought by most patients in most situations.

To summarize, there has been debate between supporters of the different approaches to education in health care contexts with a growing importance attached to approaches advocating active patient participation. In some situations lip service may be paid to autonomy although in practice there may be little fundamental change from a major objective of securing compliance. The degree to which full autonomy for patients is possible has been questioned. Patients also vary in the extent to which they seek active participation and the same individuals may not consistently adopt one particular stance on participation. While the debates about approaches can be pursued at a theoretical level, for those involved in day-to-day health care the diversity of views leads to questions and dilemmas which may demand resolution. For example:

1. Should education respond to needs expressed by the patient or should it be professionally determined?
2. Should a major aim of education in health care settings be the achievement of behaviour change and associated health outcomes?
3. To what extent should education be directed towards achieving outcomes with demonstrable economic benefits?
4. In situations where a number of professional groups contribute to health education how can differences of view about approaches be resolved?
5. Is it acceptable to let patients make their own decisions if these turn out to be contrary to professionally recommended ones?
6. Can health services accept working to outcomes determined by patients?

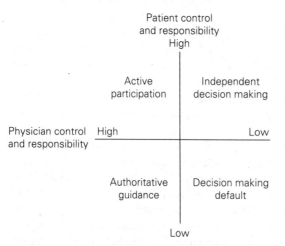

Figure 5.1 Decision making control and responsibility dimensions of client–provider relations.

THE DEVELOPMENT AND ORGANIZATION OF EDUCATION IN HEALTH CARE CONTEXTS

Initially it is convenient to discuss primary care and hospital situations separately although later it will be argued that much better co-ordination is needed between the two sectors if education is to be a more coherent activity and, in the end, a more successful one. While the importance of education for patients in hospital settings would not be challenged in terms of the proportion of patient contacts and the continuing relationships with patients, primary care is arguably the most important sector for health education. In this section we will look briefly at the historical development of education in these settings as reflected in official documents and other reports. Later in the chapter the overall effectiveness of these settings as contexts for health care will be addressed.

PRIMARY HEALTH CARE

Primary care describes all those health services provided outside the hospital sector. Globally the term primary health care is associated with the Alma Ata Declaration from which originated the goal of Health For All 2000 (WHO, 1978). Alma Ata laid down principles for the development of comprehensive primary health care (PHC) as the means by which this goal might be achieved. PHC was to be acceptable and accessible essential health care for individuals and their families, involving full community participation and at a cost that families, communities and countries could afford. It was intended that PHC should provide preventive, curative and rehabilitative services and include eight essential components, of which health education was to be the central one. The others were to be:

1. Basic sanitation and an adequate source of safe water;
2. Healthful nutrition and a secure food supply;
3. Maternal and child care, including family planning;
4. Immunization against the major infectious diseases;
5. Prevention of endemic diseases;
6. Appropriate treatment of common ailments;
7. A supply of essential medications

The first level of care would depend on the activities of community health workers, nominated by communities and given some basic training to enable them to deal with a delimited range of activities and the skills to refer upwards to the next level of care. The community or village health workers would not typically be paid for their services although support in kind would be provided by their communities and work would be undertaken alongside other roles in the community. While there have been variations in the ways in which PHC programmes have developed there has been broad implementation of the village health worker concept.

The ideas enshrined in the Alma Ata Declaration were not new and represented, it has been said, 'less a birth than an endorsement of an idea whose time, by popular consensus, had come' (Mull, 1990). While the slogan of HFA 2000 has become universal the relevance of PHC for those countries which already had well established systems of comprehensive and professionally delivered health care has not been fully acknowledged. There is to some extent a view that PHC is a strategy for developing countries and unnecessary in developed ones. Green (1987a) pointed to the confusion which still existed in some minds between primary health care and primary health care services. He argued that the UK, although a signatory to Alma Ata, had failed to provide an adequate framework for a PHC strategy and much remained to be done in order to achieve the principles of primary health care. A particularly good example of the gap between principle and practice is offered by community participation.

While there are many examples of initiatives which are true to the principle there are other situations where 'community participation' is being used as a label for activities which are more narrowly focused.

In the UK primary care services deal with nine out of ten contacts with the health services and most of these contacts are patient initiated. These services include the management of illness and a variety of activities with the well population registered with a practice. Except in emergencies and in the case of some minor injuries, access to hospital care is by referral from primary care. Ninety per cent of family doctors work in practices employing some ancillary staff and most practice in groups. The membership of primary care teams varies but it is common to have, in addition to general practitioners, practice nurses, health visitors, community nurses, district nurses and midwives.

Increasingly health education has been recognized as an essential element of professionalized primary medical care although not ascribed the same pivotal role as within PHC. The role of education will vary between countries but its development and place within the National Health Service in the UK provides an illustrative example. Over the last ten years or so a number of reports and official documents have provided comment on health education and prevention in primary care. These have included the document *Care in Action* (DHSS, 1981), reports from the Royal College of General Practitioners (RCGP, 1981a, 1981b), consultative documents (DHSS, 1986, 1987a), Project 2000 (UKCC, 1986) and government White Papers (DHSS, 1987b; DOH, 1992). *Care in Action* emphasized individual responsibility for prevention and it looked at ways that the NHS, in adopting a preventive role, could provide the information people needed to make sensible decisions about personal health. It said that health authorities should insist on commitment to policies on health promotion and preventive medicine, ensure

resources are directed to these purposes and establish priorities for programmes which meet the health interests of local populations.

The Royal College of General Practitioners (RCGP, 1981a) noted existing preventive work in primary care and identified particular subjects for health education within the normal consultation: antenatal and postnatal care; smoking; assessment of coronary risk status and family planning. Further activities which would involve co-operation with other members of the primary care team and require identification of people not necessarily presenting for consultation included primary immunization, developmental surveillance and preventive work with older people. In addition, suggestions were made for prevention through working with others in the community.

The 1986 consultative document on primary care (DHSS, 1986) identified as key objectives the promotion of health and the prevention of illness as key objectives and the subsequent *Promoting Better Health* (DHSS, 1987b) stated that the government wished to strengthen the GP's role in health promotion by:

1. Paying special fees to encourage doctors to provide health checks and necessary follow-up to patients registering for the first time with an NHS doctor;
2. Considering incentives to achieve specified target levels of vaccination, immunization and screening, as well as to meet the costs of call and recall;
3. Considering amendments to doctors' terms of service to clarify their role in the provision of health promotion services and the prevention of ill health.

While these documents use the terms 'prevention', 'health education' and 'health promotion', they contain little which goes beyond a preventive model of health education. Project 2000, which addressed the education and training needed for nursing, midwifery and health visiting, was a more wide ranging document as far as health promotion is concerned and said that in exploring future needs it was concerned to examine trends in social life, health and disease (UKCC, 1986). A reorientation in initial training towards the community was called for and health promotion should be given high priority as a topic in its own right as well as being considered separately for each care group.

The *Working for Patients* document (DHSS, 1989), which incorporated a range of reforms for the NHS, enabled GP practices, initially larger ones, to hold their own budgets. In the same year a new contract for general practitioners was introduced with the aims of 'increasing consumer choice, bringing health promotion and disease prevention within the general medical services, strengthening management and budgetary control and making remuneration more dependent on performance' (Hannay, 1992). The contract included a number of specific measures designed to encourage health promotion, including payments for the following activities: health checks for defined groups; achievement of targets for immunization and for cervical screening uptake; and health promotion clinics. Activities encouraged include well person screening, antismoking groups and clinics for the management of stress, diabetes, hypertension and asthma. The contract requires a medical examination and preventive health advice to be offered to all patients aged 16 to 74 years who have not consulted in the previous three years. The developments of health education have to compete with other costed activities and this is likely to influence the adoption of wide ranging health promotion activities.

Finally, the recent *Health of the Nation*, the first strategy document for health in Britain, has put particular emphasis on disease prevention and health promotion and prescribed targets. A range of key areas or settings are identified for health promotion activities and there is emphasis on the formation of alliances between settings in order to progress targets. The document asserts that primary and community health care services will have a major role in achieving successes and that ways will be explored of developing the existing health promotion arrangements in primary care in response to the national strategy. The focus on key targets for action and specific settings may be expected to impose a level of constraint on such health promotion activity which appears to fall outwith the target areas.

HOSPITALS

In 1991 the WHO issued a Health Promoting Hospital declaration (WHO, 1991) and hospitals have been identified as one of the key settings in *The Health of the Nation*. The latter document affirms that hospitals exist to provide treatment and care but they also offer unique opportunities for more general health promotion of patients, staff and all who come into contact with them. Prior to this focus on general health promotion policy there had been a slow development of specific health promotion policies in this setting – nutrition and smoking being common targets in some countries, joined more recently by breastfeeding. The recent WHO/UNICEF Baby Friendly Hospital Initiative asks every health care facility where babies are born to re-examine their policies in the light of current knowledge and to implement the 'Ten Steps to Successful Breastfeeding' (Donovan, 1992). The health promotion developments in hospitals represent a broadening out from the long term emphasis on specific patient education and criteria that may be used in assessing this role will be noted later.

The USA has one of the longer histories of commitment to the hospital-wide education of patients. While some of the influences which contributed to this development are general, others were more specific to the form of organization of its health care. At a 1964 conference, the American Hospital Association took the position that it should act as the nationwide agency for stimulating the development of patient education. Education was recommended as an integral part of patient care and thus a direct responsibility of hospital personnel. This conference was noted as one emphasis, together with the consumers' rights movement, for a Patient's Bill of Rights (American Hospital Association, 1972) approved by the House of Delegates in 1973 and which stated that the patient has 'the right to obtain from his physicians complete and current information concerning diagnosis and treatment in terms that he can reasonably be expected to understand'.

By 1974 the President's Committee on Health Education emphasized the importance of reorientating the health care system to the maintenance of good health and prevention rather than primarily to the treatment of acute illness. In the same year the Blue Cross Association reflected on the demands for health care systems to improve their effectiveness and efficiency and, while assuring quality of health care services, to contain rising health care costs. The cost effectiveness of patient education was noted and this has been a recurring theme in the patient education literature. A further statement by the American Hospital Association in 1981 said:

> Patient education services should enable patients and their families, when appropriate, to make informed decisions about their health, to manage their illnesses and to implement follow-up care at home.

While other countries have looked to the USA for emerging wisdom on patient education their own developments have not followed identical directions. The language of rights has been somewhat less evident in discussion and the attention to the economic benefits of patient education was less predominant (until recently) in those countries where the basis of funding for health care was different from the USA.

EVALUATION OF EDUCATION IN HEALTH CARE SETTINGS

Following the pattern of the previous chapter we will examine the effectiveness of individually focused education followed by some consideration of the factors which contribute to the overall success of education in health care settings.

As discussed earlier, education is viewed by some primarily as a means to increase patient adherence to regimens and the management of conditions while for others it is a tool for enhancing patient participation in care and diminishing the power differential between patients and professionals. A distinction between outcomes, intermediate and indirect indicators has been used in earlier chapters. This division will be adopted here although it needs to be emphasized that in the terms of one approach a measured variable may be an outcome while in another it would class as an intermediate indicator. For example, within the preventive model, decision making skills are intermediate to the making of responsible decisions associated with desired health outcomes but within the self-empowerment model these same skills would be the specified outcome. Similarly if an educational programme is responding to patients' expressed wishes for information, patient satisfaction could be an outcome measure but where it is believed to motivate desired behaviour change, measures of satisfaction become an intermediate indicator.

Table 5.3 gives some examples of indicators which can be used in evaluating all aspects of health promotion in health care settings and Table 5.4 illustrates measures which may be undertaken at the various interacting levels of activity.

In the preceding chapter a number of features of schools which had a bearing on evaluation were outlined. In the same way there are features of health care contexts which affect education and evaluation.

Table 5.3 Evaluating success

Outcomes	Intermediate indicators	Indirect indicators
Behaviours, e.g. adherence to medication, dietary change, smoking Decision making skills Active participation Campaigning for services Development and implementation of health promotion policy Cost savings Health: mortality, morbidity and subjective health measures Medication use Personality measures: self-esteem, locus of control, autonomy Anxiety Patient satisfaction Professional satisfaction	Beliefs Attitudes Decision making skills Closed-circuit television use Self-esteem Locus of control Knowledge Informed consent Behaviours	Patient education libraries Closed-circuit television provision Uptake of leaflets Provision of leaflets Shared records Professional collaboration Health education in professional training Co-ordination Education policy Planned programmes of patient education Informed consent legislation Professional motivation Professional collaboration Co-ordination of patient education activities Sharing patient record

1. In contrast to schools (where the one professional group, teachers, carry the main responsibility for the educational process) several professional groups have roles to play in both primary care and hospitals.

2. The longstanding dominance of the medical profession in health care has significance for an activity such as health education which depends on interprofessional collaboration for its full success.

3. The education of patients is increasingly seen as an activity where nurses, particularly in hospital settings, have a major role.

4. The barriers to the acceptance and implementation of educational and self-empowerment approaches may be greater than in other settings.

5. The pressures to demonstrate the effectiveness of education in cost saving terms may be strong and pervasive.

6. With the increasing practice of setting health targets, whether at international, national or regional levels, activities which fall outside the targets may be more difficult to initiate and justify.

7. While there is evidence of much expressed demand for education it is not necessarily a major or even a minor priority for all people seeking health care.

It is not possible to review activities oriented to the full range of indicators listed above. Increasingly meta-evaluations have been provided of specific areas of patient education to which the reader will be referred. We will focus on the levels of activity

Table 5.4 Levels of activity

Individual	Institution	Policy
Compliance and adherence	Patient education	Health education in
Health measures	co-ordinators	initial training for all
Personality measures	Education as routine	health professionals
Satisfaction	part of consultation	Appointment of patient
Decision making skills	in primary care	education co-ordinators
Active participation	Patient education in	Inservice education
Compliance	care of hospital patients	Health promotion policy
Health related behaviours	Provision of audio-visual	in NHS
	material, leaflets and	
	other resources	
	Health education for	
	at-risk groups in primary	
	care, etc.	
	Smoking policy	

in Table 5.4 and offer discussion of a number of indicators which either reflect the balance of work in the patient education literature or reflect particular concerns associated with ideological positions. While much evaluation literature may be reporting on single or a restricted range of indicators, it is equally important to comment on the extent to which the full range of educational needs is met in educational encounters.

INDIVIDUAL LEVEL

We will discuss a number of specific indicators and then look at examples of comprehensive programmes. As in the schools chapter, we will begin by looking at knowledge and information, followed by discussion of behavioural outcomes with particular reference to compliance and adherence which have a substantial place in patient education literature. Taking up the concerns of the empowerment model, the activities and successes in achieving patient participation will then be considered prior to comment on integrated activities.

KNOWLEDGE AND INFORMATION

There is extensive evidence of low levels of knowledge about the aspects of health which bring people into contact with health care settings. Daltroy and Liang (1993), for example, report Hull *et al.*'s finding that 65% of arthritis patients could not name their diagnosis. It is also routine for users of health care services to register their needs for information and equally routine for the literature to record shortcomings in meeting such needs. Dekkers (1980) concluded from a review of several investigations that between 30% and 40% of hospital patients are not satisfied with the information they receive. It is not only patients but also their families and friends who have informational needs. Meissner *et al.* (1990) analysed the unmet needs of the significant others of cancer patients as reflected in the calls to the Cancer Information Service in the USA. The leading three areas of information need were the same for both significant others and diagnosed patients: cancer site, treatment and referral/second opinion. Brooker (1990) has examined the unmet information needs of carers in the case of schizophrenia and concluded that a paramount need is for information about the actual condition.

Information needs can include: the wish for information on the existence, the causes and prognosis of specific diseases; the need for anticipatory guidance for hospitalization and surgery; information necessary to support rehabilitation; sources of future support both material and personal and so on. Information needs may be the specific outcome sought or may be intermediate to meeting other goals. The levels of dissatisfaction recorded with the meeting of informational needs vary with respect to a range of variables including the particular parties involved in a communication process, the area of health, the specific area of information and the country and context in question.

The failure to meet information needs satisfactorily can happen for reasons of **omission:** oversights, disruption from competing activities, inappropriate timing of informational inputs, inadequate provision of written materials; poor professional communication; or **commission:** denying informational needs and knowingly withholding information. Whether the failures are due to unintentional or intentional reasons does not necessarily affect the patients but does have implications for specifying ways of improving future practice. Korsch and Negrete's early study (1972) of 800 separate mother–doctor interactions illustrated the failure to provide adequate information. Almost half of the mothers left the consultation still unsure about what had caused their child's illness and 20% felt that the illness had been properly explained. It could, of course, be suggested that if the other 80% were satisfied this was a good outcome.

There can be one or more of a number of causes where failure occurs: that doctors had not adequately elicited or patients had not fully expressed information needs, the information conveyed was not fully tailored to needs or was inadequately communicated.

Professionals have reported difficulties in assessing patient needs. In a study of informed consent with consultants in eight countries, Taylor and Kilner (1987) reported that 40% said that it was always difficult to assess patients' desire for information.

A number of reasons have been offered for the conscious withholding of information. These include the reluctance to convey uncertainty, the difficulties associated with giving bad news and holding back information as a means of maintaining control. For example, Davis's (1963) study of parents and children with poliomyelitis reported that where the prognosis was fairly well established health professionals still maintained it was uncertain. Holding back the information served to delay the obligation to counsel and comfort. A further illustration was provided by Elian and Dean (1985) who were allowed to work with a consultant's patients as long as these patients did not find out that they had multiple sclerosis. And yet, of 167 interviewed, 83% favoured knowing their diagnosis and 137 actually did know it – 40 having received the information from a doctor rather than a consultant, 32 had diagnosed themselves and a large number had found out by accident. Only 45 had been informed by the consultant. An editorial in the edition of *The Lancet* that contained the study report said:

> ... It is indefensible on ethical and humanitarian grounds that patients should be left to make one of the most devastating discoveries in their lives by accident and without any professional support or explanation.

Providing for informed consent is an aspect of health care which requires a full sharing of information. In Taylor and Kilner's study (1987) of doctors' perspectives on informed consent, 95% of respondents saw the consent requirement as an intrusion into the doctor–patient relationship. Fifty per cent also felt that when consent was associated with participation in a randomized controlled trial the doctor's dual role as both scientist and caregiver was exposed. In their study no association was found between the legal requirements in specific countries on informed consent and the amount of information physicians actually reported giving to their patients. While some of the doctors' comments reflected a concern that the regulations for informed consent interfered with the sensitive sharing of information as and when patients were ready for it, there was also evidence of physicians' claims to rights to control information. Only 37% of respondents in the study believed that the best judge of the amount of information disclosed should be the patient.

The variations in patients' informational needs should not, of course, be overlooked or underestimated. Cassileth *et al.* (1980) examined information preferences among cancer patients. People who sought detailed information tended to be younger, as were those who wanted as much information as possible, whether good or bad news. Preferences were independent of sex.

If the exchange of information between doctors and patients is to be more effective closer studies of these interactions is required. An important study was that of Tuckett *et al.* (1985) who studied 1302 consultations between doctors and patients. Their aim was to explore the extent to which ideas were shared in the medical consultation and they started from the view that the consultation was a meeting between experts: the doctor with scarce specialist knowledge and the patient, by dint of experience, immersion in a culture and past experience, having a set of ideas about the issue of concern. The researchers examined the information that doctors chose to seek from and give to patients and the information that patients sought from or volunteered to doctors.

A main finding of the study was that the consultation was a one-sided affair: doctors and patients did not achieve a full dialogue and did not exchange ideas to any great degree. Doctors spent a fair amount of time sharing what they thought but much less

trying to share what patients thought. Doctors did little to encourage patients to present their views and often actually inhibited them, evaded what they did say, did not tailor information to the known details of patients' lives and the few efforts that were made to establish patients' ideas and explanations were brief to the point of being absent. On the other hand, patients offered little which would have triggered dialogue; as they neither made clear nor were helped to make clear their ideas, they could not receive explanations in reaction.

Only some aspects of information sharing between patients and health professionals have been mentioned here, but from the evidence noted and from other studies there is the need for the following activities if satisfactory sharing of information is to occur.

1. Helping patients to recognize and communicate their information needs;
2. Helping health professionals (especially doctors) to recognize and elicit information needs;
3. Development of positive attitudes among health professionals towards the sharing of information and providing the institutional climate and resources to facilitate such sharing;
4. Increasing the understanding of the ways that information sharing is constrained in health care contexts;
5. Identifying effective and efficient means of sharing information which are also satisfying to those concerned.

One way of enhancing information exchange in primary care is to share the patient record. This was advocated by Metcalf (1980) who said:

> The central idea is that sharing the patient record symbolizes sharing the responsibility for health – an adult to adult relationship which protects or restores the patient's autonomy or dignity.

Fischbach *et al.* (1980) reported on a pilot project of the joint production of the patient record in which they found that patients participated actively regardless of socioeconomic status. The additional information available to them had not made patients 'too directive' with providers and open disclosure had not led to malpractice or to improper self-care. Positive outcomes from sharing problem cards developed from patient records with 100 patients was also described by Tomson (1985). The sharing gave patients an opportunity to review their health needs and in some cases to correct inaccurate information: 80% were grateful for seeing the card, 88% felt cards should be shared and 51% thought that seeing their cards would help them to manage their health better.

A final example is provided by Tew and Deadman (1993) who conducted an experimental study of parent held child record cards. The experimental group were given the cards immediately after the child's birth while records for the control group were handled in the traditional way. A number of criteria were used to assess the effectiveness of the intervention.

1. The level of communication between parents and professionals and between different professional staff;
2. The accuracy of the records;
3. The ease of access and availability of records;
4. The utility of records as a vehicle for health education and promotion.

The parent held card was found to be administratively more efficient than the traditional system. The findings showed that parents in the intervention group perceived communication with professionals to be better than did those in the control group. Over 70% of professionals involved in the study developed a more positive attitude as the study progressed. Finally the quality and accuracy of information on the parent held cards was found to be of a higher standard. The system was felt to encourage a close working part-nership between parents and professionals and was later extended to school age children.

In conclusion we can report that there are many examples of successes in enhancing knowledge and information and concur with Daltroy and Liang (1993) that knowledge, while generally insufficient by itself for achieving behavioural and health outcomes, is nevertheless fundamental to patient education interventions.

BEHAVIOURAL INDICATORS – COMPLIANCE AND ADHERENCE

A rapid scan of the patient education literature conveys an impression of effort directed towards the achievement of compliance. Compliance describes the extent to which people's health behaviours are in tune with the advice of health professionals. While a great deal of literature has focused on compliance with drug regimens and other forms of treatment, with the growing attention to primary health education in health care a range of lifestyle variables are now receiving consideration. The failures in compliance have traditionally been blamed on patients and to a lesser extent on shortcomings in the communication process between health professionals and patients. The rationality of the 'health messages' communicated has been assumed and equally, the irrationality of people's failure to comply. More recently, attention has challenged this notion of irrationality and begun to focus in on the fabric of ideas around specific areas of health which form the context in which people decide whether or not to comply with recommended behaviour changes.

There is a multiplicity of evidence of failures fully to comply with medical recommendations – a figure of 50% is commonly suggested (Becker and Maiman, 1980) and a wide range of health issues have been studied in the literature. The factors which are involved in decisions to adhere to medical advice can be studied through the use of any of several theoretical models. Likewise, theoretical models can be used as the basis for planning interventions.

Nonetheless, criticism has been made of the weakness of theory in both the understanding of compliance and in designing interventions. General criticism of evaluative studies was made by Green (1987b) on the basis of a sample review. Most behavioural changes were, he said, measured by self-reporting with the attendant problems of memory and truth telling. Where intermediate measures were chosen other criticisms were levelled. Attitudes which were assessed were more often directed towards the intervention rather than to the behaviour which was the focus of the intervention. Underlying many of the studies was an implied causal pathway from education through to behaviour change.

Patient   →   Patient   →   Behaviour
education   satisfaction   change

Many articles failed to describe the educational and behavioural techniques employed. Green's main criticism was of the over-simplification of the analysis of behavioural tasks. Often little attention was given to reviewing and differentiating the behavioural and non-behavioural determinants of health problems or to giving priority to health behaviours on the basis of a critical assessment of their relative importance and changeability. A tendency to oversimplify the multiple influences of attitudes, beliefs, values, perceptions, social support, physical and financial barriers and the behaviour of health providers on patient's health also existed. These omissions and oversimplifications resulted in educational resources being concentrated equally on both trivial and important behaviours, simple and complex ones and on rare and prevalent attitudes and beliefs. The outcome was an indiscriminate allocation of scarce educational resources resulting in a poor return in outcomes relative to apparent investment of effort.

Haynes *et al.* (1987), in their review of studies of compliance with medication published in the previous ten years, looked for those which met the following criteria: relevant end points reported (behaviour and/or treatment outcomes); scientifically acceptable designs; at least 80% follow-up; six months follow-up in long term treatments; statistical analyses; and protection against false negative results. Only two studies met all criteria. One of the best studies was that of Colcher and Bass (1972) who investigated compliance with streptococcal pharyngitis medication. Patients were assigned to three groups.

1. Ten day course of oral medication with the usual instruction;
2. Ten day course plus special instructions emphasizing the need to take the full course even if symptoms subsided;
3. Compliance obviated by administering treatment in a single parenteral dose.

Condition 2 was adequate in ensuring high compliance with significantly superior results to condition 1 and with clinical results equivalent to condition 3. Other studies showed that short term compliance could be marginally but reproducibly increased by reducing the frequency of dosage to once or twice a day and by special packaging and calendars. With simple short term regimens specific instructions were generally seen to be sufficient to achieve compliance.

On the other hand, for long term regimens Haynes *et al.* concluded that, up to that date, no single intervention of any sort was sufficient to improve long term compliance. For long term regimens multiple strategies were required including: self-monitoring; home visits; tangible rewards, peer group discussion, counselling by health educator or nurse, and special pill packaging. In the combinations studied most of the successful interventions involved cues and rewards. They produce a list of actions which had been shown to work in the area of compliance with medication (Table 5.5).

Table 5.5 A short list of compliance improving actions that have been shown to work

For all regimens
Information:
  Keep the information as simple as possible
  Give clear instructions on the exact treatment regimen, preferably written

For long term regimens
  Reminders:
    Call if appointment missed
    Prescribe medication in concert with patient's daily schedule
    Stress importance of compliance at each visit
    Titrate frequency of visits to compliance need

  Rewards:
    Recognize patient's efforts to comply at each visit
    Decrease visit frequency if compliance high

  Social
    Involve the patient's spouse or other partner

While in any specific instance a number of alternative combinations of compliance improving actions may prove successful it is important, given resource issues, to identify those which are most cost effective and feasible in specific situations and for specific health conditions. Achieving compliance, for example, with TB medication in rural settings where patients may be several days' walk away from the hospital which initiates treatment will require a different strategy than in urban settings where ongoing contact with patients may be relatively straightforward. In the former setting it is important to ensure that enough of the compliance improving actions can be facilitated in this local context – probably through the involvement of village health workers.

The emphasis in many discussions of compliance is on the patient. We might usefully switch emphasis to the compliance of professionals – with the appropriate strategies which have been identified for achieving adherence to medication and other treatments. Haynes *et al.* (1987) commented that despite the knowledge that had been gained, many practitioners remained unaware of basic compliance management principles.

While there continues to be a need to understand the theory and practice of compliance the effective application of existing knowledge could improve compliance measures.

A list of guidelines, derived from the research literature for use in improving compliance in clinical practice, was later provided in the *British Journal of General Practice* (Carr, 1990):

1. Develop an appointment system which ensures minimum patient waiting time.
2. Adopt a friendly and informal conversational style which encourages patients to provide information.
3. Assess patients' beliefs about the aetiology of their complaints and their expectations concerning treatment.
4. Clarify how much information patients would like about their condition.
5. Offer an explanation of the patient's condition and the rationale for treatment.
6. Present the treatment regimen and the rationale upon which it is based in language that patients can understand and which allows them to remember what is said.

7. Help the patient appreciate the costs and benefits of compliance and non-compliance.
8. Enlist the aid of the patient's family or friends in helping the patient comply with medical advice.
9. Review compliance at each follow-up consultation.

In conclusion, we will return to the issue raised at the beginning of the section – the need to look at non-compliance from the patient's perspective and to see it not as non-rational and 'deviant' but as a rational response.

Donovan and Blake (1992), for example, examined compliance with rheumatology treatment. Advice from doctors had to compete with other advice and perceptions before patients decided what to do about treatments recommended. The people in their study did not forget or misunderstand what the doctor had said but they chose to ignore advice or alter doses: they were active in their non-compliance. The key to improving compliance – although this would effectively do away with the concept – was, they said, to develop active co-operative relationships between patients and doctors. They conclude:

> Perhaps the issue now should not be compliance, but how medical staff can understand and participate in the decisions that patients already take about their medications.

BEHAVIOURAL INDICATORS – PREVENTIVE BEHAVIOURS

The growing importance of education oriented towards primary and secondary prevention (and to a lesser extent to the promotion of positive health) within both primary care and hospital settings has been noted. The health areas selected will vary according to country and to some degree between settings. The specification of national and regional

health targets may be a particular influence in creating incentives to work in certain areas. In any review we may wish to note the nature of activities undertaken in addition to assessing successes.

When considering effectiveness it can be useful to draw on meta-evaluations. That of Simons-Morton *et al.* (1992) reviewed patient education for preventive health behaviours delivered in clinical settings from 1971 to 1989. The studies assessed met criteria for true or quasiexperimental design and were for seven areas of prevention: contraceptive use; breast self-examination and testicular self-examination; exercise and physical activity; injury prevention; nutrition; smoking, stress management and weight loss and management. One hundred and seventy-one studies were found although only 64 met acceptability criteria. The quality of the educational approaches used was also rated from one to four using criteria stated by the United States Prevention Services Task Force: relevance, individualization, feedback, reinforcement and facilitation (see below). The number of 'communication channels' used was also noted.

Smoking cessation was the preventive area represented most frequently (33% of studies), followed by education on specific nutrients, contraceptive use, weight control and injury prevention. Population or representative samples were used in 44% of studies, most commonly in smoking studies. The use of educational principles also varied according to topics. The writers concluded that enough rigorous studies had been reported to allow us to determine what types of educational approaches are most effective in general and also for certain specific behaviours but at the same time gaps in the literature did still exist. Relevant and acceptable studies in health care settings had been found for only 14 out of 21 of the preventive areas identified. On the basis of their findings the writers observed that evidence for the most effective approaches to education and counselling was sparse for some of the preventive behaviours currently recommended in the USA.

In the above review smoking cessation was found to be one of the areas well covered and a study included was that of Russell *et al.* (1988) which built on their earlier study (Russell *et al.*, 1979) demonstrating the effectiveness of smoking education within the consultation between general practitioners and patients. The 1987 study was an attempt to see if the activity previously shown to be effective could be incorporated into the daily routine with patients rather than be provided as an intrusive element for the purposes of short term study. In this later investigation, 101 general practitioners in 27 practices in London took part in a quasiexperimental study designed to examine whether a brief intervention applied to all smokers seen by practitioners and sustained on a continuous basis could in time have a cumulative effect and reduce the prevalence of smoking.

Of 21 practices in one health district, seven opted for a brief intervention with support from the smokers' clinic, four opted for the intervention without support and six acted as care controls. A further ten practices in a second district acted as further controls. Six cross-sectional surveys were carried out over three years, each consisting of all adults attending a doctor during a defined two week period. The estimated decline in self-reported smoking prevalence over the first 30 months from the start of the intervention was 5.5% in the group receiving supported intervention but only 2.0% in the group receiving the intervention alone and 2.1% and 3.0% in the control groups receiving usual care. The study results suggested that intervention on a routine basis was most effective when backed up by further support.

A final example in this section is offered by Chirwa *et al.* (1988) who carried out a review of evaluated studies of teaching about oral rehydration salt and sugar solution for use in diarrhoea in children. In addition they reported on an experimental evaluation of teaching about oral rehydration therapy in an Oral Rehydration Unit in Igbo Ora, Nigeria. Five hundred and twenty-four mothers took part in the intervention and 110 mothers who had not attended the ORT centre acted as controls. Pre- and post-tests were used and the intervention consisted of interactive small group discussion and participatory demonstration. In follow-up visits to participants' homes interviews focused on the questions included in the post-test and mothers were asked to make up the oral rehydration solution. In comparison with the control group mothers, the attenders at the ORT clinic demonstrated greater awareness, knowledge, skill and use of oral rehydration solution and other diarrhoea management concepts. Results were seen to compare favourably with those from other studies.

ACHIEVING ACTIVE PATIENT PARTICIPATION

As discussed earlier, active participation in health care and health decision making is an outcome of the self-empowerment approach and integral to consumerism in health care settings. There is evidence that people seek active participation and the importance of this was stated in a *Lancet* editorial (Slack, 1977):

> It seems to me that communication between patients and doctors should not be used to persuade patients to do what physicians want them to do, rather it should be used to outline the possible plans of action, so that patients can decide clinical matters for themselves.

At the same time Steele *et al.* (1987) have pointed out that there is little evidence that active participation is sought by most people in most situations. In seeking, therefore, to facilitate active participation the rights of patients to maintain a more passive role should also be safeguarded. From their review of the research literature Steele *et al.*

commented that the links between patient autonomy and clinical outcomes tended to be weak, ambiguous and mediated by unexamined variables. Greenfield *et al.* (1985) also questioned whether greater involvement in care was related to better health outcomes. Where comments are being made about achievement of health outcomes – whether defined by professionals or researchers – this may be missing the point of promoting active participation where the outcome ought to be defined as the opportunity and ability to take part in decision making rather than health indicators.

The previous chapter offered some discussion of decision making in school health education and outlined a 'vigilant' strategy recommended for use in situations where the choices made have important consequences and where people want to make the best choices for themselves. For such decision making to be possible in health care contexts, the right of the patient to a role in decision making has to be recognized and the process facilitated. This facilitation can involve some or all of the following: ensuring that people are aware that choices are actually available; specifying the alternatives; making information available on alternatives or enabling people to acquire it; offering counselling support in the stage of weighing the alternatives and in the post-decision period; and ensuring that patients have the personal skills necessary to be able to use their decision making competencies in the social situations of primary care and hospitals and at times when normal health may be impaired.

A number of studies have looked at aspects of decision making and active participation. Morris and Royle (1988) provided evidence that actually being offered a choice has positive outcomes. They investigated whether choice of surgery influenced levels of anxiety and depression pre- and postoperatively. A significantly higher percentage of those not offered the choice experienced clinical levels of anxiety and depression preoperatively and

up to two months postoperatively. By six months differences were not statistically significant although the trend was unaltered. Speedling and Rose (1985) focused directly on involving doctors and patients together in clinical decisions. Using a method of quantitative analysis of the probabilities of events and the weighted importance of each event's outcome, a decision tree was built up and patients attached a 'quality of life' assessment to each alternative. No specific evaluation was reported although the writers felt that the most immediate benefit from clinical decision making would be the legitimacy given to the patient's point of view and the encouragement of a more active role in the doctor–patient relationship.

After reviewing the 'active patient' concept and research studies, Steele *et al.* (1987) drew the following conclusions:

1. Because the active patient concept has been defined and operationalized in various ways it is difficult to know if apparent differences in the participation preferences of patients are genuine or reflections of assessment procedures.
2. Sample sizes in studies have been small, non-representative and cross-sectional. Future research needed to focus on the various determinants of information needs and the preferences for active involvement.
3. There was no coherent theory guiding research and an orienting framework was essential.

In conclusion we can suggest that there is scope for further research in this area.

INTEGRATED PROGRAMMES

The studies which investigate interventions directed towards specific variables, whether informational, attitudinal or behavioural, are important in building up a knowledge base on effective and efficient education in health care settings. A significant proportion of people who are in contact with primary or secondary care have some labelled condition and we are also interested, therefore, in assessing the degree to which the range of educational needs are met for specific conditions.

There have been calls for education to be a part of every contact between a patient and a health provider and a fully integrated part of health care. If this were to happen we might not wish to focus, in any depth, on each and every health condition. In general, however, developments have tended to be condition specific rather than general with resultant good planning and incorporation of education in some conditions but relative neglect in others. There are, for example, many reports of programmes for diabetes education, cancer education and heart disease prevention but rather fewer for arthritis, tuberculosis and mental health.

There has, however, been a stage of hospital care where general education provision has been developed – that of preparation for hospitalization and surgery. It was successes in this area of patient education which were persuasive in campaigns to institutionalize education as a part of health care. The impacts of education are seen to be both physical and psychological for this stage of care and a range of measures have been used including: reductions in pain, medications used, length of hospital stay and increases in satisfaction. Many studies have been carried out under experimental conditions and have tested the relative impact of alternative educational and counselling strategies. The successes have been associated with a provision of consistent education which meets patients actual needs (Breemhaar and van den Borne, 1991). Presurgical education has consisted broadly of three types of input, used singly or in combination: information about procedures to be undergone and sensations to be expected: development of mental strategies to reduce threatening cognitions; and coping behaviours – relaxation, breathing, coughing and turning.

Theoretical models have been drawn on as bases for structuring educational inputs and for providing explanations for the success of interventions but according to Breemhaar and van den Borne, there is as yet little certainty for the effectiveness of the measures adopted. A particular feature of discussions has been the relation between educational input and the development of control and these writers have recently reviewed the link. They conclude that positive effects of presurgical education can be explained by the fact that education and support increase feelings of control. Perceived control can reduce stress experienced and affect the ways in which it is managed. The positive effects of measures to increase perceived control appear, they say, to be dependent both on the tendency of individuals to ascribe influence to themselves and on the extent to which situations offer opportunities for the actual exercise of control.

Such conclusions, in line with earlier discussions, serve to remind that quick fixes of presurgical education applied uniformly are unlikely to be consistently successful. Assessments are required of the need in specific situations for patients to exercise control and of the actual opportunities for doing so. At the same time assessments of patients' wishes to exercise control and their beliefs in their efficacy to do so need also to take place. As Breemhaar and van den Borne point out, if the situation does not require control and/or the patient does not wish to exercise it, it is better to leave out the provision of detailed information and behavioural instructions and simply provide assistance in regulating emotions. When some active contribution is required patients will need to be convinced of the value of the behaviours suggested and of their own abilities to carry them out.

A meta-analysis of 191 studies (undertaken between 1963 and 1989) of the effects of psychoeducational care of surgical patients on recovery, postsurgical pain and psychological distress has recently been reported

(Devine, 1992). Devine recorded statistically reliable, small to moderate sized beneficial effects on all three areas and noted that these findings reconfirmed earlier ones. She also makes a comment on the cost implications of preoperative education. About one hour of staff nurse time per person plus booklet or AV materials ought to be sufficient for reasonably comprehensive preoperative and early postoperative care which Devine suggests is not a major investment to set against improved patient welfare and recovery.

For other specific areas of health where patient education programmes have been developed over relatively long periods, meta-evaluations are also available including: long term health problems involving drug medication (Mullen *et al.* 1985); cardiac patient education (Mullen *et al.* 1992); childbirth education (Jones, 1986); diabetes (Brown, 1990). In introducing the analysis of cardiac patient education, Mullen *et al.* (1992) note that existing evaluations have not previously been synthesized to assess the average effects or to identify which programme characteristics have the greatest impact. On the basis of an analysis of 28 controlled studies they concluded that results indicated that cardiac patient education had demonstrated measurable impact on blood pressure, mortality, exercise and diet and that other parameters were positively affected but less consistently. While the 'communication channel' did not have an effect on study outcomes the adherence to specific educational principles did.

The principles identified in this study and others (Mullen *et al.*, 1985; Simons-Morton *et al.*, 1992) were as follows.

1. **Relevance**. The relevance of content and educational methods to learner's interests and circumstances should be ensured.
2. **Individualization**. The educational programme should provide opportunities for patients to set the pace of their own learning and to receive answers to personal questions.
3. **Facilitation**. Behaviour should be facilitated by providing the means for patients and their families to take action or reduce barriers to action.
4. **Feedback**. The degree to which the patient is achieving progress should be demonstrated.
5. **Reinforcement**. The patient should be given encouragement or rewards for progress towards goals and objectives.

Clearly there is nothing unfamiliar about these principles. In a previous study Mullen *et al.* (1985) had demonstrated that for adherence to long term medication use of these principles was the strongest predictor of outcomes. Interestingly in the cardiac education analysis no differences were found in effect for the number of educational contacts or for total hours of educational contact and it was emphasized that it is not time per se but how it is spent that is important.

INSTITUTIONAL LEVEL

At the beginning of this chapter we provided some discussion of official and other documents which have addressed education in health care settings. There are invariably gaps between proposals of what might or ought to be and actual practice on the ground. In this section we offer some consideration of the overall contributions of primary care and hospitals to health education and also to health promotion. In some places existing achievements can be noted but in other areas developments have not reached the evaluation stage and comment will be offered on evidence to be sought.

PRIMARY CARE

In the UK there are now expectations that health education will form a part of services with requirements formalized in the new contract. Prior to this health education activities occurred opportunistically in the doctor–

patient consultation and in planned ways as part of other primary care services.

The views of professionals about health education and their professional skills in carrying it out are mediating factors between any policy and actual practice. Studies have examined general practitioners' views about health education and also attempted to assess the nature and extent of health education occurring prior to the new contracts. A small scale study (Calnan, Boulton and Williams, 1986) of 34 doctors with a responsibility for postgraduate and continuing education in general practice reported that all saw prevention and health education as important in general practice. The activities were seen as a new domain of medical expertise and largely practice based with few, apparently, having clear ideas of the roles they might play in health education in the community.

A larger scale study using a postal questionnaire with 1291 general practitioners (79% response rate) in the Oxford region in England (Coulter and Schofield, 1991) found very positive attitudes to roles in preventive care and health promotion. When respondents were asked to indicate, using open ended questions, difficulties they had encountered in the past or expected to encounter in the future in developing preventive activities, 82.5% mentioned at least one. The most common was lack of time (49.8%). Other barriers mentioned were: patient's lack of interest in lifestyle advice (16.2%); lack of financial incentive (15.9%); lack of interest on the part of the doctor (11.8%); too few practice staff (10.5%); inadequate records and registers (10.1%); inadequate premises (6.4%) and the lack of a computer (4.3%).

Research which has examined actual patient education in the consultation has used both observational methods and surveys. The study by Tuckett *et al.* (1985) discussed earlier concluded that prevention was discussed in only 25% of consultations. By focusing on the lifestyle issues of smoking, diet and alcohol consumption the consultations were assessed in terms of the opportunities that were provided, the discussions that occurred and the advice given. A distinction was made between education raised in connection with the presenting problem and that raised independently of it. A large proportion of consultations provided opportunities for problem related education, especially with reference to smoking although the majority of opportunities were not used. Opportunities for non-problem related education were virtually never explored.

In a separate paper Boulton and Williams (1983) commented that the way the doctors overlooked opportunities cannot be seen in neutral terms as just 'lost opportunities'. Patients may interpret and attach as much significance to comments not made as to those which are made. In Coulter and Schofield's study described above, respondents were asked to indicate the circumstances in which they would ask about smoking, diet, drinking habits and exercise and the actions that would be taken. The results can be seen in Table 5.6.

There were clear differences between the percentage who discuss topics when patients attend with relevant symptoms or for health checks and the percentage who discuss topics in routine consultations although the differences are significantly lower for smoking. Smoking is, of course, the area of prevention where the general practitioner's potential to achieve significant impact has, on the basis of the studies by Russell *et al.* (1979, 1988), been promoted. In a table of tentative estimates of quality adjusted life years (QUALYs), Maynard (in Drummond *et al.*, 1993) placed GP advice to stop smoking as the third cheapest QUALY, behind cholesterol testing and diet therapy for adults 40–69 (first) and neurosurgical intervention for head injury (second). In a recent editorial, Rose (1993) states that the decline of chronic bronchitis and lung cancer in men has resulted from the vigorous antismoking campaign by doctors. While their contribution has been important

Table 5.6 Preventive activities carried out by general practitioners: circumstances in which discussion would be initiated, records and statistics kept and likely actions

	% of GPs responding positively for:[a]			
	Smoking	*Drinking*	*Exercise*	*Diet*
Circumstances in which subjects discussed				
When patient presents with relevant symptoms	96.3	90.3	83.8	95.8
In health checks	93.7	93.6	82.1	84.1
In most adult consultations	63.5	25.9	10.8	11.6
Records and statistics kept of factors				
Recorded on >70% of patients' notes	46.3	17.4	2.4	20.6
Practice statistics	11.5	5.0	1.1	4.8
Likely actions when problem identified				
Offer simple advice	94.8	92.8	97.4	95.5
Offer leaflets	70.5	36.7	22.4	48.6
Offer specific aids[b]	80.4	27.9	40.1	88.7
Offer another consultation	54.4	71.2	11.5	75.0
Refer to practice nurse	9.6	3.5	2.9	30.2
Refer to another professional	28.6	39.7	0.8	69.1
Refer to self-help group	10.8	75.9	37.4	42.3

[a]Respondents could choose more than one option. [b]Prescription (smoking); drinking diary; information about local sports centres and recreational facilities; diet sheets

it should be seen alongside all the other antismoking activity of the last 20 years.

If education is to be effective in primary care as a whole it needs to be provided routinely by the relevant health workers. For those education and preventive activities which are required within terms of service within a particular country it becomes possible to audit activity and its impact on specified indicators. Questions have been raised about some of the areas which have, to date, been particular targets for general practice activity. Rosser and Lamberts (1990), for example, point out that serum cholesterol measurement has been widely promoted to the public in North America, the UK and other countries despite a lack of good evidence to support mass screening programmes. Their comments have been endorsed by Sheldon *et al.* (1993) who conclude from an indepth examination that untargeted cholesterol screening is not justified. More generally

there are debates about the value of population versus high risk screening – followed up with appropriate education. Although much discussion of the impact of primary care as a whole focuses on disease specific activity many would argue that it should be giving an increased proportion of time to the promotion of positive health.

Irrespective of the content of health education in primary care, effectiveness across these services as a whole will depend on the motivation of professionals to acquire and put into practice proven educational strategies. While training for health promotion is now a central component of nurse education in many countries it continues to play a minor role, apart from attention to the communication process, in the initial training of doctors.

In a recent study of the role of GPs in coronary heart disease prevention in primary care, a survey was sent to a representative sample of GPs (Killoran, *et al.*, 1993). This provided some useful findings on health promotion training undergone and perceptions of need, not only of the GPs but also of other practice staff. Twenty-six per cent of the GPs had had no health promotion training. Of the 72% who had training only 37% had received it through medical education. Training needs included practice organization and management, communication skills, clinical training and use of computers. It is the practice nurses who carry out a substantial proportion of the health promotion work in primary care. From the survey, 62% of these say that they require further training and the following areas are mentioned: personal counselling skills, planning health promotion, knowledge of risk factors and use of computers. The study identified five sets of factors that are seen to be significant in determining the level and quality of health promotion in general practice and which will have to be met if primary care is to contribute effectively to achieving *Health of the Nation* targets. They are:

1. Training in planning and organizing health promotion audit and evaluation and counselling skills. Multidisciplinary training is recommended;
2. Motivation and commitment;
3. Practice capacity for planning and organizing health promotion;
4. Audit, evaluation and research;
5. The amount of support from Family Health Service Authorities, health authorities and facilitators.

HOSPITALS

Earlier in the chapter we mentioned the Health Promoting Hospitals initiative. This network was established in Europe in the late 1980s in affiliation with the Healthy Cities network and by 1991 included 24 hospitals in 12 countries (Ashcroft and Summersgill, 1993). The notion of a health promoting hospital provides an appropriate context within which

effective health education can take place. The constituent elements have been identified (Baric, 1992) as the:

1. Creation of a healthy environment for staff and clients;
2. Integration of health promotion into all the activities of the institution (prevention, treatment, education, rehabilitation, etc.);
3. Creation of 'healthy alliances' between the hospital and other institutions resulting in a 'health promoting community' in which all the institutions are health promoting.

Five main principles have been proposed for use in assessing whether or not a hospital is 'health promoting (Ashcroft and Summersgill, 1993):

1. Health must appear on the agenda of policy makers in all sectors and at all levels of the hospital;
2. Work carried out in the hospital must be organized so as to create a healthy hospital environment;
3. Hospital personnel and patients must be empowered and enabled so that together they can have control of the elements that influence their health while in the hospital;
4. Personal and life skills of personnel and patients must be developed;
5. The hospital must extend its activities in the health care system beyond merely providing clinical and curative services.

For each of these principles specific indicators will need to be developed to monitor progress and achievement. The reports of evaluations from the early hospitals to join the network will be followed with interest.

A number of factors are known to have a bearing on the overall effectiveness of hospitals where education is concerned. We need to achieve successful activity not only in a few areas of health but across a whole hospital institution and ultimately across the hospital system in total. For institution wide successes we need: policies which specify that educational activity is provided as a total part of care; health workers who are appropriately trained to undertake the educational component of care; organizational arrangements which maximize the possibility of educational success; widescale adoption of educational activities in line with client needs and which are known to be effective and efficient; and widescale availability of appropriate educational resources. We will comment selectively on these factors.

POLICY

At the beginning of the chapter we commented on a number of policy documents which have recommended education in hospital care and more recently addressed the whole question of the health promoting potential of hospitals. The extent to which recommendations have been put into effect has varied between countries and the extent to which there have been incentives to undertake such development. Because of its perceived capacity to reduce costs patient education received early support in the USA. In other countries it was slower to develop. In the new market oriented NHS the incentive for purchasers to build health promotion into the contracts which they negotiate ought to provide a major impetus to education in hospital settings.

Evidence from some countries of the extent of patient education policies and practice was reported in a series of papers in 1990. In Canada, 37% of hospitals (Bartlett and Jonkers, 1990) had health promotion policies while 21% stated that health promotion was not part of their role. From Australia, Degeling *et al.* (1990) reported that most hospitals surveyed 'recognized the importance of patient education, but support was based on individual efforts resulting from initiatives taken in specialty areas rather than reflecting overall hospital policy'. In the USA a number of trends were having an impact on hospital patient education and in particular affecting the 'budget and administrative clout' of the co-ordinators and the increasing use of management features known to contribute to more successful programmes. As Green comments (1990): 'Hard times have forced a more systematic, co-ordinated, strategically planned and evaluated patient education program'. Finally, the Netherlands had recently seen a rapid development of the co-ordinator role with 60% of hospitals now employing people for such a role.

ORGANIZATION

The first stage in ensuring that the educational component of patient care is met is to ensure that it is specified in the care plans. The next stage is to ensure that the educational needs identified are met. In any period of hospital care patients encounter a number of different professionals, ancillary staff, other patients and also their own families and friends. All can provide contributions to their education, both formally and informally. If such varied contributions go unco-ordinated it is highly unlikely that a coherent programme will result.

At the level of the individual patient the educational component can be recorded alongside all other aspects of care. Since hospital stays are reduced in time and may only form a small percentage of the time of an illness episode it is particularly important that there is co-ordination of education between hospital and primary care. In addition to co-ordination of education for specific patients there are other levels at which co-ordination can take place – at the level of specific conditions or as a general hospital-wide activity.

The institution of patient education co-ordinators first developed in the USA but has now spread more widely. Evidence of the effectiveness of co-ordination came from a study in Michigan in the USA. Eighteen criteria for patient education were incorporated into a survey of subject based programmes. Of 281 programmes reported, 219

(78%) had either a fulltime or a part-time co-ordinator (Pack *et al.*, 1983). The mean number of criteria met by these programmes was 13.8 where there was a fulltime and 12.7 with a part-time co-ordinator but only 8.3 where there was no co-ordinator. There was some variation in the number of criteria met according to the type of co-ordinator. Where education was considered to be the prime responsibility more criteria were likely to be met than where responsibilities were diverse. If the co-ordinator had received further training, programmes tended to be more comprehensive and met more criteria.

The development of the function of patient education co-ordinator in the Netherlands was described by Fahrenfort (1990). This is instructive for those countries currently at the early stages of development of patient education. This innovation started with a research project funded for three years (later extended to five) in five hospitals. The hospitals selected had to meet certain criteria: agreement to appoint a patient education co-ordinator for the duration of the project; to have demonstrated an interest in patient education prior to applying for the grant; and the hospital management had to be supportive to the experiment and agree to external monitoring, advice and evaluation. The monitoring and evaluation were expected to address the following areas: the benefits to the development of patient education of the co-ordinator appointment; the qualifications for the co-ordinator role and the tasks to be performed; the changes in the hospital brought about by the co-ordinator; the organizational supports and barriers to development; and the long term necessity of the co-ordinator function.

At the outset of the project two views of the co-ordinator role were in evidence: hospital administrators tended to stress the public relations aspect of co-ordination and the actual co-ordinators were more interested in exploring organizational change. The co-ordinator job was not defined in detail and the people appointed had to negotiate positions for themselves – a task that took at least two years. The project reported successes in combining aspects of organizational change and the education of members of the medical staff about communication with patients.

During the period of the research project other hospitals appointed co-ordinators and by 1990 Fahrenfort estimated that 60% of the general hospitals in the Netherlands had, as noted above, fulltime or part-time co-ordinators. She commented on positive influences on the development of patient education and noted two particular trends: the emergence of the belief in patients' rights to autonomy and the development of a greater market orientation to the provision of health care. Patient education was seen to be compatible with both although Fahrenfort noted that the 'government support for patient emancipation veered towards supporting emancipation as consumerism'. She commented on potential conflicts which resulted in developing the co-ordinator role. The easily visible promotion aspects of the role can take priority over the slower and more difficult, but more important work of organizational development and change leading to: improved procedures for health professional–patient contacts; better understanding of the patient education process; support for professionals in changing their professional image; and educating patients to real autonomy. Through the institution of patient advice counters the hospital can 'show its good intentions towards patient education without actually changing anything in the way patients are informed about their own condition'. The skills of the co-ordinator will need to include those of balancing the demands for quick and visible results with the needs for the longer term organizational change, recognizing in the process that the former can frequently trigger support for the latter.

Whether or not hospitals appoint specialist patient education co-ordinators, it is necessary to monitor the progress to meeting educational needs in all areas of service. Hospital care is typically only an element in a 'patient career' which began with consultation in primary care, was followed by referral to hospital and subsequent admission and is followed up by further contact with primary care. The educational needs begin from the point of first referral to primary care and it makes sense therefore to respond to these needs from this point. A mechanism for enhancing the autonomy of the patient in the educational process would be the use of a patient held record card (Dickey, 1993). This would record the process of eliciting needs at different stages and also the nature and timing of all educational responses. Ideally the card would record, at the same time, medical interventions, etc. Use of such a device could make a contribution towards improving articulation between education in the primary and hospital sectors.

FACILITATING THE EDUCATIONAL PROCESS

Educational and counselling needs have to be defined through dialogue with patients, possibly with the use of diagnostic tools such as Patient Learning Needs Scales (Bubela *et al.*, 1990) and normative needs also taken into account before educational activities can be specified and organized. In deciding on these activities, in addition to needs, account has to be taken of other characteristics of patients and facilitators and the particular constraints of the context in question.

In this section it is not the intention to review these activities in detail but to comment on a few issues which have a bearing on meeting the educational needs of all patients across all hospital settings: timing and delivery of education; choice of educational methods; choice of educators; use of mass media.

TIMING AND DELIVERY

It is a truism to say that education and counselling are most effective if provided as near as possible to the time when need arises. In a

study by Wallace (1988) patients expressed a consistent preference for preparation (including booklets) prior to hospitalization rather than after admission. With the use of individualized care plans and the encouragement of active participation of patients in their care, there ought to be a continual monitoring of educational need and organization of appropriately timed response. Much of this response may take place on a one-to-one basis in association with other ongoing activities. In addition, there may be needs which could usefully, and cost effectively, be met through group methods.

Although the intention in many situations is to integrate education within total care it can also be organized on a separate basis or through 'hybrids' of integrated and separate elements. Bartlett (1991) cites as an example of separate educational provision the Patient Learning Centre at the University of Michigan in the USA where cancer patients are taught to perform high technology procedures. Patient self-help groups, consumer libraries and telephone information lines are also educational inputs which can be accessed without formal legitimation by caregivers. The New York University Co-operative Care Unit which employs both educational and clinical nurses is cited as an example of hybrid care. Educational nurses provide most of the formal teaching and counselling to patients and their families although clinical nurses are expected to answer patients' questions and to reinforce informations and skills.

Since many countries now give high profile to the educational skills of nurses a development of hybrid forms of organization of the educational component of care might be opposed. Given the time commitment needed, however, to develop a full understanding of the educational process and competence in diagnosing and meeting educational needs in a crowded nurse training, it may be worth considering some development of both general and specific nursing contributions to education.

EDUCATIONAL METHODS

There are a variety of ways in which cognitive, affective or skills learning objectives can be met. Some may, on the basis of evaluated studies, be more effective than others but not necessarily the most cost efficient methods or popular ones with particular groups. A cheap and simple educational method which can be available to all patients and their families may be preferred to a more complex one which requires heavy investments of health professional time and can only reach a proportion of people. An instructive example was provided by Wilson-Barnett (1988).

She discussed a study of Ozbolt Goodwin (1979) which evaluated a programmed learning booklet for use by patients following pulmonary surgery according to individual abilities and recovery rates. Adherence to this approach was shown to have significantly positive effects with patients experiencing fewer infections and periods of hospitalization.

Given the reductions in length of time of hospital stay the potential for bringing together groups of patients with equivalent needs at one point in time will be limited for many aspects of health care. There are conditions, however, where use of groups is convenient and a good way of meeting needs. An example can be offered from diabetes education. An interesting study by Basso (1991) reported on the use of structured fantasy group activity as part of education for children with diabetes. The study was not an experimental one or exposed to long term follow-up but it reported that the group activity helped children to express their feelings about diabetes and its management and their concerns about stresses in their family and peer relationships.

CHOICE OF EDUCATORS

The question of whether people other than health professionals should be involved in the educational process can be addressed. Clearly if we have a model of the autonomous patient we also accept that this goes along with some opportunities for choice of educational contacts. A common activity is to join self-help groups which can draw on a variety of non-professional input in line with members' needs.

Within institutional contexts where there is a provision of integrated patient education, there has been some assessment of the role of peer educators. These are defined by Bartlett (1985) as people who currently or formerly have experienced the illness or condition in question and have been specially recruited to participate in educational activities. The Reach to Recovery programme for women who have experienced mastectomy is a specific example of the use of peer educators. Van den Borne *et al.* (1987) reviewed studies of the effects of contacts between patients with cancer. Of the 18 studies identified, most did not meet methodological conditions necessary to draw conclusions. Four of the six studies with sound methodological design showed positive effects of contacts including: more knowledge about (breast) cancer; better movement of the arm after mastectomy and more use of breast prostheses; greater improvements in perceptions of general health and greater reductions in negative feelings. In his review, Bartlett said that early experience with the use of peer educators was encouraging but limited empirical research had been undertaken. Based on findings from existing programmes he suggested that peer educators could be used most effectively when the illness was chronic; the illness was socially stigmatizing due to physical handicaps; and/or impairment of self-concept or body image existed.

USE OF MASS MEDIA

The limitations of mass media will be assessed in a later chapter but they have an important part to play in education in health care settings. The provision of informational leaflets and booklets is a relatively cheap and easy way of meeting informational need, either through the professional–patient encounter or through education 'shops'. Some hospital and primary care settings have introduced the use of video and there has been a small growth of patient libraries in primary care.

Two things are important: generating informational materials appropriate to the range of client groups and providing opportunities for discussion of content when required. Parrinello (1984), in a an evaluation of an arterial bypass booklet, said that over 90% of respondents found the booklet helpful but those who had the opportunity to discuss it with a health worker found it of greater value.

CONCLUSIONS

This chapter has reviewed selectively some aspects of the evaluation of education in health care settings. The educational component of health care has developed at varying pace in different countries and in many remains underemphasized and underfunded. However, in the short time since the first edition of this book, the growing health promotion movement has led to a new focus on the health promoting nature of hospitals and communities in which primary care is located. It is hoped that this will lead to significant achievements across the range of indicators incorporated into health promotion audit.

At the same time there has been a shift towards a greater market orientation in the provision of health care. As happened earlier in the USA, patient education fits in with a consumerist model of the patient and is seen also to be a means to reducing costs. Some years ago Bartlett (1985) discussed some of the issues pertaining to seeing patient education as a cost saver:

> In this cost conscious environment, it is very tempting for patient educators to advocate the need for patient education primarily as a cost savings tool. In economics jargon,

patient education is being justified less as a consumable service which is valuable in its own right and more as a social investment which will reduce net costs.

Bartlett saw this strategy as perilous on two grounds. First, it undermines aspects of patient education which do not save money and may well increase costs. He believed that it would, in fact, be difficult to demonstrate a direct relationship between most informal educational activity in hospital and subsequent cost savings. Second, the emphasis on cost containment condoned a double standard. Newly proposed medical treatments and procedures may be routinely approved on the basis of medical necessity while patient education must demonstrate both its effectiveness and capacity to cut costs. Since some patient education activities are associated with cost saving it is worth making this known but education as in integrated component of every patient's care may not necessarily lead to cost saving in either the short or long term. The danger of an increasing focus on costs is to increase pressure to set educational goals which are more easily and cheaply achieved. The specific behavioural and medical outcomes associated with preventive medical approaches to health education may, therefore, be preferred to the more diffuse and probably more difficult ones associated with empowerment models.

We have noted the need for more results of evaluation – in some places because developments are new and we await evaluation, in others because there has been insufficient evaluations or those undertaken have had methodological shortcomings. At the same time the increasing availability of meta-evaluations has demonstrated effective interventions. On the basis of existing knowledge if proven interventions were routinely applied across health care settings as a whole, significant gains could be achieved. The statement made in 1985 by Bartlett still holds good:

The answers to many research questions remain cloudy and other questions remain to be formulated. Yet a considerable body of knowledge now exists upon which effective, practical and acceptable patient education programs can be developed. More research attention now needs to be directed to the question. 'Why aren't we applying the knowledge we already have?'.

REFERENCES

American Hospital Association (1972) *A Patients' Bill of Rights*, American Hospital Association, Chicago.

Ashcroft, S. and Summersgill, P. (1993) Perpetual promotion. *Health Services Journal*, **103**(5349), 29.

Baric, L. (1992) Health promoting hospitals. *Journal of the Institute of Health Education*, **30**(4), 141–8.

Bartlett, E.E. (1985) Editorial. At last, a definition. *Patient Education and Counselling*, **7**, 323–4.

Bartlett, E.E. (1991) Editorial. Integrated versus separate education. *Patient Education and Counselling*, **17**, 1–2.

Bartlett, E.E. and Jonkers, R. (1990) Editorial. Patient education – an international comparison. *Patient Education and Counselling*, **15**, 99–100.

Basso, R. (1991) A structured fantasy group experience in a children's diabetic education program. *Patient Education and Counselling*, **18**, 243–51.

Becker, M.H. and Maiman, L.A. (1980) Strategies for enhancing patient compliance. *Journal of Community Health*, **6**, 113–35.

Boulton, M. and Williams, A. (1983) Health education in the general practice consultation: doctor's advice on diet, alcohol and smoking. *Health Education Journal*, **42**, 57–63.

Breemhaar, B. and van den Borne, H.W. (1991) Effects of education and support for surgical patients: the role of perceived control. *Patient Education and Counselling*, **18**, 199–210.

Brooker, C. (1990) The health education needs of families caring for a schizophrenic relative and the potential role for community psychiatric nurses. *Journal of Advanced Nursing*, **15**, 1092–8.

Brown, S.A. (1990) Studies of educational interventions and outcomes in diabetic adults: a meta analysis revisited. *Patient Education and Counselling*, **16**, 189–215.

Bubela, N., Galloway, S., McCay, E. *et al.* (1990) The patient learning needs scale: reliability and validity. *Journal of Advanced Nursing*, **15**, 1181–7.

Calnan, M., Boulton, M. and Williams, A. (1986) Health education and general practitioners: a critical appraisal, in *The Politics of Health Education*, (eds S. Rodmell and A. Watt), Routledge and Kegan Paul, London.

Carr, A. (1990) Editorial. Compliance with medical advice. *British Journal of General Practitioners*, **40**(338), 358–60.

Cassileth, B.R., Zupka, R.V., Sutton Smith, K. and March, V. (1980) Information and participation preferences among cancer patients. *Annals of Internal Medicine*, **92**, 832–6.

Chirwa, B.U., Brieger, W.R. and Ramakrishna, J. (1988) Evaluating health education for oral rehydration therapy at a rural Nigerian health clinic. Part II. *Patient Education and Counselling*, **11**, 203–13.

Colcher, D.S. and Bass, J.W. (1972) Penicillin treatment of streptococcal pharyngitis, a comparison of schedules and the role of specific counselling. *Journal of the American Medical Association*, **222**, 657–9.

Coulter, A. and Schofield, T. (1991) Prevention in general practice: the views of doctors in the Oxford region. *British Journal of General Practice*. **41**(345), 140–3.

Daltroy, L.H. and Liang, M.H. (1993) Arthritis education: opportunities and state of the art. *Health Education Quarterly*, **20**(1), 3–16.

Davis, F. (1963) *Passage Through Crisis: Polio Victims and their Families*, Bobbs, Merrill, New York.

Degeling, D., Salkeld, G., Dowsett, J. and Fahey, P. (1990) Patient education policy and practice in Australian hospitals. *Patient Education and Counselling*, **15**, 127–38.

Dekkers, F. (1980) Patient education between right and practice (I, II, III and IV). *Medical Contact*, **35**, 640–3, 674–7, 709–12, 737–40.

Devine, E.C. (1992) Effects of psychoeducational care for adult surgical patients: a meta analysis of 191 studies. *Patient Education and Counselling*, **19**, 129–42.

Dickey, L.L. (1993) Promoting preventive care with patient-held minirecords: a review. *Patient Education and Counselling*, **20**, 37–47.

Department of Health (1992) *The Health of the Nation; a Strategy for Health in England*, HMSO, London.

Department of Health and Social Security (1981) *Care in Action: A Handbook of Policies and Priorities for the Health and Personal Social Services in England*, HMSO, London.

Department of Health and Social Security (1986) *Primary Health Care: An Agenda for Discussion*, HMSO, London.

Department of Health and Social Security (1987a) *Neighbourhood Nursing – a Focus for Care: Report of the Community Nursing Review*, HMSO, London.

Department of Health and Social Security (1987b) *Promoting Better Health: Government Programme for Improving Primary Health Care*, HMSO, London.

Department of Health and Social Security (1989) *Working for Patients*, HMSO, London.

Donovan, P. (1992) Leading the way to a baby friendly world. *HYGIE*, **XI**(2), 8–10.

Donovan, J.L. and Blake, D.R. (1992) Patient non-compliance: deviance or reasoned decision making? *Social Science and Medicine*, **34**(5), 507–13.

Drummond, M., Torrance, G. and Mason, J. (1993) Cost-effectiveness league tables. *Social Science and Medicine* **37**(1), 32–40.

Elian, M. and Dean, G. (1985) To tell or not to tell the diagnosis of multiple sclerosis. *Lancet*, **ii**, 27–8.

Fahrenfort, M. (1987) Patient emancipation by health education: an impossible goal. *Patient Education and Counselling*, **10**, 26–37.

Fahrenfort, M. (1990) Patient education in Dutch hospitals: the fruits of a decade of endeavour. *Patient Education and Counselling*, **15**, 139–50.

Fischbach, R., Sionolo-Bayog, A., Needle, A. *et al.* (1980) The patient and practitioners as co-authors of the medical record. *Patient Education and Counselling*, **2**, 1–5.

Green, A. (1987a) Is there primary health care in the UK? *Health Policy and Planning*, **2**(2), 129–37.

Green, C.A. (1987b) What can patient education learn from 10 years of compliance research? *Patient Education and Counselling*, **10**, 155–66.

Green, L.W. (1990) Hospitals and health care providers as agents of patient education. *Patient Education and Counselling*, **15**, 169–70.

Greenfield, S., Kaplan, S. and Ware, J. (1985) Expanding patient involvement in care. *Annals of Internal Medicine*, **102**, 520–8.

Hannay, D. (1992) Editorial. General practitioners' contracts: the good, the bad and the ugly. *British Journal of General Practice*, **42**(358), 178–9.

Haynes, B.R., Wang, E. and Mota Gomes, M. (1987) A critical review to improve compliance with prescribed medications. *Patient Education and Counselling*, **10**, 155–66.

Jones, L.C. (1986) A meta-analytic study of the effects of childbirth education on the parent–infant relationship. *Health Care for Women International*, **7**, 357–70.

Killoran, A., Calnan, M., Cant, S. and Williams, S. (1993) Pacemaker. *Health Service Journal*, **103** (5340), 26–7.

Korsch, B.M. and Negrete, V.F. (1972) Doctor patient communication. *Scientific American*, **227**, 66–73.

Meissner, H.I., Anderson, D.M. and Odenkirchen, J.C. (1990) Meeting information needs of significant others: use of the cancer information service. *Patient Education and Counselling*, **15**, 171–9.

Metcalf, D. (1980) Why not let patients keep their own records? *Journal of the Royal College of Practitioners*, **30**, 420.

Morris, J. and Royle, G.T. (1988) Offering patients a choice of surgery for early cancer: a reduction of anxiety and depression in patients and their husbands. *Social Science and Medicine*, **6**, 583–5.

Mull, J.D. (1990) The primary care diabetic: history, rhetoric and reality, in *Anthropology and Primary Health Care*, (eds J. Coreil and J.D. Mull), Westview Press, Oxford.

Mullen, P.D., Green, L.W. and Persinger, M.S. (1985) Clinical trials of patient education for chronic conditions: a comparative analysis of intervention types. *Preventive Medicine*, **14**, 753–81.

Mullen, P.D., Mains, D.A., and Velez, R. (1992) A meta analysis of controlled trials of cardiac patient education. *Patient Education and Counselling*, **19**, 143–62.

Ozbolt Goodwin, J. (1979) Programmed instruction for self care following pulmonary surgery. *International Journal of Nursing Studies*, **16**, 29–40.

Pack, B.E., Hendrick, R.M., Murdock, R.B. and Palma, L.M. (1983) Factors affecting criteria met by hospital based patient education programs. *Patient Education and Counselling*, **5**, 76–84.

Parrinello, K. (1984) Patients' evaluation of a teaching booklet for arterial bypass surgery. *Patient Education and Counselling*, **4**, 183–9.

President's Committee on Health Education (1974) *Report of the President's Committee on Health Education*, Department of Health, Education and Welfare, New York City.

Rose, G. (1993) Editorial. Preventive strategy and general practice. *British Journal of General Practice*, **43**(369), 138–9.

Rosser, W.W. and Lamberts, H. (1990) Do our patients receive maximum benefit from preventive care? A North American perspective. *British Journal of General Practice*, **40**(339), 426–9.

Roter, D. (1987) An exploration of health education's responsibility for a partnership model of client–provider relations. *Patient Education and Counselling*, **9**, 25–31.

Royal College of General Practitioners (1981a) *Health and Prevention in Primary Care: Reports from General Practice*, RCGP, London.

Royal College of General Practitioners (1981b) *Prevention of Psychiatric Disorders in General Practice*, RCGP, London.

Russell, M.A.H., Wilson, C., Taylor, C. and Baker, C.D. (1979) Effect of general practitioners' advice against smoking. *British Medical Journal*, **2**, 231–5.

Russell, M.A.H., Stapleton, J.A., Hajek, P. *et al* (1988) District programmes to reduce smoking: can sustained interventions by general practitioners affect prevalence? *Journal of Epidemiology and Community Health*, **42**, 111–15.

Sheldon, T., Song. F., Freemantle, N. and Mason, J. (1993) Big screen ending. *Health Service Journal*, **103**(5356), 32–3.

Simons-Morton, D.G., Mullen, P.D., Mains, D.A., Tabak, E.R. and Green, L.W. (1992) Characteristics of controlled studies of patient education and counselling for preventive health behaviours. *Patient Education and Counselling*, **19**, 173–204.

Slack, W. (1977) The patient's right to decide. *Lancet*, **11**, 240.

Speedling, E.J. and Rose, D.N. (1985) Building an effective doctor–patient relationship: from patient satisfaction to patient participation. *Social Science and Medicine*, **21**, 115–20.

Steele, D.J., Blackwell, B., Guttman, M.C. and Jackson, J.C. (1987) Beyond advocacy: a review of the active patient concept. *Patient Education and Counselling*, **10**, 3–23.

Szasz, T.S. and Hollender, M.H. (1956) The basic models of the doctor–patient relationship. *Archives of Internal Medicine*, **97**, 587–92.

Taylor, K.M. and Kilner, M. (1987) Informed consent: the physician's perspective. *Social Science and Medicine*, **24**, 135–43.

Tew, J. and Deadman, N. (1993) Parent power. *Health Service Journal*, **103**(5345), 31.

Tomson, P. (1985) Sharing problem cards with patients. *Journal of the Royal College of General Practitioners*, **35**, 534–5.

Tuckett, D., Boulton, M., Olson, C. and Williams, A. (1985) *Meetings Between Experts: An Approach to Sharing Ideas in Medical Consultations*, Tavistock Publications, London.

United Kingdom Central Council for Nursing, Midwifery and Health Visiting (1986) *Project 2000: A New Preparation for Practice*, UKCC, London.

Van den Borne, H.W., Pruyn, J.F.A. and van den Heuvel, W.J.A. (1987) Effects of contacts between cancer patients on their psychosocial problems. *Patient Education and Counselling*, **9**, 33–51.

Wallace, L.M. (1988) Psychological studies of the development and evaluation of preparatory procedures for women undergoing minor gynaecological surgery, PhD thesis, University of Birmingham.

Wilson-Barnett, J. (1988) Patient teaching or patient counselling? *Journal of Advanced Nursing*, **7**, 323–4.

World Health Organization (1978) *Primary Health Care: Report of the Conference in Primary Health Care*, WHO, Geneva.

World Health Organization (1991) *The Budapest Declaration on Health Promoting Hospitals*, WHO European Regional Office, Copenhagen.

THE MASS MEDIA IN HEALTH PROMOTION

6

Nothing is easier than leading the people on a leash. I just hold up a dazzling campaign poster and they jump through it.

Joseph Goebbels, Director, Ministry for Popular Enlightenment and propaganda (1976)

In this chapter, the mass media are viewed in the same strategic way as, for instance, community development, patient education or the schools. Just as the schools have particular characteristics and may thus make a qualitatively different impact from, say, informal education in the community, mass media have their peculiar strengths and weaknesses. Ideally they would be used as part of a comprehensive programme which employs the range of strategies and agencies described earlier in this book. All too frequently they have been used in far from splendid isolation – either because the prospect of a fully co-ordinated programme has been too daunting or, more likely, because they have been assumed to possess a power akin to that of a kind of educational 'magic bullet'. The view expressed at the head of this page is not unique to Dr Goebbels!

It should by now be clear that to ask whether health education works is to ask a meaningless question. This tenet certainly applies to the analysis of mass communication campaigns which, over the years, have been the cause of much heated debate about effectiveness and efficiency. Rather than asking whether mass media work, we should be asking what kind of effect we might expect from different kinds of media used in different situations and contexts to present different sorts of message about different subjects to different target groups. We must also ask questions about both the intended and unintended or incidental effects of mass media and examine the extent to which such effects should be taken into consideration or even deliberately manoeuvred as a tool of health promotion.

We are faced with a complex picture and yet it is possible to provide valid generalizations both at the level of communication theory and at the more pragmatic level of guidance for users. This chapter will, then, seek to illuminate certain key issues in the use of mass media. It will examine the peculiar features of the media and their different forms; it will consider the incidental and unplanned effects of media; it will discuss the essential elements of theories of mass communication and their pragmatic application in social marketing; it will ask what lessons might be learned about marketing health and will place particular emphasis on pretesting. It will conclude with a sampler of health education programmes having a major mass media component, reinforcing the general – and perhaps stunningly obvious – point that a successful community programme incorporates mass media as a subsidiary but important element within the programme as a whole.

THE MEANING OF MASS MEDIA

As the words suggest, the two key features of mass media are their mass audience and the fact that there is no interpersonal communication between the originator of the message and the mass audience: the message is mediated. It is the mass audience which is so enticing to the communicator: it offers the seductive but illusory prospect of instant influence. As de Tocqueville (1961) observed: '... nothing but a newspaper can drop the same thought into a thousand minds at the same moment'. Goebbels experienced a similar but more ambitious optimism for his propaganda ministry. With the advent of radio and television the possibility of wholesale change at national or even international level created joy in the minds of those seeking to manipulate population behaviours and alarm in the minds of those who wished to preserve the integrity of individual freedom to think and decide. However, although it is certainly possible to contact a mass audience, the second major characteristic of mass media makes it extremely unlikely that the population might be manipulated at the whim of the propagandist. In other words the fact that the message is mediated makes it impossible to gain immediate feedback of the results of the communication and thus provide a tailor-made communication which is responsive to the needs, personality and moods of the audience. As has so often been noted, the blunderbuss attributes of mass media are inconsistent with offering the 'different strokes for different folks' which are a component of an efficient influence process. Figure 6.1 makes this important point about feedback and reminds us of the difference between communication and education.

In interpersonal communication the communicator effectively codes a message for transmission to an audience (typically one person or a small group of people). The format of the message will most often be symbolic (e.g. written or spoken speech) but may be iconic, in which case pictures may be used to clarify the message. Alternatively, because it is considered likely to produce certain learned outcomes, an enactive format could be employed. This would require some form of audience participation to communicate the message and achieve the communicator's purpose. For example, role play might be used to increase awareness of a social issue or to change audience attitudes. Non-verbal communication is an important component of the whole communication package.

It is of course apparent that mass media may simulate some of the features of this

The mass media in health promotion

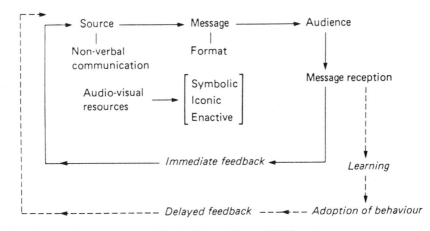

Figure 6.1 The communication process (derived from Tones, 1981).

communication process – the presenter of a television programme may be specially chosen to be credible to the audience and may seek to ensure that his or her non-verbal communication is consonant with the programme goals. Again a variety of iconic messages may be used on television or other visual media. Some attempt may be made to achieve audience participation. However, there is no way of knowing whether or not the audience has participated, has responded to the pictures or the charm of the presenter or whether, indeed, the audience has even understood the various messages let alone acted upon them. Although feedback may be provided for media producers – in the form of audience research, return of newspaper coupons, measures of population behaviour before and after programmes – there is no instant and observable response from the individuals comprising the audience. Audience phone-ins during radio programmes probably provide the closest approximation but the encounter is typically very short and excludes the majority of the listeners. Delayed feedback is no substitute for immediate feedback if anything other than the communication of relatively simple messages is to be achieved comprehensively and efficiently. Moreover, immediate feedback not only allows the communicator to repeat, clarify and vary the message, it enables him or her to look for unwanted side effects such as the arousal of excessive anxiety, a point of some ethical importance.

Most communication attempts are concerned to do more than ensure that the message has been correctly interpreted and understood. In reality their purpose is 'to generate some learned outcome: the acquisition of new information or understanding; a change in belief and attitude; the learning of a new skill and even the adoption of a new practice or change in lifestyle. It is usually acknowledged by media workers that there is a 'hierarchy of effects': it is relatively easy to 'agenda set' and communicate simple

information; it is increasingly difficult to change attitudes, teach complex skills and persuade people to adopt new behaviours, especially where these involve exertion, discomfort or the abandoning of pleasure! The various intermediate indicators of programme success which were described in Chapter 3 and the model underlying these relate to this communication dilemma for the mass media. In order to achieve the more difficult and often long term outcomes, the requirements of immediate feedback and the personalizing of approaches make it difficult for mass media to compete with interpersonal education.

Before proceeding to clarify further the capabilities of different forms of media, we should note the distinction between mass media and the various media devices used as adjuncts to interpersonal communication and education. The film used as an audio-visual aid to a lecture or as a trigger for group discussion may appear superficially similar to a mass media television programme. In effect the film is a learning resource which is part of the iconic and enactive format of the communication; it is directly controlled by the communicator without loss of the important feedback principle. A good example of such use is provided by the work of Evans and McAlister based on McGuire's inoculation theory (McGuire, 1973; Evans *et al.*, 1978; McAlister and Hughes, 1979). These studies utilized film or video as part of a programme designed to inoculate young people against social pressures to smoke. By and large, film was effective in producing behavioural outcomes only when accompanied by other techniques such as peer-led teaching and structured role play. McAlister *et al.* (1980) were able to claim that students receiving this media-aided interpersonal teaching were recruited to smoking at less than half the rate of controls not receiving the programme. Similar results using life skills training in the field of substance misuse provide evidence of the importance of interpersonal education in the problematic arena of persuading the young

'... to eschew deeply satisfying activities which are validated by peer and other social pressures'. The effectiveness of mass media-based smoking programmes should be judged against this alternative – or rather complementary – approach (Botvin *et al.*, 1984).

It is interesting in this general context to consider the special case of programmed learning. At first glance a programmed text or programme designed for use in audio-visual would appear to have characteristics of both a resource to be used as part of interpersonal education and at the same time share some of the features of mass media. A programme could, for instance, be used totally outside the interpersonal encounter, either on a self-access, student-centred basis or through mass distribution as a book. Since properly validated programmes are highly efficient teaching devices, this would appear to give the lie to earlier assertions about the limitations of mass media. The fact is, of course, that a programmed text or related device has (i) been designed for a specific audience (cf. the notion of market segmentation below) and (ii) through the proper process of validation and standardization, it incorporates the principle of immediate feedback in its construction (providing the student with 'IKR' – immediate knowledge of results). The dissemination of such programmes with their intrinsic capacity to interact with the audience might well combine the advantages of interpersonal education with the attractions of reaching a mass audience. The implications for open learning and distance learning are self-evident although a discussion of these is beyond the scope of this book. Reference to this tactic does, however, remind us of the heterogeneous nature of mass media, a fact we must consider before seeking to make generalizations.

MEDIA VARIETIES

It is apparent that mass media vary considerably in their potential and capabilities,

despite the common characteristics discussed above. They differ in form and format: leaflets and posters are substantially different from the electronic media of television and radio. They differ in their potential for reaching audiences and in the nature of the audience they reach: local radio listeners have different characteristics from readers of quality national press; in the UK Open University and Channel Four documentaries will appeal to viewers who may not be addicted to soap opera. They differ in their credibility and trustworthiness. Fuglesang (1981) offered a salutory reminder that modern media technology is relevant only to about 20% of the world population who can read and write and have access to electronic media. Folk media using, for example, puppets and the oral tradition of proverb and storytelling replace the technology and mass audience of western society. However, the focus of this book is on developed countries and three examples will illustrate the different potential of various forms of media.

The first example illustrates the superiority of cinema advertising compared with what many would regard as the most powerful medium – television. Douglas (1984), in a guide to advertising, reminds us that cinema not only offers higher quality sound and image definition than television but also differs in audience composition and involvement (in addition to the fact that it is possible to advertise 'illicit' products in the cinema which it is not possible to present on television, at least in many countries). Douglas cites Marplan research which compared recall of a hitherto unknown product after exposure to cinema and television advertising. Young women who had seen the commercials were interviewed on the following day. Recall of the main point of the commercial by the cinema audience was 26% compared with 9% by the television audience. In the context of discussion about what we might expect from media exposure, it is interesting to note that spontaneous recall was only 2% for the television audience (but 8% for the cinema audience). Recall after prompting went up a further 36% for television audiences compared with 56% for cinema audiences. Douglas ascribed this superiority to the greater impact produced by screen size, better sound and image quality and absence of distractions.

The second example offers evidence of the kind of result which might be expected from one of the trusty stock-in-trade media devices of the health promoter – the exhibition. Research carried out by the Transport and Road Research Laboratory (TRRL) in 1970 recorded numbers of people attending road safety exhibitions, audience characteristics and their source of information about the exhibition, their progress round the exhibition and the time spent at each exhibit or display. The TRRL adduced the following principles:

1. Attendance at even the best road safety exhibitions is unlikely to exceed 1000 per day. It is often much less than this. The prospects of getting at ... (major target group) ... are therefore extremely poor.
2. Local press publicity can increase the attendance by at least 50%.
3. The audience at exhibitions appears to be a broad cross-section of the population ... it has not been possible to find whether they ... are in most need of propaganda.
4. When going round exhibitions visitors tend to spend very short times at exhibits. The average time spent at many exhibits is less than one minute. None of the visitors see all the exhibits, many see less than half. Animated exhibits attract a lot of attention, but often distract visitors from the static displays.

The third example concerns credibility. It is an axiom of attitude theory that beliefs and attitudes are unlikely to change if the source of the communication is perceived to be untrustworthy, lack expertise or other forms of authority. A similar point is made in communication of innovations theory by the principle of homophily. It is therefore interesting to ask whether different forms of mass media are more acceptable than others and whether these are more or less credible than alternative forms of interpersonal communication. Budd and McCron (1979) interviewed 692 adults from Central England and, among other things, invited them to indicate how far they would trust information about changing one's life for the sake of one's health derived from each of 12 sources. These sources included medical personnel, lay people and media. The family doctor received the highest rating (an average score of 3.51 on a four point scale). The four lowest ratings (1.8, 1.72, 1.69 and 1.68 respectively) were accorded to a magazine article, television advert, newspaper article and, last of all, a friend or neighbour. Radio and television documentaries scored at an intermediate level (2.43; 2.39) but were boosted by having doctor involvement! Even the humble poster was rated third most credible when displayed in a GP's surgery or waiting room.

A more recent study (Kerr and Charles, 1983) makes a related point. However, while television advertising – especially about health – was treated with scepticism and mistrust, women's magazines and certain television personalities were often considered more credible than some health professionals, at any rate on the subject of feeding a family.

INCIDENTAL AND PLANNED EFFECTS OF MEDIA

Before considering what the generalizations from mass communication theory have to offer for health education practice, we must note a further dimension to the classification of mass media effects. Whereas the main concern of health education is the development of programmes deliberately designed to influence audience characteristics, it is important to recognize that mass media may well have incidental and often unpredicted effects. Rather like the hidden curriculum in the school setting, these incidental effects may have to be taken into account as possibly unhealthy pressures or canalized in the interests of health promotion.

The fact that mass media can have a dramatic and unforeseen impact has been fully recognized since Cantril (1958) documented the sizeable panic produced among the citizenry by Orson Welles' production of H.G. Wells' *War of the Worlds* in the 1930s. Less dramatic but more insidious is the way in which press and television report health issues. Even the recording of cancer cure is likely to be couched in terms which reinforce the general alarm and pessimism conjured up by the very term. Wellings (1986) makes a similar point about the public's processing of media reporting of the 1983 'pill scare'. Draper and his colleagues made related points about the ways in which the very grammar of television reporting tends to introduce bias which, for example, favours the supremacy of high technology medicine at the expense of the less glamorous but potentially more beneficial preventive and health promotion measures (Best *et al.*, 1977).

Again the incidental presentation of health issues in entertainment programmes and soap opera may foster misleading images and attitudes. Characterization may serve to validate images of unhealthy lifestyles as part of a norm-sending process. The portrayal of alcohol on television conveys a norm of heavy drinking and associates consumption of alcohol with benefits rather than costs (Hansen, 1986; Institute for Alcohol Studies, 1985).

The impact of advertising unhealthy products is a highly contentious political issue. Advocates of advertising, not unsurprisingly, stress its social benefits and minimize the negative effect on recruitment (Henry and Waterson, 1981). The effect of cigarette promotion on children has been the subject of research (Piepe *et al.*, 1986; Chapman and Fitzgerald, 1982; Charlton, 1986; Aitken *et al.*,

1987). Although it is not yet possible to demonstrate unequivocally that there is a causal relationship between advertising, sponsorship and smoking recruitment, it seems likely that children who smoke are generally aware of cigarette advertising and sponsorship than non-smokers and more favourably disposed to the brands. What is clear is that such advertising and sponsorship establishes a hidden curriculum which legitimizes smoking and denotes its continuing acceptability.

We will now, however, turn to the deliberate use of mass media to produce desired learning outcomes, focusing particularly on their potential for producing behaviour change and the adoption of approved practices.

MASS COMMUNICATION THEORY

An analysis of research and theory into the effects of mass media suggests a shift in opinion over the years from an apparently magical belief in their omnipotence (fostered perhaps by a mixture of Dr Goebbels and Vance Packard) to an almost totally opposite assertion that mass media will not produce any significant changes in actual behaviour, especially in the difficult domain of health. A more cautiously optimistic view is currently prevalent. Day, in a foreword to Douglas (1984), describes colourfully the emotion generated by the debate about the effectiveness of media advertising:

> Advertising has always been wreathed in metaphysical mists. From the time of the first medicine-man selling snake oil from the back of the stagecoach, to the self-induced hypnosis created by so-called 'subliminal' advertising, to the about-to-be wonders of global commercials via satellite, there has always been a need on the part of some people, at least, to believe in the talismanic properties of advertising and its supposed power to 'manipulate' its audience.

Day adds, 'I have yet to see the evidence that advertising unsupported by product performance has ever had more than a temporary effect in persuading anyone to do anything against their own best interests'.

This view is consistent with the orthodoxy which came to replace the early 'direct effects' or 'hypodermic' models of media influence. According to the latter the community presented itself as a compliant patient for its injection. If the injection did not work either a different medicine was called for or a larger dose! The influence of Katz and Lazarsfeld (1955) and Lazarsfeld and Merton (1975) led to a kind of 'null effects' model in which mass media were considered to have a minimal impact. Katz and Lazarsfeld proposed their two-step hypothesis of influence according to which the adoption of behaviours by a social group or community resulted from interpersonal interaction with opinion leaders who were (i) more receptive of media information than the mass of people, and (ii) were sought out for advice by the community and were thus relatively influential. Lazarsfeld and Merton further argued that mass media would not induce change unless one or more conditions were met: 'monopolization', i.e. where there are no contrary influences and messages; 'canalization', i.e. where a particular message or recommendation for action plugs into existing motivations and preferences; and 'supplementation', i.e. where interpersonal efforts supplement media-based messages. Klapper's influential (1960) review consolidated this general view of media limitations. Reinforcement rather than conversion was the prime role of the media:

> Within a given audience exposed to particular communications, reinforcement, or at least constancy of opinion, is typically found to be the dominant effect (of mass media), minor change as in intensity of opinion is found to be the next most common; and conversion is typically found to be the most rare
>
> *(cited in Wallach, 1980, p. 15)*

Mendelsohn's (1968) conceptualization of mass media replaces the image of the hypodermic with that of an aerosol:

> Rather than being a hypodermic needle, we now begin to look at mass communication as a sort of aerosol spray. As you spray it on the surface, some of it hits the target: most of it drifts away; and very little of it penetrates.

It is worth noting in passing that Mendelsohn does acknowledge the possibility that at least some of the message hits the target even though presumably very little actually results in desired behaviour change.

The audience has, so far, been represented as a relatively passive entity which is more or less difficult to influence – depending on whether it is the hypodermic or the aerosol which is wielded. It is, however, misleading to consider the recipients of the message as either undifferentiated or passive. As was noted in an earlier chapter, communication of innovations theory classifies the community into categories in accordance with their relative openness to change. This analysis is useful in that it not only views the audience as a heterogeneous group but also relates readiness to adopt innovations to the perceived characteristics of the new idea or practice and the likely costs or benefits which might result from adoption. In other words, the recipients of mass media messages neither passively accept nor reject the influence but rather analyse and interpret it in an active fashion, typically in the context of interpersonal interactions with family or friends. Mendelsohn (1980) makes a distinction between 'Homo mechanicus' and 'Homo volens', the latter being an '... active organism who often seeks out usable information – the dynamic individual who uses only that information he or she needs from the media while disregarding the useless stuff'.

This latter approach has elsewhere been referred to as a uses and gratifications model, suggesting as it does that the active recipient of media messages selects from those messages what (s)he needs to gratify current motivation. As Dorn and South (1983) have pointed out, this interpretation is very acceptable to the promoters of unhealthy products since it denies accusations of manipulation of a naïve and gullible public! They also note how this conflicts with both right and left wing theories of media manipulating the populace. Right wing mass manipulative models view people as being often naïve and feckless and therefore corruptible by unhealthy media influences. Left wing theories view the mass of people as being subjected to control by a capitalist elite which uses its ownership of media to exploit its audience.

Budd and McCron (1979) emphasize that mass media influences cannot and should not be isolated from a social context in which they:

> ... interact and sometimes compete with, other sources of information and influences in complex ways, and that the individual selects, and compares from these diverse sources to construe a meaningful explanation for himself about particular issues which may, or may not, be in line with the intention behind any or all sources of information available to him.

The social context can also be interpreted in terms of what Dorn and South (1983) refer to as a 'consensual paradigm', i.e. media collude with and encapsulate, in cliché and stereotype, social norms, exemplified earlier by reference to the norm-sending role of soap opera and news reporting. Dorn (1981) further draws our attention to his preferred class cultural model which urges health educators to take account of the subcultural constructions of meaning of, for example, different social classes and ethnic groups. Ball-Rokeach and de Fleur (1976) propose a dependency model involving a tripartite relationship between media, audience and society. An interesting implication of the theory is that:

> ... when people's social realities are entirely adequate ... media messages may have little or no alteration effects ... In contrast, when people do not have social realities that provide adequate frameworks for understanding, acting and escaping, and when audiences are dependent in these ways on media information received, such messages may have a number of alteration effects.

It should by now be clear that it is not enough to say that mass media can or cannot readily influence audience behaviour. It is also apparent that the media influence process is a complex one. One simple fact can, however, be stated: in normal circumstances, mass media will not easily change people's behaviour unless individual motivation and normative influences are favourable. McKinlay's lament (1979) on the failure of mass media to promote health is eminently explicable when this simple fact is taken into account.

> How embarrassingly ineffective are our mass media efforts in the health field (e.g. alcoholism, obesity, drug abuse, safe driving, pollution, etc.) when compared with many of the tax-exempt promotional efforts on behalf of the illness generating activities of large-scale corporations. It is a fact that we are demonstrably more effective in persuading people to purchase items they never dreamed they would need, or to pursue at risk courses of action, than we are in preventing or halting such behaviour.

The comparison which McKinlay makes between commercial advertising and health marketing is particularly apposite at a time when health educators are urged to learn from the superior expertise of commerce and adopt the social marketing approach. The relevance of social marketing will therefore now be considered. In particular it should be possible to see how recommended approaches articulate with communication theory as discussed above. Moreover, if we are to make sound judgements about the evaluation of mass media in health promotion, we should understand the kinds of expectations of success inherent in social marketing as well as noting the rules pertaining to efficient management of educational interventions using media.

HEALTH EDUCATION AS SOCIAL MARKETING

Marsden and Peterfreund (1984) argued that adoption of marketing principles would provide public health departments with a guide and incentive to help them '... shed a bureaucratic tradition and a lacklustre image which compromises their ability to provide services and to function as authoritative sources of health information'. Others, who have perhaps interpreted health promotion rather narrowly as a profile-raising excursion into energetic media-backed publicity, look to commerce for tips on how to sell health (see, for instance, Docherty (1981); Player (1986). However, Bonaguro and Miaoulis (1983) outlined a marketing approach to Green's well-known PRECEDE* model asserting that the goals of marketing and health promotion are similar. Since one of the major aims of this chapter is to examine what kinds of success we might realistically expect from mass media-based health education, it is clearly important to look critically at these claims for the social marketing approach. Do we have a new panacea or, more modestly, what insights can we gain from the best commercial practice for the marketing of health?

First of all, we should note that the notion of health marketing is not that recent a discovery. In 1977 Lovelock commented on the value of marketing concepts and strategies for health marketers. He also referred the reader to earlier work by Kotler (1975)

and Zaltman *et al.* (1972). More recently, Solomon (1981) identified ten key marketing concepts having relevance for health promotion through public communication campaigns:

1. The marketing philosophy;
2. The 'four Ps' of marketing;
3. Hierarchies of communication effects;
4. Audience segmentation;
5. Understanding all the relevant markets;
6. Information and rapid feedback systems;
7. Interpersonal and mass communication interactions;
8. Utilization of commercial resources;
9. Understanding the competition;
10. Expectations of success.

These ten concepts will serve as a basis for discussing what we might learn from commercial approaches to marketing but in order to assess their relevance we should be in no doubt about the fundamental differences between the selling of commercial products and the selling of health.

As McCron and Budd (1987) have pointed out, the question of advertising effectiveness is shrouded in myth yet the popular view is not only that advertising is powerful but it must work because businesses spend so much money on it. It is, in fact, salutary to note the difference in expectations of success between businesses and those who look for quick results from health education! This is, however, only one of the distinctions between the commercial and public domains. These differences may be summarized as follows.

1. There is clearly a considerable difference in the size of budgets typically available to commercial and public domain communicators.
2. Commercial advertisers would normally set much lower standards for success

---

*For details of this, the reader is referred to Green, L.W. and Kreuter, M.W. (1991) *Health Promotion Planning: An educational and environmental approach* (2nd edition), Mayfield, Toronto.

than commissioning health education programmes. Whereas the latter would expect evidence of behaviour change – preferably dramatic – the former would have much lower ambitions and might not expect any change in, for example, sales at all. During the late 1970s a well known chain of bakers spent some £300 000 on ten television commercials. These were thought to have been a great triumph even though there had been no increase in volume sales. The firm was content to maintain their market in the context of a general rise in bread consumption! (Reported in *Daily Mail*, 13 February, 1980.)

3. A more important distinction between the marketing of health and commercial products is the fundamental difference in the nature of the products on offer. The commercial product offers the customer gratification of some existing need; if the customer does not like the product, the manufacturer will produce something he or she does like or will change its image. The highly successful campaign to sell the chocolate bar 'Yorkie' was in the last analysis based on people's liking for chocolate. The campaign's success lay in appropriate manipulation of brand image to appeal to psychological needs other than the taste gratification. By contrast health education is trying frequently trying to sell a product which commercial advertisers would consider no-one in their right mind would buy! Potential customers are not uncommonly urged to stop doing something they find enjoyable and start doing something unpleasant or difficult. Playing with brand imagery is of course possible (as we noted in the section on pretesting) but this involves the adding of 'psychographic icing' to an often rather unpalatable cake.

What is more, the product which is being promoted by health education is frequently intangible and offers gratifi-

cation at some indeterminate time in the (often distant) future. This almost exactly reverses the pattern of commercial sales technique which promises immediate gratification, often on credit.

4. A further important distinction concerns ethical considerations. While commercial advertising is now constrained to avoid blatant lying, it is by its very nature economical with the truth. Education, by definition, should be concerned with helping people make informed decisions (although there are proponents of a persuasive prevention model who are eager to use advertising techniques to manipulate and coerce). Again health education should be concerned with avoiding unwanted side effects such as anxiety or unresolved dissonance. Commercial advertising is also concerned to avoid negative images and connotations which are likely to have an immediate impact on sales figures. However it is much easier to do this since the basic message is invariably positive: our product will meet your needs and make you feel good. Again, health education cannot, ethically, make a decision to ignore or abandon the equivalent of an unprofitable market. Indeed disadvantaged groups and other resistants to the sales talk often form the main market.

5. Finally, because commercial advertising can rely on the pre-existence of audience motivation, the change in the audience which it seeks to produce is often limited to brand awareness and the creation of a positive attitude to the particular product. The behavioural response is relatively simple – the purchase of a product which in all probability differs from previously purchased products only in its packaging, physical or psychological. Health education seeks to change deeply seated attitudes and even values and sometimes to produce the adoption of often complex behaviours.

The very real differences between the marketing of health and commercial products should, however, not blind us to the lessons to be learned from good commercial marketing practice. Indeed, perhaps the most important lesson is that the products on sale are very different! We will use Solomon's ten-point analysis as a basis for the discussion.

1. MARKET PHILOSOPHY

The first point worthy of note has to do with the concept of 'market philosophy' which is based on the idea of 'exchange', i.e. that there should be equity between marketer and consumer: the prime goal is to meet consumer needs (real or imagined); the customer is always right! As Marsden and Peterfreund (1984) reminded us, the cavalier presentation of health services would make the commercial marketer blush. Apart from the obvious need (in the words of the Ottawa Conference) to reorient health services, the way in which some health educators patronize their clients can be counterproductive. Mendelsohn (1980) makes the point very forcibly:

> Among the 'needs' we all have is not to be bombarded with information we already have or do not have any use for (e.g. information asserting that excessive drinking may be bad for us); not to be commanded to do something that is vague and unachievable without explicit simple instructions regarding its achievement (e.g. 'drive carefully'); not to be unreasonably frightened (e.g. any drinking during pregnancy, no matter how moderate, will surely result in the birth of a monster); and not to be insulted by the health communicator who implies that everyone the communicator is trying to address is (1) ignorant ... (2) ... sinfully 'irresponsible' in that they don't give a damn about their own lives/or the lives of others; and (3) they are slothfully 'apathetic' in not immediately doing with-

out question what the communicator commands them to do.

An important question concerns the definition of consumer 'needs'. As we will see, community development urges us to base our programmes on 'felt needs'; frequently these needs do not match the epidemiological reality and require a complex negotiation with the client group which is beyond the scope of mass media.

2. FOUR Ps – PRODUCT, PRICE, PLACE, PROMOTION

Solomon's second point was concerned with the four Ps, namely product, price, place and promotion – what others have called the 'marketing mix'. There are clear messages for the health educator: the (health) product should be tangible, attractive and accessible. While some health promotions meet all three of these criteria, many others are unnecessarily vague. For example, the sale of condoms or wholemeal bread involves tangible products which are relatively accessible and which may be attractively packaged, but general messages to 'take more exercise' or 'look after yourself' are less tangible and, for a majority of people, inaccessible and downright unattractive. The relative lack of attractiveness of the product has already been noted but the notion of accessibility is of interest. While there may be an element of physical accessibility in health promotions (e.g. access to clinic; availability of healthy food) the question of psychological accessibility may be overlooked. It is clear that many people wish to adopt a healthier lifestyle but lack skills and support to do so. The lack of these facilities effectively renders the desired change inaccessible (see earlier references to the Health Action Model).

The matter of price is self-evident. In health promotion the cost is more likely to be psychosocial than financial. It is only necessary to remind the reader of the central part which the notion of costs and barriers plays in the Health Belief Model (discussed in Chapter 3).

Place and promotion may be considered together. Place emphasizes the importance of distribution of the goods and retail outlets. Promotion reminds us that advertising is only one element of the marketing mix. The relevance of both of these will be taken up later when we consider the seventh of the ten points.

3. HIERARCHY OF COMMUNICATION EFFECTS

The third concept refers to the 'hierarchy of communication effects'. This describes the importance of recognizing what was called in Chapter 3 the causal chain between input and output. Commercial marketing acknowledges that success becomes increasingly difficult to achieve as we move from measures of simple market penetration to behaviour change. McGuire (1981) comments on this 'distal measure fallacy' and points our nicely the different criteria of success used by the public and commercial sectors:

> All too often the communicator evaluates the campaign or its component parts in terms of a response step early in the chain, quite distant from the later step (no. 10) that actually constitutes the criterion of success. The public communication campaigner should look with horror upon the practice in the commercial advertising industry of buying 50 billion dollars' worth of time and space each year solely on the Step 1 (exposure) criterion of Neilsen ratings or circulation figures as if all that counts is reaching the public.

Despite McGuire's objection and for reasons stated earlier, because of pre-existing motivations of the public, market penetration may be all that is necessary to sell products.

4. AUDIENCE SEGMENTATION

The fourth concept is that of audience segmentation. It is concerned with the idea of market aggregation and argues that media campaigns will be more effective insofar as they can move towards disaggregation. In other words if messages and channels can be devised which appeal to different homogeneous subsets of the population, more effective and efficient results will be achieved. It is worth observing in passing that interpersonal communication is based on what would be called total market disaggregation, i.e. the condition achieved by interpersonal approaches which supply 'different strokes for different folks'.

The criteria for segmentation range from the cruder geographic and demographic variables, e.g. targeting lower social class groups via popular press, to more sophisticated measures of personality (sometimes referred to in advertising parlance as 'psychographics'). Stein (1986) ascribed part of the success of a cancer information service to its targeting of four groups: smokers who want to quit, persons over 50, cancer patients and their families, and blacks. Mendelsohn (1986) described an effective crime prevention campaign which found it impossible to refine its message delivery to reach specific groups. Nonetheless the blunderbuss approach adopted appeared to work but produced different effects in different segments of the audience. For instance, in relation to demographic variables, affluent people (at proportionately lower risk) made greater gains in intention to engage in neighbourhood crime prevention activity than did the higher risk less affluent groups. On the other hand lower income groups showed a greater readiness to report suspicious looking people to the police. In respect of psychographic criteria, the campaign appeared to have resulted in greater overall levels of preventive competence among those who initially believed themselves to be relatively less able to safeguard themselves and their property. The attitudes of those perceiving themselves initially to be less at risk of crime were more likely to have been influenced by the campaign than those perceiving themselves to be more vulnerable. The latter group, however, were more likely to act and follow the specific crime reduction recommendations made by the programme.

Lavigne *et al.* (1986) viewed market segmentation as a central feature of their APPLAUSE project (Appropriate public presentations for learning about alcohol and other drugs using segmentation effects). This illustrates particularly well how pretesting of population groups and individuals forms an integral part of programme planning. Lavigne *et al.* subdivided their market segment of parents into two further high and low risk groups and listed demographic and psychographic characteristics. For instance, the high risk group were more likely to be blue collar and male, having negative attitudes to legal and social controls over alcohol use and being less likely to believe that parents influence their children's behaviour. They were also more likely to engage in risky drinking behaviours and to have experienced health and social consequences of drinking. This segmentation allowed the project team to develop strategies designed to take account of these intergroup differences.

Apart from the self-evident value of identifying and pretesting key market segments, perhaps the main principle to be extracted from the points made above is the difficulty faced by mass media in achieving precisely tailored programmes; such fine tuning must be left to interpersonal interactions.

5. MARKET UNDERSTANDING

The fifth of Solomon's recommendations is to understand the market. In effect this is an injunction to recognize the existence of secondary markets which might facilitate or inhibit access to and the success of programmes in influencing the primary target groups. On a simple level we might invite media workers to 'look for the gatekeeper'. If a programme depends on the display of posters in clinics and the nurse or doctor in charge is upset by the poster presentation no amount of pretesting on the target group will prevent disappointment. The poster will not be displayed!

6. FEEDBACK

Solomon's sixth recommendation concerns the evaluation process. In short he urges that each programme, in addition to summative, should incorporate formative/process evaluation to allow the programme to be modified through the provision of rapid feedback of results.

7. INTERPERSONAL AND MASS COMMUNICATION INTERACTION

His seventh point centres on the interaction of interpersonal and mass communication. It is virtually axiomatic that mass communication may be enhanced by interpersonal education. Commercial practice has recognized this guiding principle in its firm separation of advertising from the broader promotion/marketing function and, more specifically, in its recognition of the importance of the retail outlet in influencing customer purchasing patterns.

8. COMMERCIAL RESOURCES

Here, Solomon makes the point that those marketing health should utilize commercial resources where possible. There is readily available commercial expertise (e.g. market research firms) which may have greater expertise than, say, a small health education department. The firm (suggests Solomon) may even provide their services at discount rate or even for nothing – in order to improve their own brand image!

9. COMPETITION

When marketing health, it is essential to understand the competition and produce a better product! The competition for health education consists primarily of the antihealth lobby and its political supporters. One of the most interesting recent attempts to learn from this maxim is described by Chesterfield-Evans and O'Connor (1986) who report on the Australian BUGAP campaign (Billboard utilizing graffitists against unhealthy promotions). Chapman's (1986) *Lung Goodbye* offers the would-be subversive a handy set of tactics to combat the powerful Goliath of the tobacco industry.

10. EXPECTATIONS

In planning a campaign, it is necessary to formulate realistic targets and not be cajoled into colluding with unrealistic expectations of success.

THE LESSONS OF SOCIAL MARKETING AND MASS COMMUNICATION THEORY

Having reviewed social marketing theory's recommendations for success and noted the extent to which this is compatible with the different orientation of health education, we should now be in a position to relate this review to general mass communication theory and ask what we might legitimately expect from mass media in health promotion. We should, therefore, note the complexity of interpersonal communication and the learning process and limit our expectations. We should note the particularly difficult task of selling health and curtail our expectation of success even further. Mass media will not normally be able to achieve certain health educational goals.

1. They will not convey complex messages and create understanding of the often complicated issues related to health and disease, such as the interplay of risk factors in coronary heart disease.

2. They will not readily teach complex motor or social interaction skills, such as breast self-examination or the capacity to deal assertively with interpersonal pressures.

3. They will not produce attitude change in resistants nor will they provide the support necessary for motivated individuals who wish to change their behaviour in adverse physical and social circumstances.

On the other hand mass media will deliver simple messages and, where people are already motivated, this may trigger often dramatic changes in behaviour. Provided that audience penetration can be achieved (the simplest measure of media effectiveness), mass media can be stunningly successful in their agenda-setting function. As has been frequently noted, it is difficult to tell people what to think but very much easier to tell them what to think about. Unfortunately this powerful agenda-setting function which is so very relevant to the radical, critical consciousness raising role described in Chapter 1 cannot be used on the powerful medium of television because of its political unpalatability.

Mass media will, clearly, only achieve their potential if programmes are constructed in accordance with good communication practice, many of which have been discussed in the context of social marketing. It is worth adding that good communication practice will also take account of the models described in Chapter 3 and utilize the well accepted principles of attitude theory. The communication model at the beginning of this chapter provides a framework which has been fully elaborated by McGuire (1973), Albert (1981) and Flay (1981), all of whom provide analyses based on the Hovland–Yale model which emphasizes *inter alia* the importance of source and message factors in achieving attitude change.

Two other broad recommendations may be made. The first of these has to do with

Solomon's observations (point seven in his list) about the interaction of media communication and interpersonal communication. This offers the generalization that mass media will be more effective in achieving goals other than agenda-setting the more they manage to enlist interpersonal support (and thus lose their medialike characteristics). This is of course integral to the use of educational media (such as Open University) which attempt to create viewing groups to offer mutual support and to enlist the interpersonal and pedagogical skills of local tutors.

The generalization, as we have seen, is a major tenet of communication of innovations theory and the two-step hypothesis discussed earlier in this chapter. Chaffee (1981), in an interesting analysis of political campaigns, makes a similar point. He argues that about one fifth of a community pay little attention to politics; one third are politically active communicators but about one half of the total population follow politics in a relatively passive fashion via the media and '... are moved to interpersonal discussion only on the occasion of a highly salient, unanticipated or ambiguous political event'. It is the interpersonal discussion which influences political attitudes. Chaffee supports this view with the observation that watching the Watergate hearings on television was less important than discussing them in accounting for any changes in political attitude. He goes on to make a point of especial relevance for our understanding of the potential of mass media for influencing attitude and behaviour. Media are most effective on their own when (i) there is low audience involvement in the matter under discussion, (ii) there is little difference in available choices and (iii) the message is unopposed.

Liu (1981) provides an intriguing examination of mass campaigns in communist China and reminds us that the Chinese have always stressed the importance of training activists to support their mass media campaigns. Flay

et al. (1986, 1987) discuss the synergy of media and interpersonal education from the opposite perspective and show how media in the form of television programmes can boost the effect of school-based education and trigger further interpersonal influence in the form of parental involvement.

The second recommendation for effective media practice seeks to underline the importance of pretesting of health education programme. Although this is related to the notion of audience segmentation, pretesting received little prominence in Solomon's discussion. It will receive much greater emphasis here not only merely because of its importance as part of effective practice but because of the way in which it illuminates the process of evaluation generally and the importance of the various intermediate indicators discussed in Chapter 3.

A SELECTIVE REVIEW OF MEDIA STUDIES: GENERAL OBSERVATIONS

The mass media strategy is in one important respect different from the remaining delivery strategies discussed in this book. Although each of these has its own idiosyncracies and flavour, mass media differ fundamentally in the lack of personal contact between educator and audience. The media strategy is therefore of particular interest, especially since it promises so much but, in many people's view, delivers relatively little. This latter part of the chapter will therefore present evidence which should help us decide what we might realistically expect from mass media. In judging this evidence, we must of course bear in mind the general principles, stated in the first part of the book, that the quality of evidence will depend on (i) the definition of success employed therein, (ii) the extent to which appropriate research designs have been used, and (iii) the choice of particular methods based on intelligent use of learning and communication theory. The latter point will not, of course, apply to the mass media strategy except insofar as media are used to represent particular tactics such as face-to-face interaction (e.g. a video of a counselling session) or group work (e.g. a film of a smoking cessation clinic). In such instances learning tactics are being employed at second hand. The only other situation where choice of appropriate teaching methods is important in the context of mass media use is when the latter are supplemented by auxiliary interpersonal methods.

Particular varieties of media do of course have different capabilities and characteristics as we have seen above and the review which follows will provide separate evidence of the potential of some of these for achieving different kinds of outcome. More particularly, we will consider the use of posters and leaflets and compare these, implicitly or explicitly, with the arguably more powerful electronic media – radio and television. In addition, we will examine the capabilities of mass media for dealing with some specific health problems including a particularly problematic issue, that of substance misuse.

What then might we say about mass media efficiency? Can we generalize or must we again say it depends on the type of media, subject matter and target group? As indicated in the introduction to this book, Gatherer *et al.* (1979) have provided one of the most recent attempts to provide a comprehensive answer to the question, 'Is health education effective?'. As a result of analysing 49 reported evaluations of mass media programmes, they concluded that mass media were in fact inferior to individual instruction and groups. Seven out of eleven of their cases demonstrated some changes in knowledge (of the order of 6% and typically shortlasting); two out of two studies demonstrated some attitude shift (of between 3% and 6% – though four studies recorded an attitude change in the wrong direction); 20 out of 30 studies showed some behaviour change. As regards this latter category, Gatherer *et al.* note that behaviour

change is most likely where a single action is required (e.g. clinic attendance or use of a phone-in service); it tends to be relatively short-lived and change is less likely to occur when general changes in behaviour pattern are required.

Atkin (1981) also provides a review of campaign effectiveness; his analysis was not intended to be the kind of comprehensive catalogue which Gatherer *et al.* compiled but provides a rather more thorough and sophisticated analysis of the reasons why certain campaigns were or were not effective. He commented, for instance, on the failure of a campaign to teach Cincinnati residents about the United Nations. Neither knowledge gain nor effective change resulted from a '… heavy flow of multi-media messages'. According to Atkin, lack of success was due to excessive quantity of information at the expense of quality. He ascribed other failures to the use of unpopular media channels and lack of audience penetration; use of vague messages rather than making specific recommendations; poor audience segmentation; generating audience reaction through hard-sell techniques, and failure to take account of the audience's latitude of acceptance.

On the other hand when learning theory and the principles of effective media communication were taken into account, programmes have been demonstrably successful. Atkin cites a programme on sexually transmitted diseases called 'VD Blues' (Greenberg and Gantz, 1976) which attracted a wide audience, increased their perception of the seriousness of the problem, enhanced knowledge levels – especially about mode of transmission and cure – and apparently resulted in thousands of people visiting VD clinics after the programme. He also referred to a successful programme described by Mendelsohn (1973) which utilized a quiz format to communicate information about a National Driver Test Program. This had an estimated audience of 30 million viewers, generated over a million letters and '…

stimulated thousands to enrol in driver improvement courses'.

There are other well documented examples of successful media programmes which should satisfy critics. For instance, Farhar-Pilgrim and Shoemaker (1981) described a series of campaigns designed to influence Americans' extravagant use of energy. Applying communication of innovations theory, they concluded that proper design which took account of audience motivation could produce very acceptable results. They demonstrated, for example, a good level of penetration – their messages reached 83% of city adults an average of 14 times. The target group seemed to be more willing to pay for energy saving devices (the percentage varied between 5% and 17%). Moreover, an increase in sales of such devices was recorded and a higher proportion of the target group undertook various energy saving practices such as installing shower flow control devices than a comparison group: the adoption rate was between 16% and 27% higher than the comparison, depending on the device in question. While this example might not appear to be directly relevant to health education practice, it does illustrate that campaigns which ask people to take action for the collective good can be effective provided that appropriate appeals are made to self-interest (in this case, financial gain).

Bell *et al.* (1985), in their review of research in health education (1948–1983), also report examples of effectiveness. For instance, an assessment of the Glasgow rickets campaign claimed an eightfold increase in demand for vitamin D supplements for older Asian children together with a 33% increase in requests for paediatric drops (Dunnigan *et al.*, 1981). The review also included England and Oxley's study (1980) which reported a halving of the rate of head infestation among a population of 147 385 children after a regional campaign. Again, Bell *et al.* record the success of a programme in increasing the level of rubella vaccination which involved general prac-

titioner support of a national publicity campaign directed at women in the practice population. Within the study population, 1187 women responded to a request to attend for screening and 106 of the 133 who were eligible for immunization accepted this (Hutchinson and Thompson, 1982).

Turning now to the use of educational broadcasting, it is clear that properly constructed programmes can have a wide range of desirable effects. Rogers (1973) showed how the BBC 'Merry-Go-Round' sex education programme (when used in the context of classroom teaching) could change beliefs and attitudes. Children who experienced the programmes not only increased their knowledge of sexual vocabulary but also developed different attitudes to nudity, reproduction and toilet habits: in other words they acquired a greater and more healthy openness in relation to sexuality.

Again McCron and Dean's (1983) thorough evaluation of a series of programmes produced by Channel 4 Television on health matters ('Well Being') revealed a wide range of beneficial outcomes. They summarized some of these effective outcomes as follows:

> ... in television terms, a relatively successful programme attracting a considerable audience, which showed a relatively high appreciation of the programmes ... follow-up activities ... were useful in ... promoting a degree of audience feedback and participation ... programmes promoted thinking and encouraged the development of new understandings.

A review by Gordon (1967) of a traditional mass media-centred campaign also reveals how a mix of radio, TV, posters and pamphlets can have a behavioural outcome. A mix of 800 posters, 50 000 leaflets, mass mailing of letters to groups and clubs, press releases, press advertising, 11 radio spots and the involvement of three TV stations generated attendance at a Baltimore diabetes clinic on the three following days in the following proportions: day one, n = 512; day two, n = 790; day three, n = 1350. Interviews with those attending the clinic seemed to confirm that attendance had been primarily due to media information (64% press; 14% radio; 8% TV; remainder interpersonal contact). As the author notes, '... large groups of individuals stand ready to take action on any given issue and merely lack the information or cue to make the action possible'.

Certainly in this case, media triggered action. It would, however, be patently wrong to say this would happen for any given issue. Indeed, analysis of the examples of the media programmes above will in all cases indicate the presence of a key condition: pre-existing audience motivation; time and professional presentation necessary for communication of complex information; adjunct of interpersonal pressure, etc. However, it is rather difficult to find an easy explanation of the apparent success of a media-based intervention by the Indian Cancer Society which claimed to have doubled attendances at its six Bombay clinics specializing in the early detection of cancers. This would have been expected, a priori, to have been a difficult task. The journal article provides insufficient detail from which to determine which important preconditions seem responsible for overcoming the important affective barriers which often militate against successful cancer education (Ajit, 1982). Following the ten points of social marketing, the charitable involvement of an advertising agency might indeed, as claimed, have provided the skills and expertise necessary for a sensitive campaign! On the other hand, it may be the case that developing countries are more susceptible generally to mass media interventions and/or that it is easier to utilize community networks to enhance the impact of mass media. Alternatively, it may be that in western, urbanized society health education is more concerned with requiring the abandoning of pleasures and addictions associated with affluence whereas the major barriers in developing

countries have to do with cultural misconceptions and associated issues. Whatever the reason, there seems to be consistent evidence of successful media interventions in these countries. For instance, Jenkins (1983) reviews 17 projects: most reveal some significant changes and many of these are behavioural. These include a 3% decline in population growth rate (Costa Rica); an improvement in breastfeeding from 25% to over 50% (Micronesia, Yap Islands); 75% of all under-fives vaccinated on one day (Nicaragua); an increase from 0% to 24% adding oil to meals to enhance the energy content after a radio campaign (Philippines); an increase from 20% to 59% having latrines (Tanzania).

Evidence of the effectiveness of family planning campaigns have normally come from developing countries. Taplin (1981) reported that six projects 'improved contraceptive availability, increased sales of products, spread knowledge and stimulated wider use of methods promoted...'. A campaign in Esfahan increased pill accepters by 54% and total contraceptive use by 64% over a six-month period. Again, the impact of China's family planning programme is legendary and, as Liu (1981) indicated, this combined a blend of media and interpersonal persuasion. By 1972, 79% of China's population was using contraception; the rate of population increase was reduced from 23 per 1000 in 1963 to 4.7 per 1000 in 1974.

The International Quarterly of Community Health Education (Vol. 5, pp. 149–66, 1985) included a study by Cernada and Lu (1982) in a list of articles, selected by health educators, of the most worthwhile publications of the 1970s. This described a mass media demonstration project which provided evidence of successful penetration, knowledge and attitude change and an increase in low cost contraceptive practice. It could, of course, be argued that it is relatively easy to sell at least some varieties of family planning practice: health educators are offering a tangible product together with real benefits in terms of reduction of anxiety and economic pressures while minimizing loss of gratification. Relatively few thoroughly evaluated studies of family planning education are available for western countries, possibly because the service does not really need promoting! Those that are available seem to indicate reasonable levels of success. For instance, a study of a press/poster/leaflet campaign in Lambeth in 1972–3 increased numbers of new patients at clinics by 68%, total attendances by 26% and clinic sessions by 46%. A similar programme in Holland aimed at young people under the age of 18 succeeded in trebling numbers of clinic visitors at a time of year when attendance figures normally dropped. Both studies are reported by Smith (1978).

One final point will be made about the use of mass media in developing countries. It will be recalled that the major single benefit – perhaps the sole benefit – of mass media is their capacity to reach a mass audience and to do so relatively cheaply. As Leslie (1981) indicates in her review of mass media and nutrition education, '... the most firm conclusion suggested by the evaluations is that mass media health and nutrition education projects can reach large numbers of people (up to several million) in a relatively short period of time. The evaluations also indicate that, although there is a considerable range in costs among projects it is possible to achieve this outreach at a cost as low as $0.01 per person.' She goes on to point out that between 10% and 50% of the audience remember the main nutrition message and that when a specific nutrition message has been designed, there is '... a reasonable expectation that the target audience could modify their behaviour accordingly and ... a reasonable expectation that this modified behaviour could bring about an improvement in health or nutrition status ...'.

This chapter will be concluded by considering three situations where particular aspects of mass media or the kind of message they convey will determine the likelihood of success. In this way a major theme of this

book will be reiterated: it is of relatively little value making generalizations about effectiveness without a careful analysis of goals, strategies and methodology. First, we will consider the influence of media characteristics by considering and comparing the use of leaflets and posters. Secondly, we will look at a functionally different kind of health education problem – persuading individuals to use seat belts. Thirdly, we will consider goals and content by reviewing particularly problematical issues for health education – the misuse of substances. This will include comments about drugs generally and alcohol and smoking in particular.

POSTERS AND LEAFLETS

Before considering the potential of these two popular devices, we should reiterate the distinction made earlier between the use of media as mass media and the use of media as audio-visual aids or learning resources. It is almost a truism to say that the appropriate use of an audio-visual aid will enhance any given teaching method. For instance Burt *et al.* (1974) described a successful piece of patient education in which interpersonal education by medical and nursing staff delivered to survivors of acute myocardial infarction was supplemented by written advice and pamphlets. Sixty-two per cent of the smokers in the experimental group had remained non-smokers for between one and three years compared with 27.5% in a control group. This study did not quantify separately the relative contribution of the written materials. However, Russell *et al.* (1979) were able to show that leaflets added a couple of percentage points to the effectiveness of the verbal advice provided by a doctor.

The use of leaflets as mass media – i.e. without interpersonal support – is more problematical. Tapper-Jones and Davis (1985) documented a detailed and comprehensive survey of a sample of Welsh general practitioners' use of leaflets. The study demonstrated clearly that leaflet use was widespread in primary medical care: the vast majority of doctors used leaflets and/or other teaching aids. Of the sample of 176 GPs, 91% used diet sheets, 85.5% a variety of hand-drawn diagrams, 58.5% various leaflets, 39% pre-printed diagrams, 26% plastic models, 19% a patient counselling compendium, 15.5% 'Family Doctor' booklets and 3.5% 'some other aid'. The major suppliers of the leaflets were, first of all, various pharmaceutical companies and, second, the Health Education Council. Interestingly, GPs rated television as the most effective means of communication followed by 'personal advice from doctors – the reverse of Budd and McCron's (1979) observation of patients' rating of credibility!

The study by Russell *et al.* cited above led to the development of a specially tailored booklet containing advice on giving up smoking. This was dispatched to all GPs in England and Wales. Its fate serves to illustrate some of the limitations of the leaflet and will now be considered in the context of social marketing's notion of a 'hierarchy of effects'. We should first note that a leaflet must often be delivered to a 'gatekeeper' who will make it available to the prime user. The leaflet must be acceptable to the prime user and its message must then impinge on the consciousness of the target population: people must pick up the leaflets, read them, pay attention to the messages contained therein and, if they have been properly pre-tested, they should understand their content. Hopefully, they may also believe the message and this belief may in turn contribute towards the development of a favourable attitude to a healthy outcome which may then predispose the learner to adopt some behaviour or, possibly, to change some unhealthy practice, assuming, of course, that the social and physical environment will support and not inhibit such a course of action!

Spencer (1984) attempted to track the GUS ('Give Up Smoking') leaflets mentioned above. His survey revealed that 57% of the sample did not remember having received the booklets. Of those who did recall having received them, 72% found them acceptable and 39% had used them. However, only one in three of this user group appeared to have used the booklets in the prescribed fashion, i.e. as a consultation aid requiring the GP to provide a personalized message for the patient in the context of interpersonal advice and exhortation about stopping smoking. Posters accompanied the booklets and 69% of the 43% of doctors who had any recollection of receiving the kit claimed to have displayed the poster in the practice premises.

The ubiquitous and frequently maligned poster has been subjected to many appraisals, most of which demonstrate very low effectiveness when used without interpersonal support. Posters are, almost by definition, designed to convey persuasive messages without such adjuvant support (by contrast with a chart which is meant to be used as a teaching aid). Grant (1972) studied the impact of two differently styled posters urging women to have a cervical smear. These were prominently displayed in a number of clinics and women were interviewed in order to determine what they recalled of the posters. Relatively few could recall the posters (although one designed in a question-and-answer format was superior to the other). Significantly the women who were most aware of the posters had already had a smear test; their recall doubtless reflected self-congratulatory selective attention! A similar study by Cole and Holland (1980) reported that only 16 out of 198 women could remember accurately two posters displayed in a health centre waiting room. Over 90% did not read available leaflets or take one home.

A particularly optimistic attempt to use posters was described by Auger *et al.* (1972). Both posters and mobiles were used in a hospital setting to influence smoking behaviour. While the researchers did not imagine that a poster could influence the smoking habit, they thought that smokers in canteen areas might be persuaded not to smoke in that given situation or perhaps to extinguish their cigarettes. An ingenious form of indicator of success was employed: base line 'debris indices' were developed by counting and measuring cigarette butts before and after the poster/mobile display. The results? No change! It should be noted, in passing, that this study predates the substantial normative shift away from smoking and the prevalence of non-smoking policies in hospitals, restaurants and the like. It might well be the case that posters would have some trigger effect if used today in a similar context.

The Transport and Road Research Laboratory has carried out several experimental studies of media impact. One study demonstrated that by taking learning theory into account and sequencing the information presented in a poster, a significant improvement in correct interpretations of safe road crossing practices could be produced in children of various ages. While 36% of all children aged five to seven misinterpreted all messages on a draft poster, only 9% got the messages wrong on the revised 'sequenced' poster. Clearly, as the designers noted, understanding is only weakly related to road-crossing behaviour; nonetheless, the same organization demonstrated that posters used by the roadside could actually influence driving practices. After displaying double crown size posters for a week in six sites, the number of overtaking actions fell from 1866 to 1355 and the proportion of risky overtaking declined from 9% to 4.5%. However, posters used in a similar way had no effect on more complex driving behaviours such as keeping an adequate distance between cars on the M4 at Slough! (TRRL, 1967, 1972; BBC, 1982).

The final example to be discussed in this section on posters and leaflets is a well designed and extensively monitored campaign to prevent children's accidents. It is particularly interesting in that it: (i) used booklets in conjunction with a series of television programmes, (ii) its measure of effectiveness encompassed most of the kinds of indicator examined in Chapter 3 and (iii), because it appealed to caretakers of young children, motivation to take action must have been relatively high, certainly by comparison with programmes which required the audience to undertake uncomfortable activities or forgo gratification. The campaign consisted of three components: a ten programme television series lasting ten minutes per programme and employing a popular television personality as presenter; a 36-page booklet; a community initiative which sought to establish local 'Play It Safe' groups consisting of a variety of lay and professional people concerned with safety. The impact of the programme has been thoroughly documented (BBC, 1982; Jackson, 1983). The effectiveness of the TV programme will be summarized before analysing the separate effect of the booklets. Results will be described in accordance with the 'chain of indicators' ranging from awareness through to behaviour change.

First, audience penetration was good. Some 8 million people on average watched each programme (15.5% of the viewing population over the age of four). By the end of the series 59% of adults and 40% of children had seen at least one programme. The viewing figures indicated a representative social class distribution; as it was hoped to reach lower socio-economic groups, audience segmentation was thus satisfactory. Second, viewers had a positive attitude to the programmes: 96% of viewers found them interesting; 47% found them 'very helpful' and a further 37% considered them 'quite helpful'. More important, however, for the achievement of campaign goals is the audience attitude to the preventive measures which the programmes attempted to promote. In seeking to gain insight into these outcome measures and the intermediate variables which influenced them, some 2000 people were interviewed before and after the campaign. A sample of viewers was also compared with a matched group of non-viewers and their beliefs, attitudes and reported changes in practice were compared. The results can be summarized as follows.

1. Viewers tended to have more favourable reactions on four measures of six general attitudes to child safety;
2. Viewers were more likely than non-viewers to accept the probability of specific accidents occurring in eight out of 11 test situations;
3. Viewers were also more likely than non-viewers to believe that parents could do something to prevent the 11 accident situations described in the booklets. Whereas neither of the differences in (1) and (2) were statistically significant, two of these efficacy beliefs did meet the criterion of statistical success.

Third, in respect of actions taken, viewers were on average more likely to have translated positive attitude into practice. Of a possible list of 15 specific safety actions, viewers took 5.97 actions compared with non-viewers' 5.44. Again, this difference was not significant statistically. However, when a separate analysis of viewers who were 'responsible for children every day' was carried out, the differences in this category and in the categories listed above did reach a level of significance. In other words, the section of the target group which perceived the direct relevance of the recommendations was influenced significantly to a greater or lesser extent. Whether a difference of 0.9 safety actions taken is considered a success clearly depends on expectations of a mass media campaign!

Turning next to the contribution of the booklet, the following information was provided by the BBC's research department. Between December 1981 and the end of March 1982, a total of 1.5 million copies had been distributed, a figure which included 45 000 individual requests. Research into the population reached by the booklet indicated that some 11% of a total of 1926 adults interviewed had seen the publication and 4% claimed to have read it. By comparison, 15% of a sample of 1080 programme viewers had seen the booklet and 6% claimed to have read it. Predictably the proportion of lower socio-economic groups having written for the booklet, seen it or read it was smaller than middle class groups. Some 75% of the 1080 viewers claimed to have read all of the booklet and 71% of these claimed to have read it thoroughly. Ninety-seven per cent were pleased with the publication and found it useful. Fifty-nine per cent considered it taught them 'a lot of things I didn't know' but 76% believed that 'sensible parents would already follow most of the advice in the booklet'. What of actions taken? Although there may well be overclaiming, it does seem to be the case that the booklet had prompted actions among at least some readers. For example, 16% of booklet readers (which, remember, is 16% of the 4% of the population who claimed to have read it) stated that they now took more precautions in the kitchen; 15% were more careful with medicines and dangerous liquids; 10% took safety action concerning glass; 6% took more fire precautions and checked electrical safety; 4% secured windows, made stairs safer and secured cupboards.

A further interesting observation may be made about the impact of the total campaign. Some 15 local groups had been formed before the TV series was actually shown as a result of advance publicity and liaison work. This additional source of interpersonal support might be expected to maximize the impact of the campaign proper. In fact a study in an inner city area by Colver *et al.* (1982) showed that 55% of the working class families interviewed did not watch any of the TV programmes and only 9% of a group specially encouraged to watch the series took any of the 15 safety actions. However, when a comparable group received a home visit and were given specific advice, some 60% actually took some kind of action.

The evaluations of posters and leaflets discussed above clearly make the point that the peculiar features of given media will influence the likelihood of a successful outcome. However, these intrinsic factors will compete with other components of the whole influence process making prediction difficult if not impossible: for instance the success of the 'Play It Safe' booklets was affected by the context of the TV programmes, by the audience's beliefs about children's vulnerability to accident and, above all, by the addition of interpersonal education in Colver's study. Sometimes the anticipated benefits of given media may not materialize. For example, Harris (1983) reported on the failure of a local radio-based campaign to persuade the community to take on responsibility for preventing hypothermia in elderly relatives and neighbours. One of the key indicators – whether or not elderly people living alone had been visited in the previous seven days – seemed to show that there had been a 9% decline in visits after the programmes! At first glance, the 'folksy' nature and community orientation of local radio might have made it particularly suitable for this kind of campaign. Although hypothermia might not seem to be a particularly problematical health topic – most people would not be expected to be hostile to helping old people – the subject matter of many programmes offers an almost desperate challenge to the ingenuity of those seeking to produce change through mass media.

In the next section of this chapter, the results of a particularly rigorous study will be presented which seem to the author to indicate just what unsupported mass media can achieve under difficult but not impossible circumstances – promoting the wearing of seat belts. The concluding section of this chapter will review an acknowledged problem area, that of substance abuse in general. It will comment on drug education, identifying the prevention of alcohol misuse as especially difficult compared with tobacco smoking.

SEAT BELTS

In 1973, Levens and Rodnight assembled evidence of the effectiveness of a series of controlled area experiments in the use of mass media to promote seat belt wearing in Britain. The value of the study rests on the following facts:

1. Evidence of important driver/front seat passenger characteristics is presented;
2. Precise details of media input and their cost are provided;
3. Objective evidence of specific behaviours is described;
4. We can be as confident as anyone can that the results of media programmes can be ascribed to the input rather than other 'contaminating' events.

First, the pretesting of driver characteristics revealed the following useful data: drivers appeared already to be motivated to wear seat belts. Some 85% of those interviewed claimed to have a positive attitude to seat belt wearing, believing that this would cut down injuries. It seemed that despite this attitude many drivers did not 'belt up' and it was not possible to rely on reported use of belts since drivers consistently overestimated it. The number claiming to wear seat belts more than half the time was 57% but observed levels of wearing were only 17%. Any measure of programme effectiveness must therefore try to use observation rather than self-report.

Further research into the failure of drivers to use seat belts, despite their generally favourable attitude, suggested that this might be due to beliefs that although belts would reduce accidents, drivers were not susceptible to such accidents in a variety of situations (despite objective evidence to the contrary). In health belief model (HBM) terms, the target group clearly believed in the effectiveness of seat belts but were ambivalent about susceptibility and seriousness. At all events a programme was devised which used three appeals: 'appeal to the head', 'appeal to the heart' and 'appeal to the nervous system'. In other words a logical/factual approach compared with an emotional approach and an approach which tried to instil a habit so that seat belt wearing became routinized. Qualitative research indicated that this latter was probably the most effective and the slogan 'Klunk, Klick! Every Trip', presented by someone having high source credibility, was considered to have provided a mnemonic. The implication of this being that in HBM terms, the main perceived cost was merely the effort involved in establishing a routine (apart, of course, from the 15% who were implacably opposed on ideological grounds!).

The programmes were then launched in different regions in Britain utilizing different levels of expenditure, mostly on television advertising but supported by poster display. The results were carefully monitored by observing levels of seat belt wearing at a variety of sampling points. The rate of wearing increased in each of the regions sampled and to some extent reflected the level of media expenditure. There did seem, however, to be a decay effect with the exception of the final area where the trend seemed to be upward, perhaps indicating the start of a normative shift. The extent of the effect is summarized by Levens and Rodnight as follows.

> It is possible, within a media expenditure range corresponding to a national equivalent of from £235 000 to £720 000 (1972 prices) to raise the level of seat belt wearing by a percentage ranging from 3% to 16% (from a basic 14%–15% start point) and to do so within a period of three weeks.

They concluded that a burst of advertising over three weeks followed by supportive posters for a further three weeks would be the most cost effective way of proceeding. If we return to our earlier comment about the expectations of commercial advertisers, the changes produced would represent a very high level of success. However, the researchers do observe that having reached such a level

any further effects could not be achieved by more mass media work. Using the level of seat belt wearing prevalent in Australian states (where, at the time, legislation had been introduced) as a yardstick (i.e. 75% wearing), they concluded, 'The probable cost of bridging the gap between 32% and 75% wearing by persuasive advertising alone…could never be justified in benefit terms'.

In Britain, the need for such media-based health education has disappeared with the advent of legal compulsion. It is worth noting, as an aside, that although education failed to increase the level of wearing much above 30%, its agenda-setting function facilitated the enactment of health policy as described in Chapter 1. In other parts of the world, health education is still needed to protect vehicle occupants. In this context it is interesting to note how a broad-based media plus community programme in North Carolina followed good commercial practice and offered various incentives to drivers wearing seat belts (in the form of prizes and the opportunity to draw a winning lottery ticket). The programme was successful in raising the level of wearing from 24% to 41% in six months and sustaining it at 36% after a further six months (Gemming *et al.*, 1984). Let us compare this level of success with programmes which seek to modify substance abuse and influence levels of drug and alcohol use and smoking.

SUBSTANCE ABUSE

By comparing with safety education, family planning and many of the other topics receiving consideration above, attempts to deal with the problems of substance abuse seem to be doomed to failure, especially if the sole mode of attack is mass media campaigns. In short, the task would seem to involve persuading individuals to forsake habits which give them pleasure and to which they may be addicted – in one sense or another – or which meet some important psychological or social need. The significant of these motivational barriers will be apparent when we consider examples of campaigns designed to promote smoking cessation and foster sensible drinking. First, however, we will consider a recent attempt to use mass media to influence illegal drug use.

EXPERT OPINION

Despite expert opinion and Home Office policy, the UK government made a decision to launch a mass media campaign costing some £2 million directed at heroin misuse. The amount of money involved may be put into some kind of perspective by noting that the major national health education agency's total budget at the time amounted to some £10 million. It is highly probable that the hidden goals of the campaign were to be seen to be doing something to deal with a problem of doubtful magnitude but which created a good deal of moral outrage and indignation. At any rate, an evaluation was commissioned by government. In assessing the results of this evaluation, four questions have to be asked.

1. Should £2 million have been spent on the programme?
2. Were any real changes detectable in the target audience at the end of the campaign?
3. If there were any such changes, could they reasonable be attributed to the campaign?
4. In the event of real changes being observed, were these really significant rather than merely statistically significant, i.e. might they make any contribution to the reduction of drug misuse?

Of course, a priori, the money should not have been spent in that way. First, epidemiologically the problem of heroin use did not justify such an expenditure. Second, the accepted wisdom of drug education asserted that programmes should not use unsupported mass media nor should they focus on one specific drug. However, to many people's surprise, the evaluation appeared to indicate that against all the odds there was a significant and relevant change in beliefs and attitudes (since heroin use was so unusual there was no possibility of measuring any actual behaviour change). It is not possible here to provide a detailed and critical analysis of the research (for fuller discussion see Tones 1986) but several valuable conclusions for media use generally may be drawn. First, it was apparent that the campaign had been very successful in penetrating the market (which comprised young people aged 13–20) and in achieving levels of awareness which ranged from 80% to 98%, depending on the assessment criteria used. It thus supported the general axiom that properly constructed programmes can indeed raise awareness successfully. The second point which can be made is that it is increasingly difficult to find adequate control groups for national media programmes and therefore any observed results cannot be unequivocally ascribed to the programme itself. This was unfortunate since there did appear to be statistically significant changes in a series of measures of belief, attitude and intention which appeared to indicate a general hardening of attitude towards heroin use. However, because a control group was lacking and because the perfectly acceptable practice of using randomly selected but separate population subsamples to measure attitudes, etc. before and after the campaign had been used, it was possible to argue that the observed changes might have been due to pre-existing differences in the samples, even though these should have been removed by the process of random selection. Such an argument would have looked suspiciously like rationalization on the part of opponents of mass media drug education had it not been for several anomalies in the results. For instance, there seemed to be a tendency for the precampaign sample to have a generally less cautious approach to life than the postcampaign samples: the precampaign group appeared more likely to argue with parents and a higher proportion claimed that they would 'stand by their friends whatever they did'. These general attitudes could hardly have been influenced by a campaign dealing with a specific drug and the apparent hardening of attitudes could be ascribed to the fact that the postcampaign samples were generally more cautious, god-fearing and already opposed to hard drugs!

However, a much more important point can be made about the heroin campaign. Let us assume that the claimed shift in attitudes and beliefs was genuine. What impact could this be expected to have on the likelihood of a group of young people resisting the offer of hard drugs? Apart from the fact that beliefs about the effect of heroin on the body would probably be challenged when the young people in question actually engaged with a heroin using subculture, such beliefs and associated attitudes would be insignificant in real terms in the context of the various other alleged influences on drug misuse such as unemployment, social deprivation, home background and socialization, personality factors, self-esteem, machismo, rebelliousness, curiosity, social interaction skills, peer pressure, cultural norms, availability of drugs and beliefs about the gratifications provided. In the face of these factors, the potential of mass media for influencing drug related behaviour must be small. An alternative government strategy which allocated a similar amount of money to provide for about 100 drug co-ordinators for education authorities for a year would appear to be much more cost effective, even if it did not cater for the sense of moral outrage of the populace! However, let us move on to consider our most popular drug – alcohol.

ALCOHOL

At first blush – and under the influence of a stereotyped view of desperate junkies unable to 'kick their habit' – we might expect alcohol education to offer greater opportunities for effective intervention than the heroin campaign discussed above. In fact one of the biggest challenges to health promotion is posed by alcohol. The reasons are perhaps self-evident: unlike smoking, the health education message is relatively complex. It seeks to promote 'moderate' or 'sensible' drinking and requires the individual to calculate relative strengths of different liquor; it requires judgement and decision making. Moreover, the use of alcohol is strongly supported by social norms while smoking is becoming an increasingly deviant behaviour. The vast majority of smokers acknowledge the negative aspects of their habit and claim that they would like to give up, seeking only a magic formula and appropriate support to help them do so. The tobacco manufacturers are under constant attack while the brewing industry has a much more positive image. On the other hand, like smoking, alcohol consumption provides considerable gratification, both physical and social. It is thus hardly surprising that examples of effective alcohol education are almost non-existent, particularly in the context of media campaigns and community wide programmes.

The effectiveness and efficiency of alcohol education programmes have been comprehensively reviewed. In addition to the general reviews of Gatherer *et al.* (1979) and Bell *et al.* (1985), Kinder (1975) analysed some 66 studies on drug and alcohol education published between 1963 and 1973. Blane and Hewitt (1977, 1980) also produced state-of-the-art reviews of mass media. More recently Dorn and South (1983) provided a critical appraisal of 404 publications. The conclusions to be derived from all of these reviews may be summarized as follows.

1. There have been relatively few methodologically sound evaluations (perhaps with the exception of a few studies of drink-driving).
2. Expenditure on health education has been completely insignificant compared with the promotion of alcohol. Such campaigns as there have been have tended to

have limited geographical coverage and to have been broadcast at inappropriate times. As Dorn and South observe, 'For every £1000 which is paid in liquor duty and tax in the UK, 43 pence is spent on education about alcohol and its effects. In 1980 over £76 million was spent on drink advertising.'

The pro-alcohol messages conveyed directly and indirectly by media indicate both its social acceptability and its high level prevalence.

3. A social marketing approach incorporating thorough pretesting should be used by health educators.

4. There is a need for locally oriented community programmes having a strong interpersonal education component.

5. Alcohol education programmes frequently produce a change in knowledge and occasionally attitude but rarely influence drinking behaviour.

To some extent these observations might be made about most health education issues; it just happens that influencing alcohol consumption is especially difficult. We will now illustrate the points above and other mass media issues discussed earlier by reviewing selectively a few of the plethora of studies in this area. The first of these are concerned with the incidental effects of mass media.

The incidental, 'norm-sending' aspects of mass media were mentioned earlier in this chapter and reference was made to Hansen's (1986) work on media images of alcohol. Several published studies underline the importance of this norm-sending role of media in relation to alcohol. The following are cited by Dorn and South (1983). Block (1965) described the ways in which press reporting stereotyped and stigmatized the alcoholic. A series of investigations by Breed and Defoe (1978; 1979a; 1979b; 1980a; 1980b; 1981) examined not only the portrayal of alcohol in magazine advertising but also in press reports, prime time television sitcoms, comic books and campus magazines. Gerbner (1981) pointed out the higher prevalence of alcohol images in top-rated programmes. King (1979) predated Hansen's observations by demonstrating similar types of presentation in British 'soaps'. Finn (1980) reminded us of the wide variety of mass media by reporting a content analysis of greeting cards which again perpetuated the negative stereotyped images of the alcohol abuser.

One of the possible mechanisms whereby these incidental effects may be produced is that of modelling. Both Caudill and Marlatt (1975) and Garlington and Dericco (1979) have argued that media models may influence the drinking rates of male students.

The norms conveyed through media presentations are essentially unrealistic. These mythical messages suggest that:

1. Everyone drinks heavily (i.e. at a rate per unit time far in excess of real life drinking).

2. Drinking is associated with sexual prowess, romance, enjoyable social occasions, power and commercial success and generally occurs in upmarket situations.

3. Few negative consequences are shown. Drinkers remain clearheaded, do not have accidents, stay slim and healthy or, alternatively, may be seen as antiheroes. These latter provide a celebration of cosy self-gratification and folksy moderation in the face of attempts by fanatical zealots who try to impose unattainable ideals of health and fitness on the populace at large.

4. 'Problem drinkers' are presented only in the caricatured form of skid row down-and-outs.

Following the theoretical discussion at the start of this chapter, it is not, of course, intended to suggest that this background of 'normative noise' will necessarily have any direct effect on people's drinking. It does, however, following the principles of 'uses and gratifications', provide people with the 'evidence' to justify their current practices and resist the pressures of health education. In the face of this background 'noise' conveying the normality and desirability of heavy alcohol consumption, it is perhaps some consolation that media credibility is relatively low (at any rate when it can be seen to attempt to influence). As indicated earlier, Budd and McCron (1979) demonstrated a low level of trust in health messages generally when delivered by mass media. This situation, not surprisingly, appears to apply to drugs and alcohol also. For instance Dembo *et al.* (1977) reported that high school students perceived television and radio as having low credibility compared with other media and with interpersonal sources of information. It is not, however, clear whether the incidental presentation of health related information is subject to the same degree of sceptical appraisal. It is probably wise to assume that it is not.

The implications of the work described above for health promotion are clear but not necessarily easy to achieve. At the level of policy, the controllers of broadcast media must be prevailed upon to ensure that the consequences of alcohol consumption are more realistically portrayed. At the level of individual health education, the natural scepticism of the viewing public must be nurtured by increasing awareness of media conventions and developing critical appraisal skills. Given the relative ineffectiveness of mass media in fostering 'sensible drinking' this aspect of health promotion merits increasing emphasis.

Turning now to these more deliberate attempts to influence people's knowledge, attitudes and practices with regard to alcohol, we might first ask about the trade's success in persuading individuals to start drinking and increase their level of consumption. As indicated earlier (Henry and Waterson, 1981), the advertisers of alcohol modestly deny having any effects on recruitment, asserting that they offer a public service by allowing the existing drinker to select from available beverages, i.e. the goal is brand-switching. Several attempts have been made to give the

lie to this assertion and demonstrate that advertising does have an effect on consumption. While it does seem likely that preferences for different kinds of alcohol (e.g. beer versus spirits) may be influenced (Brown, 1978), it is difficult to find sound evidence that restrictions on advertising will reduce consumption (Ogbourne and Smart, 1980) or show anything other than weak econometric associations. In the absence of such evidence, it becomes more difficult to urge governmental action. If there is an effect, it is clearly of a much lower order than the impact of such structural factors as fiscal, economic and legislative measures (Bourgeois and Barnes, 1979). However, even if advertising does not in fact increase total consumption, the norm-sending function should be sufficient to justify pressure for controls.

Again, if it is indeed true that advertisers with their vast advertising budget really cannot influence consumption, the chances for health education of reducing total consumption would, a priori, appear to be slight. Published research supports this view but also demonstrates the anticipated 'hierarchy of effects', i.e. that it is relatively easy to create awareness but increasingly difficult to influence recall, attitudes and behaviour. Some indication of this is provided by Maloney and Hersey's (1984) detailed account of an intensive marketing strategy to transmit alcohol public service advertisements (PSAs) nationwide (in the USA). Messages were aimed principally at women and youth. Assessment of the campaign reach (penetration) as measured by the proportion of the target audience likely to be watching television at a given time of day multiplied by the market share of a particular television station indicated that the PSAs reached on average 31.8% of all adults, 22% of the female target group and 19% of young people. However, according to the authors, commercial practice suggests that product purchase requires at least three exposures to an advertisement which in turn means a level of campaign reach of 42% of an audience. Although the average penetration was 22%, there were in fact 13 markets where more than 42% of the primary targets were exposed to the PSAs and three where the exposure was 60% or more.

And so, given a sufficient level of media expenditure, the first goal of awareness can clearly be attained. Two case studies will now be considered in order to illustrate what might be expected from media campaigns which try to surpass this relatively limited goal. The first was launched in the north east of England and the second in California.

The Tyne-Tees Alcohol Campaign was piloted in 1974 (HEC, 1983) and, in the view of many people, had unrealistic objectives of producing changes in consumption in a region noted for its heavy drinking. After a series of changes and developments the campaigns continued into the 1980s. At a meeting to assess its effects (HEC, 1982) eight key findings were listed. These illustrate what might realistically be expected from such a campaign:

1. People in the north east were aware of their regional attitudes to alcohol being 'different'.
2. People in the north east were more inclined to believe alcohol was a problem, though they were inclined to think of it as caused by other problems.
3. People in the north east were more aware of sources of help.
4. More than 70% recalled the campaign and there were significant levels of recall of specific messages.
5. One in eight people claimed that it had some influence on their thinking about alcohol.
6. Safe drinking levels were believed to be lower in the north east than in Leicester (a comparison region).
7. There was more awareness of 'equivalents' in the north east than in Leicester.
8. There might be some antagonism building up towards health education messages.

The programme in California, which we will now consider, is of special interest because it was designed particularly to take account of known limitations of mass media. It was called the 'Winners' programme (indicating its attempt to promote a positive image) and is described by Wallack and Barrows (1983). It ran for three years at a total cost of some $2.5 million. It was located in three sites: one acted as a control; one received a media-only programme and the third received media plus an additional community based effort (thus seeking to emulate the Stanford Heart Disease Prevention Programme). Programme goals were as follows: awareness raising and provision of information; attitude change and subsequently changes in actual drinking behaviours; medical indicators – viz. cirrhosis rates (after an appropriate time lapse) and social indicators in the form of drunk driving rates, arrests for disorderly conduct, etc. It was considered that success would lead to cost benefits and an overall reduction in per capita consumption.

The target was adults aged 18–35 and after the first year it was hoped that other groups might be influenced.

The media programme included: three 30-second television commercials, three 60-second radio slots; press advertisements; 110 billboard displays. The media mix was calculated to reach 90% of the target group on an average of 35 occasions. The message content emphasized positive advantages of lower consumption, presenting images of the moderate drinker as happy, in control, sociable and macho. Women were depicted as self-assured and in control.

It is interesting to note how political factors almost immediately affected the programme planning. The Wine Institute exerted pressure which delayed the programme to the extent that there was a 40% lower exposure than had been originally planned.

The community programme was designed to incorporate an interpersonal element. Some 14 453 people attended meetings; 67 000 pieces of programme material (balloons, badges, etc.) were distributed; various publicity events were arranged; teacher training programmes were developed. According to the authors, however, the community programme did not meet expectations in that there was little integration with media inputs and a planned recruitment of volunteers who might hold home meetings did not materialize.

The results follow the now expected pattern: good levels of awareness, some attitude change and no behaviour change. For detailed results, readers are referred to the original article. However, the following will serve to indicate the nature and scale of the changes achieved.

1. There was a high level of slogan recognition (79% in adult group, 86% in youth group). As with many other results these tended to be more pronounced in the media plus community area and greater than in the control community.
2. There was a generally high level of correct interpretation of the messages (e.g. 70% adult; 84% youth) and 20% of adults and 30% of youth scored at least eight out of 12 on a scale of overall comprehension. The problem of lack of feedback potential of media was, however, to be observed in that some 25% believed that one of the PSAs was promoting alcohol – even after pretesting and subsequent change!
3. Recall was generally good (50% adults; 72% youth).
4. In general there was a disappointing level of change in the affective area. For example, awareness of alcohol problems and concern about these problems showed relatively slight increases as did concern about own level of drinking (e.g. 8% adults and 2% youth). On an attitude scale containing 13 statements relating to advertising of alcohol, drunkenness, etc., there was only one significant change (and that was in the adult group).
5. As for behavioural outcome, 15% of those who recognized the 'Winners' slogans reported a reduction in drinking or claimed they intended to do so, but there was no supporting evidence of this. There was no change in other items which attempted to measure quantity and frequency of drinking nor was there any change in a seven category drinking problem scale.

In short, it is clear that even in a very well constructed and evaluated programme which takes account of the dictates of social marketing, there is no evidence of behaviour change. It could, of course, happen that the campaign's impact on knowledge and awareness might, in the context of future developments, make the success of such hypothetical developments more likely. Wallack and Barrows (1983) described the situation thus:

> The California Prevention Demonstration was unique in many ways, but in terms of the types of outcomes that were produced it was quite typical. The major evaluation findings of increased awareness, some gain in knowledge and no attitude or behaviour change is consistent with a myriad of other mass media programs and prevention efforts in general.

The authors argued that Lazarsfeld and Merton's views (1975) were even more applicable to the current scenario than they were 40 years ago. They strongly assert the points made in the first chapter of this book, that mass media programmes in difficult areas like alcohol use will only be effective when complemented by significant public policy measures. As it is:

> Mass media campaigns and other kinds of individual-oriented interventions are safe because they virtually never challenge any powerful vested interests. Such interventions implicitly state that the problem is in the person and not in the system. Yet as we have suggested above, the person and the

system are inseparable; you cannot address one without also addressing the other.

The results of workplace interventions, to be discussed in the next chapter, would bear out these views. However, research on mass media work in smoking yields much more impressive results, particularly when combined with interpersonal efforts and based on sound learning theory. The reasons for any such success compared with alcohol interventions were suggested earlier. For the moment, we will briefly consider some of the results of evaluations of programmes designed to foster smoking cessation.

SMOKING

Before commenting on the effectiveness of mass media in combating smoking, we must note that just as alcohol use and misuse has its own peculiarities as a public health problem, the special characteristics of smoking must be taken into account before judgements are made. First of all, there are two qualitatively different smoking prevention tasks: the prevention of recruitment differs from the promotion of smoking cessation. The motives which underlie young people's adoption of the habit are not at all similar to the motivation which may prevent adult (or even young people) quitting. For young people tobacco and its pharmacology are largely irrelevant; smoking serves a symbolic purpose and meets instrumental needs, gratifying the values associated with machismo, toughness, precocity and the like. It also provides a valuable adjunct to self-presentation and social interaction. While some of these aspects may also be important to the adult smoker, the cigarette's role in affect control becomes much more prominent.

The educational tasks demanded by these two different prevention goals are thus distinct. In simple terms, the aims of preventing the onset of smoking involve the creation of a negative attitude to the habit and, more importantly, providing substitute gratification in the form of life skills, etc. On the other hand, since the majority of smokers already appear to have a negative attitude to their habit, the major preventive goal is to provide a trigger to cessation followed by support to minimize the chance of relapse. The very nature of these different educational objectives means that the mass media have been seen as more appropriate to the smoking cessation exercise rather than to preventing recruitment (although, as we have seen, television may be a useful supplement to school-based programmes which seek to prevent recruitment to smoking). As we will see, the effectiveness of mass media in stimulating cessation (the only justifiable goal) has depended on the extent to which support can be provided or mobilized and this in turn has meant borrowing interpersonal techniques.

Two kinds of intervention will be described below. The first of these involves mere consciousness raising about the importance of stopping smoking, with or without the provision of more detailed information and mailed supporting literature. The second involves a more thorough television presentation incorporating several sessions and based on social learning theory. Typical of the former situation is the UK National No Smoking Day.

Reid (1985) describes the relative effectiveness of two successive no smoking days in 1984 and 1985. Apart from providing results which reveal the antismoking potential of this sort of publicity tactic, the hierarchy of effects is nicely illustrated. For instance, after pre-publicity designed to co-ordinate national health education efforts, on the day itself some 716 press reports were recorded together with 424 mentions on television or radio. Over a 14 day period there were 13 national radio or television slots and an estimated 134 hours of broadcasting (including in 1985 mentions on the popular 'soaps' 'Brookside' and 'Coronation Street').

Public awareness was high and amounted to some 79% of the population. There was local support from over 100 health education units as well as other organizations such as schools, hospitals, etc. In terms of acceptability, 70% of an interview sample agreed that the day was a good idea and only 7% were firmly opposed.

In order to determine the impact on smoking, a survey of 2000 adults was carried out in 130 sampling points throughout the country. The results were as follows: of 2000 adults, 735 were smokers; 95 (13%) reported trying to give up and five succeeded in giving up for the day. A further study of 4000 adults three months later provided corroboration of the first survey. Eleven per cent reported they had tried to give up smoking on National No Smoking Day; 9% claimed to have been successful for two months before relapsing. However only three out of the 4000 were still non-smokers after three months (and only one of these claimed that this was due to the day itself!).

Was this a success or a failure? The cost incurred was £50 000 and included expenditure on 250 000 posters and 300 000 smokers' contracts. At any rate, it was decided to repeat the day in 1985 with an increased budget (£100 000). Although no information was presented on cessation rates, it was clear that awareness was again high: some 76% had heard of the programme on television and 6.5% of smokers claimed to have given up for the day. An interesting indicator is provided of the booster effect of local involvement: some 22 000 people used a telephone to 'Dial a Tip' but 14 000 of these were from Plymouth where two local television personalities committed themselves to stop smoking during the week. It is clearly unwise to set unrealistic behavioural standards for a publicity venture such as National No Smoking Day. Rather it should be viewed as an agenda-setting exercise which might to some degree counteract the norm-sending messages transmitted by the tobacco advertisers and may even act as an ultimate trigger to a small number of individuals who have been screwing up their courage to abandon their habit!

A more extensive but to some extent more abortive media venture was reported by Raw and de Plight (1981). A 15 minute programme was presented at prime time in a regular documentary slot. It had a 'hard-hitting evangelical style' ('... we want to make a frontal attack on smoking ... we're going to send you every known device to make you give it up and stop killing yourself'). That section of the public who were already motivated to quit and were waiting for the 'magic bullet' responded eagerly. Four thousand calls were received in 30 minutes and eventually some 600 000 people wrote in for the kit which was to help them stop smoking. Unfortunately only 20 000 kits were available. The public was not impressed!

Eventually a more limited kit was sent out to a sample of 20 000 applicants together with a questionnaire. The response rate was 12%. Of the 1752 who returned usable questionnaires: 1602 said they intended to stop smoking; 747 tried to stop; 57 succeeded for between two and three months; 41 were still not smoking after six months and 14 were abstinent at one year. The success rate among those who returned the questionnaires was thus 0.79%. It should, however, be noted that 46% had found the kit unhelpful.

Other studies of similar ventures have met with greater success: for instance Cuckle and Vunakis (1984) studied a random sample of 4492 subjects out of half a million who requested a postal smoking cessation kit after a television programme on the hazards of smoking. Compared with a control group, cessation after one year was superior in the experimental group (11% versus 16%). Interestingly but not surprisingly validation via salivary continine measurement revealed lower results but there was still a statistically significant difference (7% versus 9%). These results are not dissimilar to those found by O'Byrne and Crawley (1981) after an Irish programme. Some 5% of kit recipients claimed to have stopped smoking between three and five months after the campaign. The superiority of the American figures presumably reflects the greater normative 'push' to non-smoking in the USA compared with Eire. Normative factors would have to be considered also in the comprehensive and well-documented study by Puska *et al.* (1979) in Finland.

In the general context of the North Karelian Heart Disease Prevention Project a smoking cessation course was presented on television in 1978. It was launched at a national press conference and was supported by extensive press reporting. The major voluntary organizations also informed their members about the programme and a serious attempt was made to encourage smokers to follow the programme in organized groups. Lay leaders of these groups were provided with support materials. The programme lasted four weeks; there were seven sessions broadcast during the evening and lasting 45 minutes each. The programmes were designed to incorporate interpersonal methods in that a group of ten smokers were featured in the studio and sessions were led by two experts. The techniques used by smoking cessation clinics were employed. In other words the mass media strategy was about as thorough as it could be: there was intensive and comprehensive coverage on the one available television channel; it was supported by additional publicity in the context of a regional programme which had raised awareness of the national heart disease problem; it employed interpersonal methods on screen and encouraged group support in local neighbourhoods. How well did it do? The results showed that 39.5% of men saw between one and three of the broadcast sessions (figures for women were 38.7%); 4.2% of men and 7.3% of women saw all seven. As for the impact on smoking, a survey carried out one year after the final programme revealed that 17% of smokers followed the programme but did not try to stop and 1.4% stopped smoking but started again. Only 0.8% of those who were smoking at the start of the series were non-smokers

after one year. Analysis of those who followed the programmes in a support group yielded the following results. In North Karelia 404 people were in these organized groups; 320 completed the course. Of those who completed the course, 21% succeeded in stopping smoking for a period of at least six months.

One of the most thorough and effective programmes employing mass media to promote smoking cessation is described by Best (1980). This used not only mass media but employed the principles of behaviour modification in the form of 'self-management' components previously used in face-to-face clinics. Six programmes were broadcast on consecutive weeks between 7.00–7.30 p.m. The potential audience was some 20 000 adults (in Washington DC). Viewers were invited to write in for the self-help guide mentioned above and each television programme was linked to a chapter in the booklet. Those who applied for the booklet served as the subjects of the evaluation.

At the end of the series, 86.5% of the survey group returned a completed questionnaire; 64.2% returned a second questionnaire at three months and 71.4% returned a questionnaire at six months. Cessation rates at these times were: 11.5%; 14.7% and 17.6% respectively.

How should we assess the results of both the Finnish exercise and the intervention described by Best? Puska *et al.* made the observation that although the programme achieved a rate of success which was small percentage-wise, some 10 000 smokers countrywide might have stopped smoking with the aid of the programme and that is a lot of smokers in absolute terms. Best commented that the spontaneous quit rate (in the USA) was probably 5%; long term success rates for smoking cessation clinics are of the order of 15–20% (perhaps higher if supplemented by prescription of nicotine chewing gum); face-to-face behaviour modification methods utilized by Best achieved 50% at six months. By these criteria the 17.6% achieved by his television programmes are good. In terms of cost effectiveness, he calculated that the face-to-face method cost $200 per success; smoking clinics cost $250 or more while, because of the large audience reached by media, the television series cost some $48 per documented abstinence (at six months).

One final point will be made about the use of mass media and smoking prevention. While it is clear that education about smoking generally and education delivered by mass media in particular are undoubtedly more effective than alcohol education, we should bear in mind Wallack's observations about the importance of structural social change in supporting education. Engleman (1983) describes this synergism between publicity, education and legal/fiscal measures in influencing smoking rates. He argues that not only has education itself had an impact on smoking, but it has also been responsible for such increases in taxation on cigarettes as have been imposed in recent years. He refers to the USA and argues that had it not been for the first Surgeon General's Report in 1964 and the subsequent education and publicity, smoking would have been 22% greater than it was in 1975. Since that time the reductions have continued, although it seems likely that as we move into the asymptote, further progress will be increasingly difficult and mass media will have an increasing role to play in stimulating policy change rather than persuading individuals to quit. At the same time the main thrust of smoking education must be targeted on young people, mainly in the schools and utilizing appropriate interpersonal educational strategies.

Because of the controversial nature of mass media, this chapter has looked in some depth at the issues involved and the requirements of effective media work. The conclusion to be drawn is that mass media can serve a very useful purpose in health education when properly designed and when their inherent limitations are recognized. In general, greater success will be achieved when mass media are used in support of community-wide pro-grammes – a point which will receive reinforcement when we consider the various heart health programmes in the final chapter. Before doing this we will give a rather less extensive review of a strategy which is increasing in popularity and which has peculiar features of interest. This strategy concerns the delivery of health education in the workplace.

REFERENCES

Aitken, P.P., Leathar, D.S., O'Hagan, F.J. and Squair, S.I. (1987) Children's awareness of cigarette advertisements and brand imagery. *British Journal of Addiction*, **82**, 615–22.

Ajit, T.C. (1982) A life worth living. *Public Relations*, Winter, 3–5.

Albert, W.H. (1981) General models of persuasive influence for health education, in *Health Education and the Media*, (eds D.S. Leathar, G.B. Hastings and J.K. Davies), Pergamon, London.

Atkin, C.K. (1981) Mass media information campaign effectiveness, in *Public Communication Campaigns*, (eds R.E. Rice and W.J. Paisley), Sage Publications, Beverly Hills.

Auger, T.J., Wright, T.J. and Simpson, R.H. (1972) Posters as smoking deterrents. *Journal of Applied Psychology*, **56**, 169–71.

Ball-Rokeach, S.J. and de Fleur, M.L. (1976) A dependency model of mass media effects. *Communication Research*, **3**, 3–21.

Bell, J. *et al.* (1985) *Annotated Bibliography of Health Education Research Completed in Britain from 1948–1978 and 1979–1983*, Scottish Health Education Group, Edinburgh.

Best, J.A. (1980) Mass media, self-management and smoking modification, in *Behavioral Medicine: Changing Health Lifestyles*, (eds P.O. Davidson and S.M. Davidson), Brunner/Mazel, New York.

Best, G., Dennis, J. and Draper, P. (1977) *Health, the Mass Media and the National Health Service*, Unit for the Study of Health Policy, London.

Blane, H.T. and Hewitt, L.E. (1977) *Mass Media, Public Education and Alcohol: a State-of-the-Art Review*, National Institute on Alcohol Abuse and Alcoholism, Rockville, Maryland.

Blane, H.T. and Hewitt, L.E. (1980) Alcohol, public education and mass media: an overview. *Alcohol, Health and Research World*, **5**, 2–16.

Block, M. (1965) *Alcoholism: Its Facets and Phases*, University Press, Oxford.

Bonaguro, J.A. and Miaoulis, G. (1983) Marketing – a tool for health education planning. *Health Education*, January/February, 6–11.

Botvin, G.J. *et al.* (1984) A cognitive–behavioural approach to substance abuse prevention. *Addictive Behaviors*, **9**, 134–47.

Bourgeois, J.C. and Barnes, J.G. (1979) Does advertising increase alcohol consumption? *Journal of Advertising Research*, **19**, 19–29.

Breed, W. and Defoe, J.R. (1978) Bringing alcohol into the open. *Columbia Journalism Review*, **18**, 18–19.

Breed, W. and Defoe, J.R. (1979a) Drinking on television: a comparison of alcohol use to the use of coffee, tea, soft drinks, water and cigarettes. *The Bottom Line*, **2**, 28–9.

Breed, W. and Defoe, J.R. (1979b) Themes in magazine alcohol advertisements: a critique. *Journal of Drug Issues*, **9**, 511–22.

Breed, W. and Defoe, J.R. (1980a) Mass media, alcohol and drugs: a new trend. *Journal of Drug Issues*, **9**, 511–22.

Breed, W. and Defoe, J.R. (1980b) The mass media and alcohol education: a new direction. *Journal of Alcohol and Drug Education*, **25**, 48–58.

Breed, W. and Defoe, J.R. (1981) The portrayal of the drinking process on prime-time television. *Journal of Communication*, **31**, 48–58.

British Broadcasting Corporation (1982) *'Play It Safe': Child Accident Prevention Campaign*, BBC Broadcasting Research Special Report, November, BBC, London.

Brown, R.A. (1978) Educating young people about alcohol use in New Zealand: whose side are we on? *British Journal of Alcohol and Alcoholism*, **13**, 199–201.

Budd, J. and McCron, R. (1979) *Communication and Health Education, A Preliminary Study*, Health Education Council, London.

Burt, A. *et al.* (1974) Stopping smoking after myocardial infarction. *Lancet*, **i**, 304–6.

Cantril, H. (1958) The invasion from Mars, in *Readings in Social Psychology*, (eds E.E. Maccoby, T.M. Newcomb and E.L. Hartley), Henry Holt, New York, pp. 291–300.

Caudill, B.D. and Marlatt, C. (1975) Modelling influences in social drinking: an experimental analogue. *Journal of Consulting and Clinical Psychology*, **43**, 405–15.

Cernada, G.P. and Lu, L.P. (1982) The Kaohsiung Study. *Studies in Family Planning*, **3**, 198–203.

Chaffee, S. (1981) Mass media in political campaigns: an expanding role, in *Public Communica-tion Campaigns*, (eds R.E. Rice and W.J. Paisley), Sage Publications, Beverly Hills.

Chapman, S. (1986) *The Lung Goodbye: A Manual of Tactics for Counteracting the Tobacco Industry in the 1980s*, 2nd edn, International Organization of Consumers' Unions, The Hague, Netherlands.

Chapman, S. and Fitzgerald, B. (1982) Brand preference and advertising recall in adolescent smokers: some implications for health promotion. *American Journal of Public Health*, **72**, 491–4.

Charlton, A. (1986) Children's advertisement-awareness related to their views on smoking. *Health Education Journal*, **45**, 75–8.

Chesterfield-Evans, A. and O'Connor, G. (1986) Billboard utilizing graffitists against unhealthy promotions (BUGAP) – its philosophy and rationale and their application in health promotion, in *Health Education and the Media*, (eds D.S. Leathar, G.B. Hastings and J.K. Davies), Pergamon, London.

Cole, R. and Holland, S. (1980) Recall of health education display materials. *Health Education Journal*, **39**, 74–9.

Colver, A.P., Hutchinson, P.J. and Judson, E.C. (1982) Promoting children's home safety. *British Medical Journal*, **285**, 1177–80.

Cuckle, H.S. and Vunakis, H.V. (1984) The effectiveness of a postal smoking cessation kit. *Community Medicine*, **6**, 210–15.

De Tocqueville, A. (1961) *Democracy in America*, Schocken Books, New York, (p. 134), cited by Paisley, W.J. (1981) Public communications campaigns: the American experience, in *Public Communication Campaigns*, (eds R.E. Rice and W.J. Paisley), Sage Publications, Beverly Hills.

Dembo, R., Miran, M., Babst, D.V. and Schmeidler, J. (1977) The believability of the media as sources of information on drugs. *International Journal of Addictions*, **12**, 959–69.

Docherty, S.C. (1981) Sports sponsorship – a first step in marketing health? in *Health Education and the Media*, (eds D.S. Leathar *et al.*), Pergamon, London.

Dorn, N. (1981) Communication with the working class requires recognition of a working class: a materialist approach, in *Health Education and the Media*, (eds D.S. Leathar *et al.*), Pergamon, London.

Dorn, N. and South, N. (1983) *Message in a Bottle*, Gower, Aldershot.

Douglas, T. (1984) *The Complete Guide to Advertising*, Macmillan, London.

Dunnigan, M.G. *et al.* (1981) Policy for the prevention of Asian rickets in Britain: a preliminary assessment of the Glasgow rickets campaign. *British Medical Journal*, **282**, 357–60.

England, P.M. and Oxley, D.E. (1980) Head infestation in Humberside: a health control exercise. *Health Education Journal*, **39**, 23–5.

Engleman, S.R. (1983) *The Impact of Anti-smoking Mass Media Publicity*, Health Education Council, London.

Evans, R.I., Rozelle, R.M. and Mittlemark, M.B. (1978) Deterring the onset of smoking in children. *Journal of Applied Social Psychology*, **8**, 126–35.

Farhar-Pilgrim, B. and Shoemaker, F.F. (1981) Campaigns to affect energy behavior, in *Public Communication Campaigns* (eds R.E. Rice and W.J. Paisley), Sage Publications, Beverly Hills.

Finn, P. (1980) Attitudes toward drinking conveyed in studio greeting cards. *American Journal of Public Health*, **70**, 826–9.

Flay, B.R. (1981) On improving the chances of mass media health promotion programs causing meaningful changes in behavior, in *Health Education by Television and Radio*, (ed. M. Meyer), K.G. Saur, München.

Flay, B.R. *et al.* (1986) Reaching children with mass media health promotion programs: the relative effectiveness of an advertising campaign in a community-based program and a school-based program, in *Health Education and the Media* (eds D.S. Leathar, G.B. Hastings and J.K. Davies), Pergamon, London.

Flay, B.R. *et al.* (1987) Implementation effectiveness trial of a social influences smoking prevention programme using schools and television. *Health Education Research*, **2**, 385–400.

Fuglesang, A. (1981) Folk media and folk messages, in *Health Education by Television and Radio*, (ed. M. Meyer), KG Saur, München.

Garlington, W. and Dericco, D. (1979) The effect of modelling on drinking rate. *Journal of Applied Behavior Analysis*, **10**, 207–11.

Gatherer, A., Parfit, J., Porter, E. and Vessey, M. (1979) *Is Health Education Effective?* Health Education Council, London.

Gemming, M.G., Runyan, C.W. and Campbell, B.J. (1984) A community health education approach to occupant protection. *Health Education Quarterly*, **11**, 147–58.

Gerbner, G. *et al.* (1981) Health and medicine on television – special report. *New England Journal of Medicine*, **305**, 90–4.

Gordon, E. (1967) Evaluation of communications media in two health projects in Baltimore. *Public Health Reports*, **82**, 651–5.

Grant, A.S. (1972) What's the use of posters? *Journal of the Institute of Health Education*, **10**, 7–11.

Greenberg, B.S. and Gantz, W. (1976) Public television and taboo topics: the impact of 'VD Blues'. *Public Telecommunications Review*, **4**, 59–64.

Hansen, A. (1986) The portrayal of alcohol on television. *Health Education Journal*, **45**, 127–31.

Harris, J. (1983) *Interpretive Summary of Hypothermia Campaign Evaluations, Winter of 1982/3*, Health Education Council, London.

Health Education Council (1982) *Report of a Meeting held on 29th April, 1982: The Tyne-Tees Alcohol Education Campaign*, Health Education Council, London.

Health Education Council (1983) *The Tyne-Tees Alcohol Education Campaign*, Health Education Council, London.

Henry, H.W. and Waterson, M.J. (1981) The case for advertising alcohol and tobacco products, in *Health Education and the Media*, (eds D.S. Leathar *et al.*), Pergamon, London.

Hutchinson, A. and Thompson, J. (1982) Rubella prevention: two methods compared. *British Medical Journal*, **284**, 1087–9.

Institute for Alcohol Studies (1985) *The Presentation of Alcohol in the Mass Media*, Report of a seminar, January 1985. Institute for Alcohol Studies, 12 Caxton Street, London.

Jackson, R.H. (1983) 'Play It Safe': a campaign for the prevention of children's accidents. *Community Development Journal*, **18**, 172–6.

Jenkins, J. (1983) *Mass Media for Health Education*, International Extension College, Cambridge.

Katz, E. and Lazarsfeld, P. (1955) *Personal Influence: the Part Played by People in the Flow of Mass Communication*, Free Press, Glencoe, Ill.

Kerr, M. and Charles, N. (1983) *Attitudes to the Feeding and Nutrition of Young Children*, Health Education Council, London.

Kinder, B.N. (1975) Attitudes toward alcohol and drug abuse: experimental data, mass media research and methodological considerations. *International Journal of Addictions*, **10**, 1035–54.

King, R. (1979) Drinking and drunkenness in 'Crossroads' and 'Coronation Street', in *Images of Alcoholism*, (eds J. Cook and M. Lewington), British Film Institute, London.

Klapper, J.T. (1960) *The Effects of Mass Communication*, Free Press, Glencoe, Ill.

Kotler, P. (1975) *Marketing for Non-Profit Organizations*, Prentice Hall, New York.

Lavigne, A.S., Albert, W. and Simmons, M. (1986) The application of market segmentation in alcohol and drug education: the APPLAUSE project, in *Health Education and the Media*, (eds D.S. Leathar, G.B. Hastings and J.K. Davies), Pergamon, London.

Lazarsfeld, P.F. and Merton, R.K. (1975) Mass communication, popular taste and organised social action, in *Mass Communications*, (ed. W. Schramm), University of Illinois Press, Urbana, Ill.

Leslie, J. (1981) Evaluation of mass media for health and nutrition education, in *Health Education by Television and Radio*, (ed. M. Meyer), K.G. Saur, München.

Levens, G.E. and Rodnight, E. (1973) *The Application of Research in the Planning and Evaluation of Road Safety Publicity*, Proceedings of the European Society for Opinion in Marketing (Budapest) Conference, pp. 197–227.

Liu, A.P. (1981) Mass campaigns in the People's Republic of China, in *Public Communication Campaigns*, (eds R.E. Rice and W.J. Paisley), Sage Publications, Beverly Hills.

Lovelock, C.H. (1977) Concepts and strategies for health marketers. *Hospital and Health Services Administration*, Fall, 50–63.

Maloney, S.K. and Hersey, J.C. (1984) Getting messages on the air: findings from the 1982 alcohol abuse prevention campaign. *Health Education Quarterly*, **11**, 273–92.

Marsden, G. and Peterfreund, N. (1984) Marketing public health services. *International Quarterly of Community Health Education*, **5**, 53–71.

McAlister, A. *et al.* (1980) Pilot study of smoking, alcohol and drug abuse prevention. *American Journal of Public Health*, **70**, 719–21.

McAlister, A. and Hughes, M. (1979) Playing the (role) part. *Audio-Visual Communcations*, **22**, 650–8.

McCron, R. and Budd, J. (1987) Mass communication and health education, in *Health Education: Perspectives and Choices*, (ed. I. Sutherland), National Extension College, Cambridge.

McCron, R. and Dean, E. (1983) *Well Being – An Evaluation*, Channel 4 Television Broadcast Support Services, London.

McGuire, W.J. (1973) Persuasion, resistance and attitude change, in *Handbook of Communication*, (eds I. De Sola Pool *et al.*) Rand McNally, Skokie, Ill.

McGuire, W.J. (1981) Theoretical foundations of campaigns, in *Public Communication Campaigns*, (eds R.E. Rice and W.J. Paisley), Sage Publications, Beverly Hills.

McKinlay, J.B. (1979) A case for refocusing upstream: the political economy of illness, in *Patients, Physicians and Illness*, (ed. E.G. Jaco), Free Press, New York, p. 12.

Mendelsohn, H. (1968) Which shall it be: mass education or mass persuasion for health? *American Journal of Public Health*, **58**, 131–7.

Mendelsohn, H. (1973) Some reasons why information campaigns can succeed. *Public Information Quarterly*, **37**, 50–61.

Mendelsohn, H. (1980) *Comments on the Relevance of Empirical Research as a Basis for Public Education Strategies in the Area of Alcohol Consumption*, Dept. of Mass Communication, University of Denver.

Mendelsohn, H. (1986) Lessons from a national media prevention campaign, in *Health Education and the Media*, (eds D.S. Leathar, G.B. Hastings and J.K. Davies), Pergamon, London.

O'Byrne, D.J. and Crawley, H.D. (1981) Conquest smoking cessation campaign 1980 – an evaluation, in *Health Education and the Media* (eds D.S. Leathar, G.B. Hastings and J.K. Davies), Pergamon, London.

Ogbourne, A.C. and Smart, R.G. (1980) Will restrictions on alcohol advertising reduce alcohol consumption? *British Journal of Addictions*, **75**, 293–6.

Piepe, A. *et al.* (1986) Does sponsored sport lead to smoking among children? *Health Education Journal*, **45**, 145–8.

Player, D.A. (1986) Health promotion through sponsorship: the state of the art, in *Health Education and the Media II*, (eds D.S. Leathar, *et al.*), Pergamon, London.

Puska, P. *et al.* (1979) A comprehensive television smoking cessation programme in Finland. *International Journal of Health Education*, Supplement to Vol. **XXII**, No. 4.

Raw, M. and de Plight, J.V. (1981) Can television help people stop smoking? in *Health Education and the Media*, (eds D.S. Leathar, G.B. Hastings and J.K. Davies), Pergamon, London.

Reid, D. (1985) National No Smoking Day, in *Smoking Control*, (eds J. Crofton and M. Wood), Health Education Council, London.

Rhodes, A. (1976) *Propaganda: the Art of Persuasion*, *World War II*, Angus and Robertson, London.

Rogers, R.S. (1973) The effects of televised sex education at the primary school level. *Health Education Journal*, **32**, 87–93.

Russell, M.A.H., Wilson, C., Taylor, C. and Baker, C.D. (1979) Effect of General Practitioner's advice against smoking. *British Medical Journal*, **2**, 231–5.

Smith, W. (1978) *Campaigning for Choice; Family Planning Association Project Report No. 1*, Family Planning Association, London.

Solomon, D.S. (1981) A social marketing perspective on campaigns, in *Public Communication Campaigns*, (eds R.E. Rice and W.J. Paisley), Sage, Beverly Hills.

Spencer, J. (1984) *General Practitioners' Views of the 'Give Up Smoking (GUS) Kit'*, Health Education Council, London.

Stein, J.A. (1986) The cancer information service: marketing a large-scale national information program through media, in *Media in Health Education II*, (eds D.S.Leathar *et al.*), Pergamon, London.

Taplin, S. (1981) Family planning campaigns, in *Public Communication Campaigns*, (eds R.E. Rice and W.J. Paisley), Sage Publications, Beverly Hills.

Tapper-Jones, L. and Harvard Davis, R. (1985) *A Project to Develop Publications to Support Health Education Within the General Practice Consultation*, Health Education Council, London.

Tones, B.K. (1981) The use and abuse of mass media in health promotion, in *Health Education and The Media*, (eds D.S. Leathar, G.B. Hastings and J.K. Davies), Pergamon, London.

Tones, B.K. (1986) Preventing drug misuse: the case for breadth, balance and coherence. *Health Education Journal*, **45**, 223–30.

Transport and Road Research Laboratory (1967 and 1972) *Testing a Children's Poster* (Report SRU 2), and *Improving Driving by the Use of Posters Beside Roads* (Report SRU 28), TRRL, Crowthorne, Berkshire.

Transport and Road Research Laboratory (1970) *Design of Road Safety Exhibitions*, Leaflet SRU 6, May, 1970.

Wallach, L.M. (1980) *Mass Media Campaigns: the Odds Against Finding Behavior Change*, University of California Social Research Group, School of Public Health, Berkeley, CA.

Wallack, L. and Barrows, D.C. (1983) Evaluating primary prevention: the California 'Winners' alcohol program. *International Quarterly of Community Health Education*, **3**, 307–36.

Wellings, K. (1986) Help or hype: an analysis of media coverage of the 1983 'pill scare', in *Health Education and the Media II*, (eds D.S. Leathar *et al.*), Pergamon, London.

Zaltman, G., Kotler, P. and Kaufman, I. (eds) (1972) *Creating Social Change*, Holt Rinehart and Winston, New York.

HEALTH PROMOTION IN THE WORKPLACE

7

The workplace provides an interesting challenge to health educators – a challenge which has been accepted rather more readily in North America than in Europe. Knobel (1983) has estimated that it is possible to reach 85% of the US population via the worksite and, for this reason alone, delivering health education to the workforce is of great strategic importance within the grand overall design of health promotion. Apart from this intrinsic merit, workplace health promotion has been included in the book because it exemplifies rather well two main propositions. First it illustrates conflicting philosophies rooted in the often different needs of key participants – workers and bosses. For management, success will normally be judged by hard economic indicators while for many radical health promoters, well-being may actually be incompatible with the profit motive! The workers' perceived needs are likely to be located somewhere between these two extremes.

Second, the workplace offers a tangible example of the ways in which success – however defined – is dependent on the synergy of individual behaviour and structural–organizational factors. For instance, smoking cessation programmes will be facilitated by a comprehensive workplace smoking policy. Similarly, the teaching of stress management skills without prior examination of the inherent stress-generating nature of work itself is neither efficient nor ethical.

This chapter will therefore seek to address the following questions: why deliver health education in the workplace? It is clearly assumed to be worthwhile (at least in North America!) but who is the real beneficiary? What can we expect from work-based health promotion? How successful is it? What is its potential for enhancing well-being and preventing disease? What are its limitations?

In seeking to answer these questions we will need to consider two key issues: (i) the relationship between health and work; and (ii) the ways in which the different motives of the various actors in the workplace situation (management, workers, trade unionists, health professionals and health educators) relate to criteria for programme success. Having done this, we will consider worksite programmes by category in order to illuminate some of the philosophical differences dividing health education workers and to provide a basis for a selective review of the extent of programme provision and effectiveness.

WORK AND HEALTH

The relationship between work and health is paradoxical. It stimulates vigorous debate and strikes a sensitive political nerve. On the one hand those of a Marxist persuasion may view work as a capitalist device to exploit the proletariat. At the risk of cheapening this point of view we might pose an oft-quoted rhetorical question: if work is so good, why don't the very wealthy do more of it? Bosquet (1977) has expressed the point with some force:

So deep is the frustration engendered by work than the incidence of heart attacks among manual workers is higher than that in any other stratum of society. People 'die from work' not because it is noxious or dangerous ... but because it is intrinsically 'killing'.

A more common (and better documented) standpoint is that unemployment rather than work is health-damaging. Indeed, the evidence has been so extensively and comprehensively assembled and presented that the relationship between unemployment and mental, physical and social disease will be taken as axiomatic for present purposes. However, in terms of the models of health education outlined in Chapter 1, both the above perspectives would favour a radical approach which sought to raise consciousness and stimulate social and political change in order to remedy what are viewed as serious social problems. Measures of success would therefore relate to the extent to which such social and political change actually occurs.

Less common but no less radical in its way is a third approach to the issue of health and work. It is concerned with the nature of work in a 'postindustrial society' (Hopson and Scally, 1981) which is characterized by chronic unemployment, reduction of the working week, job-sharing, early retirement, part-time employment and an increase in discretionary time and leisure. Preparation for a post-industrial society requires the same skills and competences needed to handle 'Future Shock' (Toffler, 1970). In other words the task of health and social education is not merely to provide an extensive preparation for greater leisure but will also involve fundamental questioning of the work ethic and the new, or rather rediscovered, enterprise culture. Since the futurologists' predictions of the nature of work will require a variety of social and personal skills associated with flexibility, resilience and proactivity, the appropriate

health education model is that which develops self-empowered decision making.

In the context of the hard and pragmatic concerns which are typically associated with workplace health promotion, the above approach might seem somewhat fanciful. However, the importance of considering fundamental questions of this kind was acknowledged by a conference on Health Promotion in the Working World organized by WHO (1987). This postulated several futuristic scenarios:

1. Business as usual. Assumes full employment will once again be achieved and this will be the predominant form of work with the associated consumption of goods and services and the centrality of paid work to individual self-esteem.
2. Hyperexpansionist. Postulates chronic unemployment as described earlier. Society will consist of two groups – employed and unemployed. The former will consist of a cadre of elite professionals using capital intensive technology.
3. Sane, humane, ecological. Again, assumes chronic unemployment but posits a radical change in values which allows other useful activities to receive appropriate recognition and payment in addition to traditional paid work. Paid and unpaid work will be equally divided between men and women. Households and neighbourhoods will be the workplaces and production centres in society.
4. Variations on some of these themes were also proposed including 'Eco-Utopia' (small decentralized, self-sufficient eco settlements) and 'Findhorn' (characterized by spirituality and inner growth). By contrast 'Chinatown' postulated a population explosion with multimillion metropolises; alternatively the 'Dallas' scenario predicted a western-dominated competitive Darwinistic imperialism in which, presumably, the North American rationale for worksite health promotion would be even more popular!

Returning to the present, the more conventional analysis of work and health sees the workplace as a source of pathogens of one kind or another ranging from general work-produced stress to specific industrial hazards such as accidents, cancers and the like. Stress is of particular interest because it illustrates so well the conflicting perspectives of more radical health educators and the employers whom they accuse of 'victim blaming'. The number of identified work stressors is legion. The World Health Organization (1987) lists poor physical working conditions, shift work, job overload and job underload, role conflict, role insecurity, promotion blockage, two-career families, lack of opportunity for participation in decision making, etc.

A more recent study by Braun and Hollander (1987) examined job stress among employees in the Federal Republic of Germany. They showed that high job demands and low job decision latitude were related to stress. The study implications could be either to teach stress management skills or to alter the structure of the work situation. Although not in principle incompatible, the choice of one or other of these alternatives is, as we shall see, likely to reveal ideological differences in approach to workplace health promotion. A successful 'victim blaming' strategy would be revealed by the acquisition of, say, relaxation skills or a reduced level of stress on an appropriate scale; the success of a more radical approach would be measured by actual environmental changes or intermediate indicators of progress towards such change.

DIFFERENT PERSPECTIVES ON SUCCESS

As will have been apparent from the discussion of health and work, successful worksite health promotion will be interpreted differently by the various actors: academics, futurologists, community physicians, public health workers and social scientists will have different value systems from employers and workers, although doubtless common ground exists. The health educator's perspective may well be dominated by the prospect of gaining access to a substantial proportion of the adult population. The choice of strategies will in part be dictated by the two principles of access and availability of skilled and credible health educators. Access to a generally hard-to-reach population is an outstanding feature of the workplace. It has been estimated in the USA that some 85% of the population may be contacted in this way, a proportion which compares very favourably with the 75% contact which the practice population has with a general practitioner every three years and the 15 000 hours spent by students in school. The question of credibility and competence is, however, a different matter. Logically we would look to the occupational health service to deliver health education but this, of course, depends on the existence of such a service! McEwan (1987) noted that in 1977 about '... 85% of all firms (in the UK), employing about 34% of the workforce, had no occupational health service other than first-aiders employed less than ten hours a week ...'. Buck (1982), after a small scale survey of firms in a district health authority in northern England, was more optimistic. Occupational health staff reported that their two most frequent types of health work were first, treatment and second, environmental visiting. Fifty-five of the 59 respondents recognized the existence of opportunities for health education in the treatment situation and 29 commented that opportunities arose 'often' or 'sometimes' in their visits to the working environment. Clearly recognition of opportunity did not mean that they actually took advantage of the situation to provide health education. Moreover since the response rate was only 47% it would not be unreasonable to expect a distinct lack of commitment in the non-respondents!

A national survey in the USA by Vojtecky *et al.* (1985) provides a useful indication of the involvement of occupational health services in health promotion. A sample of 1953 was drawn from a sampling frame of 11 000 occupational health professionals. Again there was a low response rate of 34% so observations should be treated with caution. Five categories of health professional were identified: industrial hygienists, doctors, nurses, health educators and others. The proportion of total work time which the groups claimed to spend on health education was respectively 33%, 22%, 38%, 89% and 23%. Major programme categories were health promotion, accident prevention and hazard protection. The proportion of each professional group having involvement with broader health promotion work ranged from 31% (industrial hygienists) to 98% (nurses). A wide range of teaching methods were used with the health educators using the broadest spectrum (50% using ten of 13 listed methods). Interestingly, when the groups were asked to say whether their objectives were primarily changes in knowledge, attitude or practice, it was the health educator group which seemed more determined to change behaviours (80%) whereas 50% of nurses were concerned only to provide knowledge. Whether this indicates a difference in philosophy or whether nurses tended to assume that knowledge would automatically lead to behaviour change is not clear. Notwithstanding the relatively small response rate, the situation appears distinctly

more healthy than in Europe, although the researchers lament the fact that only 62% of the occupational health professionals delivering health education had had any specific training in doing so.

THE MANAGEMENT PERSPECTIVE

The motivation of managers in respect of workplace health promotion may be summarized in two words: economic self-interest. This viewpoint is sharply illustrated by a comment attributed to Xerox top management that the loss of one executive from preventable illness would cost the organization $600 000 (Cooper, 1985). It should be noted that the received wisdom that health promotion in the worksite will in fact save money has not gone unchallenged. Walsh (1988) cites three sceptics (Russell, 1986; Warner, 1987; Schelling, 1986) in her own critique of workplace programmes. Nonetheless the general feeling appears to be that appropriate educational and promotion programmes will result in increased productivity and sales and generate a reduction in costs. The rationale for these programmes in terms of productivity and cost reduction is summarized in Table 7.1.

Clearly some of these arguments are peculiar to the US health care delivery system

Table 7.1 A summary of the main benefits of worksite health promotion programmes in North America in relation to productivity and cost reduction

Increased productivity
1. Reduction in sickness absence
2. Reduced absenteeism
3. Increase in worker morale
4. Presentation of a good corporate image*
5. Attracting competent staff in a competitive market situation

Reduction in costs
1. Decrease in accidents and associated compensation claims
2. Decline in health insurance costs as a result of lower demand for inpatient care, reduced treatment costs and fewer disability and death benefits
3. Decline in staff replacement and training costs as a result of lower staff turnover

* According to Conrad (1988a) this desirable image is acquired by 'capitalizing on cultural wellness'!

with its emphasis on private health insurance. We are reminded, however, of the significance of these costs by Alexander (1988):

> During the past decade, large corporations have become increasingly concerned that providing health care benefits no longer constitutes an incidental cost of doing business. In 1961, such benefits were 25.5% of payroll. By 1981, they were 41.2%. Between 1987 and 1980 corporate health insurance premiums escalated markedly from $43 billion to $63 billion. The most notable impact on the manufacturing sector was documented for General Motors, which in 1977 was believed to have added $176 to the cost of every car and truck to offset the $825 million it spent during the same year for employee benefits. A recent survey of a sample of Fortune 500 companies and the largest 250 industrials suggested that health insurance costs will equal profits after taxes in about 8 years.

The attractiveness of an effective health promotion service and the victim blaming nature of the programmes become understandable in the light of these statistics. The economic motivation of managers is thus hardly surprising and is supported by Davis *et al.*'s (1984) investigation of worksite health promotion in Colorado. Companies surveyed which had established programmes were asked to provide reasons for having started health promotion activities; companies interested in starting were also asked to indicated their motivation for so doing. Survey results are shown in Table 7.2. The economic motivation underlying decisions is self-evident, particularly for those companies contemplating adoption.

THE WORKER PERSPECTIVE

The worker perspective has probably received less consideration than that of management, presumably because of an assumption that workers might welcome interventions designed to enhance their well-being whereas managers would have to be subjected to a 'sales pitch'. It is doubtless true that trade unions will welcome moves which can be shown to be for their members' benefit and workers will respond to the same initiatives, particularly if these happen in 'management time'! Several studies in North America have sought to ascertain the reasons for worker participation. For example, Conrad (1988b) identified a major concern with fitness and

Table 7.2 Reasons given by companies for starting health promotion and disease prevention programmes (from Davis *et al.*, 1984)

Reason	Companies with existing programmes (%)	Companies interested in starting programmes (%)
To improve health and reduce health problems	82	68
To improve employee morale	59	52
To reduce health care costs	57	67
To reduce turnover and absenteeism	51	57
To improve productivity	50	64
Response to employee demand or interest	33	20
To be part of innovative trend	32	11
To improve public image	20	18

weight control. Spilman (1988) noted gender differences in motivation which were consistent with generally recognized views about women's health; for instance, a general high participation rate, concern with weight loss for cosmetic reasons, concern with their nurturant roles as unpaid family health care workers. Kotarba and Bentley (1988) described motivation to participate in a workplace wellness programme in terms of either a '... commitment to wellness, or as a vehicle for experimenting with or establishing a new style of self, the identity of a "well person" so highly valued in contemporary western culture'. This latter observation will serve as a cautionary note: worker motivation is clearly culture-bound and will reflect general health norms. There can be no guarantee that the UK workforce will identify with the North American healthist pursuit of 'high level wellness'! Indeed, suspicion about management motives might well predominate. Moreover, in the context of our earlier discussion of health and work, the workforce in Britain is more likely to be concerned about unemployment than even exposure to hazardous substances let alone participation in the pursuit for fitness in order to reduce management overheads!

TYPES OF WORKSITE PROGRAMME

Before commenting on the relative effectiveness of health promotion in the workplace, it is as well to consider the variety of activity incorporated under the general rubric and examine the main sources of controversy generated by certain of these activities. The definition of workplace health promotion is in no way esoteric. Parkinson *et al.* (1982) refer to a '... combination of educational, organizational and environmental activities designed to support behaviour conducive to the health of employees and their families'. Davis *et al.* (1984) provide an operational definition in their criteria for deciding whether or not a given firm had a health promotion

programme. 'A company was considered to have a HPDP (health promotion and disease prevention) programme if it provided health screenings, classes or preventive health services on an ongoing basis.' The philosophical basis which determines evaluative criteria, however, is less readily handled.

Alexander (1988), in an article on the 'ideological construction of risk', points out this philosophical underpinning. Not only is health promotion predicated on a need by '... the American state and almost all sectors of capital to curtail their share of the social wage ...', but '... corporate managers choose selectively from a body of theoretical knowledge regarding illness and disease etiology in a way that restores sanctity to the individual, eschews history and social complexity and legitimates existing social relations'. No apology is made for making a further reference to the inherent tendency for workplace health promotion to focus on the individual at the expense of general social structures and particular organizational influences on health and illness. McEwan (1987) is also concerned to make this point and cites Navarro (1976) who not only asserted the economic and political aetiology of alienation of the individual in society, occupational diseases generally and cancer in particular, but also pointed out how the power balance in western industrialized society inevitably favours the individualistic approach of traditional health education.

> ... one of today's most active state policies at the central government level in most western capitalist countries is to encourage and stimulate these health programs, such as health education, that are aimed at bringing about changes in the individual but not in the economic or political environment.

It is interesting to note that while much of the disease affecting the working class in Engels' time was supposedly due to the poor moral fibre of the workmen and their families, today the poor health conditions of that class and the majority of the population are assumed to be due to the lack of concern for their own health and their poor health education. In both cases, the solution to our public lack of health is *individual* prevention and *individual* therapy.

Walsh (1988) notes the 'healthist' aspect of the American fitness programmes. 'Could it be', she asks, 'that health promotion is a lifestyle enclave in the worksite and if so is it deflecting energy from collective efforts to improve the quality of worklife for all?' Gordon (1987) also notes the victim blaming tendency but in addition comments on the possibility of ethical difficulties relating to confidentiality and trust in workbased medical practitioners and, more importantly for our purpose here, the intrinsic tendency to exert explicit or implicit pressure on workers to participate in health promotion programmes. Such coercion – however benevolent – together with an associated 'top-down' approach, is not only inconsistent with WHO's principles of health promotion but militates against the spirit of the British Health and Safety at Work Act (1974) which emphasizes responsibility, self-regulation and participation, all of which processes are consistent with WHO's view of health promotion. However, let us turn now to a categorization of major kinds of work related health promotion programmes.

Consistent with the earlier discussion of health and work, we might usefully identify a variety of programme which is concerned to educate about work. Perhaps the best recognized of these has a radical intent and is concerned to raise critical consciousness about working conditions either in a specific workplace or in a particular category of workplace – for example, chemical industries. Freudenberg's (1981) description of attempts to activate the workforce and pressurize employers to provide a healthier environment and compensate workers for industrial diseases illustrates this approach nicely.

Education about work is also an integral part of personal and social education and includes vocational guidance and career choice. Many programmes would also seek to have students think critically about workplace conditions and the implications, say, of working on an assembly line for health and well-being. The underlying rationale is one of fostering self-empowered choice.

Education designed to empower the workforce is relatively rare, for obvious reasons! It is, therefore, worth reporting on a Canadian mental health initiative (Novick, 1987). The Mental Health and the Workplace Project is unusual in that it acknowledges the importance of environmental variables both within and without the workplace. The programme philosophy is fundamentally concerned with self-empowerment. Novick, chairperson of the project, describes a 'New Work Agenda into the Nineties' based on the following assumptions:

1. Employment is a form of work which is done for remuneration as well as for psychological and social benefits.
2. Persistently high levels of unemployment are detrimental to the health and well-being of Canadian citizens and are unacceptable waste of human resources.
3. A lack of more secure, stable, quality employment opportunities is increasing the stress and anxiety of working Canadians.

It acknowledges the 'future shock scenario', noting that groups '… previously excluded or only marginally employed (e.g. women, youth, disabled people) are making their claim for fair access to the workplace'. Wide income disparities between high paid and low paid workers and the polarization between a low skilled underclass and a high skilled elite must be taken into account by a programme concerned to educate about work. The importance of balancing employment with family life, life in the community and personal development must be recognized.

Six propositions are finally made by Novick.

1. Employment should be structured and organized in ways that are compatible with and reinforcing to the quality of Canadian family life.
2. Working life should include opportunities for continuing learning for job advancement, work skill development, retirement and general personal betterment.
3. There should be recognition of the importance of alternative forms of work, such as household, voluntarism, recreational and cultural activities as well as paid forms of work.
4. All Canadians should have access to a fair share of meaningful and dignifying employment during their adult lives.
5. People should have more worklife choices in terms of how they arrange their employment time weekly, monthly and yearly in order to complement other pursuits and interests which they have.
6. Real worklife choices must entail provisions for both income security and employment stability within a framework for economic renewal.

The approach of 'Worklife Education' is perhaps summarized in the view that, 'The workplace is a community. All of its members should be empowered to care better for themselves and for each other.' This self-empowerment approach is substantially different in emphasis from mainstream workplace programmes in which disease prevention and health protection provide the main justification for intervention (with or without the cost benefit implication).

The next category for consideration is, then, that which embodies traditional health and safety goals. It is concerned to identify and educate those at high risk – either for personal health problems such as coronary heart disease (CHD) or in the context of a specific occupation. More recently, broader based health promotion programmes have focused on general health and fitness. All three approaches are consistent with agreed goals of an occupational health service as McEwan (1987) points out in these terms.

1. Protecting the workers against any health hazard which may arise out of their work or the conditions in which it is carried on;
2. Contributing towards the workers' physical and mental adjustment, in particular by the adaptation of the work to the workers and their assignment of job for which they are suited;
3. Contributing to the establishment and maintenance of the highest possible degree of physical and mental well-being of the workers.

Examples of these programmes are readily available. For instance Ippolito-Shepherd *et al.* (1987) describe an agricultural occupational health education programme in Latin America; Schenk *et al.* (1987) present results of research into rubber industry workers' beliefs and attitudes about safety which might be used to devise risk reduction health education interventions. In the UK a general health and fitness programme originally developed by the Health Education Council for adult learners has been translated into the workplace. This 'Look After Yourself' (LAY) programme involves teaching about exercise, relaxation, healthy eating and other lifestyle health factors (Daines *et al.*, 1986). It is made available to the workplace on request; its goal is to train tutors within the work situation so that the programme becomes routinized. Although not substantially different from worksite health promotion in general, there is one well recognized category of intervention which merits separate consideration.

Although there is considerable overlap between the two, health promotion programmes may be distinguished from one well recognized category of worksite intervention, particularly in North America. This category is usually referred to as an Employee Assistance Programme (EAP). Roman and Blum (1988) provide a useful comparison between EAPs and Health Promotion Programmes (HPPs). They offer two definitions of EAPs:

> ... mechanisms to increase the chances for continued employment of individuals whose job performance and personal functioning are adversely impacted by problems of substance abuse, psychiatric illness, family difficulties or other personal problems.
>
> *(Roman and Blum, 1987)*

> ... job-based programs operating within a work organization for purposes of identifying 'troubled employees', motivating them to resolve their troubles, and providing access to counselling or treatment for those employees who need these services.
>
> *(Sonnenstuhl and Trice, 1986)*

It is immediately clear from these definitions that EAPs are concerned with secondary prevention whereas other health promotion programmes would tend to focus on primary prevention. Roman and Blum also observe that whereas trade unions (in the USA) are probably suspicious of HPPs, they almost unanimously support EAPs. They, additionally, note that both HPPs and EAPs are 'mission-driven' ('The zealotry that accompanies many HPPs is often matched by the zeal with which EAP practitioners view the urgency of recovery from alcoholism ...')! A key difference between both types of programme centres on the potential stigma associated with EAPs compared with HPPs. Clearly EAPs require confidentiality and a conviction by workforce and unions that admitting to problems will not lead to job loss. This latter point is of especial importance for the implementation of alcohol policies in the workplace. Indeed the development of worksite policies may be considered a separate category of health promotion exercise, at least in the UK.

HEALTH POLICIES IN THE WORKPLACE

The notion of a health policy is of particular importance in any discussion of health pro-

motion. Indeed, as has been noted on more than one occasion, health promotion is usefully defined as a combination of education and policy. A prerequisite for a maximally effective intervention is the existence of an appropriate environment and the establishment of a policy centres on the creation of such an environment in conjunction with various kinds of health education. Typically policy development has centred on alcohol, smoking, fitness and nutrition (often in the context of preventing CHD) and, less often, stress reduction. The elements of a workplace smoking policy will be briefly adumbrated below prior to considering implications for indicators of effectiveness (for further details see Jenkins *et al.* (1987)).

First, a smoking policy would have the following environmental goals; a ban on smoking in areas where special safety or health hazards exist; at least 50% of cafeteria areas would be designated non-smoking provided that smoke did not affect the non-smoking zone; all common areas would be non-smoking; smoking areas would be provided for smokers; smoking cessation facilities would also be made available. Appropriate signs would be displayed; information would be disseminated to the management and workforce; the policy would apply to all members of staff; there would be no discrimination against anyone exercising their rights under the policy.

Second, generally agreed steps are involved in implementing policy as follows.

1. Establishment of a working party;
2. Definition of objectives;
3. Survey of employee attitudes and request for suggestions for policy implementation;
4. Construction of draft policy;
5. Consultation exercise;
6. Adoption of agreed policy by senior management;
7. Implementation
   (a) Creation of non-smoking environment

(b) Provision of help for smokers
(c) Institution of measures for policing and maintaining policy provisions.

IMPLICATIONS FOR EVALUATION MEASURES

Evaluation measures for policy development are simple to define. In terms of outcome, success would be determined by the extent to which the various environmental goals listed above had been achieved. In relation to process evaluation, the seven implementation steps would be monitored and the illumination thus gained would be used to enhance efficiency and ensure steady progress to the next stage.

In the more general context, success would be ultimately determined by the philosophical orientation. Cost containment goals would be measured by hard cash saved and productivity or, in terms of intermediate indicators, by the extent to which appropriate lifestyle/behaviour change had occurred or there had been a change in underlying and associated knowledge, beliefs, attitudes, etc. Radical or self-empowerment goals would again be evaluated in the ways discussed in Chapter 1 and 2, e.g. in relation to worker participation in union activities, in enhanced consciousness, in the acquisition of self-efficacy beliefs and skills.

A recurrent theme in this book is the importance of ensuring that the philosophy is complemented by appropriate technology. Unless the conditions appropriate to the adoption of innovations are supplied, an effective workplace programme will not materialize. Unless approved educational methods are used, learning will not occur. A discussion of both of these requirements in relation to the worksite is beyond the scope of this chapter but it is clear that the workplace has its own special needs, not least of which is the adoption of teaching methods appropriate to the adult learner. An example of programme planning which seeks to meet adult learning requirements is provided by Manning (1983/4).

Finally we will provide a selective review of studies of the effectiveness of health promotion in the workplace commencing with some observations about the extent of provision.

HEALTH PROMOTION IN THE WORKPLACE: A SELECTIVE REVIEW

In 1970, in the USA, an Occupational Safety and Health Act was enacted '... to assure so far as possible every working man and woman in the nation safe and healthful working conditions and to preserve our human resources ...'. The achievement of this goal was to be ensured by, *inter alia*, '... education and training programs in the recognition, avoidance, and prevention of unsafe or unhealthful working conditions ...' (Vojtecky *et al.*, 1985). In Britain similar legislation in the form of the Health and Safety at Work Act was introduced in 1974. Symington, in a conference on Health Promotion in the Workplace (1987), commented on this Act and the Employment Protection Act which followed it in 1975, and argued that while they were primarily concerned with health and safety issues, '... this new awareness ... provides a climate and a platform from which health promotion activities of a general nature can thrive'. He went on to point out that while not required by the Acts, screening programmes, alcohol and smoking policies emerged as a useful byproduct. While this is undoubtedly true, the fact is that developments in Britain have not kept pace with those in North America. Indeed it is interesting to note an assertion by Webb at the same conference that after 20 years of decline in work related diseases and injuries, '... figures for recent years show an alarming rise from 70.4 per 100 000 employees in 1981 to 87.0 per 100 000 in 1984'. He goes on to speculate that '... some workers are paying in health terms for the economic changes of recent years'.

At the time of writing no comprehensive survey of UK workplace health promotion activities is available. However, examples of good practice in Scotland were presented in the conference report referred to above: these included programmes operated by seven commercial organizations, various district councils on alcoholism, trade unions, health education departments, the employment medical advisory service and local health boards. Topic areas discussed were safety, alcohol, exercise, nutrition, smoking, mental health, women's health and heart disease.

It will by now be clear that the situation in North America is very different. Fuchs *et al.* (1985) commented on the escalation of interest between 1975 and 1985. They provided a selective review of 11 key textbooks, referred to 30 journal articles on general health promotion at work and listed 101 topic-specific articles together with 25 exemplars of more popular magazine pieces. The distribution of topics by popularity is as listed in Table 7.3. If these figures are representative, it is clear that the impact of safety legislation has been less than the more general health promotion movement – with, of course, its implication for cost containment!

Davis *et al.* (1984) recorded an even greater range of topics in their survey of Californian workplaces. Between 16% and 72% of companies provided a wide range of screening services. These were, in ascending order of popularity; cervical cancer; colon/rectal cancer; diabetes; pulmonary function; annual medical examination; work related problems; height and weight; general risk appraisal; high blood pressure; pre-employment medical examination.

Between 30% and 78% offered a wide range of information programmes. Again in ascending order of popularity, these were; seat belt use; cervical cancer; breast self-examination; cancer prevention; work related injury; low back pain; high blood pressure; alcohol and drug abuse; nutrition; smoking; stress; exercise.

Various services (e.g. group instruction; individual counselling; referral to community resources) were on offer with provision ranging from 28% of firms to 80%. Services provided were: industrial alcoholism programme; employee assistance; self-defence for women; low back pain; smoking cessation; weight management; stress management; exercise.

Hollander and Lengermann (1988) carried out a systematic survey of Fortune 500 companies (i.e. 500 largest US firms) to determine the nature and extent of health promotion provision (in 1984). The response rate was approximately 50%. Of these, two thirds had a worksite programme and two thirds reported plans to expand these. One third of those not having programmes planned to initiate health promotion activities. In general, the larger firms were more likely to have programmes which also tended to be more extensive. The number of health promotion activities reported ranged from 5.7 to 8.9.

Walsh (1988) cited an unpublished manuscript of the Office of Disease Prevention and Health Promotion which reported a 1985 national survey of private sector employers having 50 or more personnel. This recorded at least one health promotion activity at nearly 66% of establishments; larger establishments tended to have many more programmes.

Table 7.3 The most popular worksite health promotion programmes (after Fuchs *et al.*, (1985)

Rank order	Topic	Number of references
1	Exercise programmes	33
2	Hypertension and CHD	19
3	Drugs and alcohol	17
4	Stress management	12
5	Smoking	8
6	Weight reduction	5
7	Safety	4
8	Cancer screening	3

It would seem unlikely from the survey data presented above that health and safety legislation alone would be responsible for the accelerating provision of health promotion programmes in the USA. A more realistic estimate would be based on the general cultural pressure towards fitness and wellness along with the belief in the cost effectiveness of interventions. Doubtless further impetus has been provided by the particular reference to worksite health promotion in the Surgeon General's report, *Healthy People* (US Dept of Health, 1979), which comments on the worksite as a locus for health education and health promotion.

> The worksite may provide an appropriate setting for health promotion as well as health protection activities. A number of companies have already shown leadership in providing employee fitness programs and encouraging worker participation, but more can be done.

The report also urged advertisers to be aware of their key role in influencing consumer behaviour and noted that advertising, '... particularly for food products, over-the-counter drugs, tobacco, and alcohol – has generally not been supportive of health promotion objectives'.

The report was published in 1979 and aspects of worksite health promotion were subsequently incorporated into the influential *Objectives for the Nation* (US Dept of Health, 1980) in 1980. Since then the appropriateness of the setting has indeed been increasingly recognized. But what of success? To what extent has the faith of employers been justified?

First, there is little doubt that if appropriate educational techniques are used, the impact of particular interventions can be positive, even in behavioural terms. For instance, Street (1987) describes two safety education interventions (Foster, 1983; Denyer, 1986). The first revealed a pre-post programme difference in knowledge, beliefs and attitudes towards wearing hearing protection. Moreover after the intervention, fewer people stated that they 'never used hearing protection'. However, the familiar gap between attitude and practice was noticeable in the reported results: Whereas some 80% of the group agreed that it was important to protect their hearing, only 65% stated that they actually wore protectors most of the time.

The second programme was concerned with eye protection. It employed relevant precursor 'educational diagnosis' of the target group and added a 'policy element' to the education in the form of threatened disciplinary action for non-compliance. Actual injuries fell over an eight week period from 72 to six.

However, rather more substantial and extensive justification for large scale investments of money and effort in workplace programmes would be expected if programmes were to continue. Davis *et al.*'s study (1984) indicates that those employers operating health promotion programmes think that they work. Perceptions of benefits accruing are reproduced in Table 7.4.

Of course employer perceptions may well have been biased by wishful thinking! However, their views on reduced absenteeism may well be justified if Blair *et al.*'s (1986a)

Table 7.4 Employers' perceptions of the benefits of worksite health promotion programmes (from Davis *et al.* (1984)

Category health promotion	Perceived as benefit by (%)
Improved morale	81
Improved health	52
Improved productivity	46
Reduced illness and injury	46
Reduced turnover of staff and absenteeism	40
Reduced medical care utilization	30
Reduced health care costs	23
Attracted better calibre applicants	17

study is generally applicable. After an intensive ten week programme of fitness teaching, there were not only significant differences in physiological and clinical characteristics in the 3846 participants receiving the instruction but there were also, on average, 1.25 days less absenteeism in the group. The researchers calculate that the programme had therefore resulted in savings of $149 578!

Many other reviews have reported similar kinds of success. Knobel (1983) reported a reduction in disability costs for each $1000 of total wage payments from $13.28 in 1976 to $9.43 in 1978 at Southern Bell. This cost saving was ascribed to a co-ordinated prevention and promotion programme.

Knobel also commented on the Campbell Soup company programme which resulted in the removal of approximately 20 polyps each year at a cost of $6500 with estimated annual reductions of $100 000 in direct insurance payments.

The company detects and treats between 60% and 90% of hypertensives thus avoiding over a ten year period an estimated $130 000 in hospitalization, rehabilitation and disability costs.

Northern Natural Gas reported reduced absenteeism by approximately five working days a year after a fitness programme. School administrators and teachers, according to Knobel, had 17% reduced absenteeism after a programme of exercise, stress management and nutrition teaching. A nine-component health promotion programme, which cost New York Telephone approximately $2.8 million in 1980, generated savings of $5.5 million from reduced absenteeism and treatment costs.

Blair *et al.* (1986b) described the programme at Johnson and Johnson whose 'Live for Life' scheme includes health risk appraisal, fitness, diet and nutrition, smoking cessation, hypertension control, stress management, weight control and general health education. Over a two year period 20% of women and 30% of men had adopted

vigorous exercise compared with 7% and 19% of a control group of company employees. Overall fitness and sense of well-being had also apparently improved. And again the 'bottom line' calculation: there were fewer hospital admissions and inpatient days in Johnson and Johnson employees and an estimated annual inpatient cost increase of $43 compared with $76 for non-programme employees (Bly *et al.*, 1986).

The Canada Life Assurance Company's Fitness and Lifestyle Project (Shephard *et al.*, 1982) provided similar evidence of success. A saving of more than 0.5 hospital days per employee was claimed which was associated with a financial saving of $84.5 per employee year.

Sloan (1987), in reviewing several of the projects mentioned above, presents a critique of the prevailing paradigm in North America. He reminds us again that '... some obvious alternative and complementary approaches are overlooked'. In particular he mentions the psychological and organizational climate of work. It should, perhaps, also be noted that there are instances where the worksite does not appear to generate successful results! For instance smoking cessation programmes may well achieve worse results than alternative modes of delivery and Klesges *et al.* (1987) reported only 17% mean success rate at six months. Jason *et al.* (1987) reported that work-based support groups increased the effectiveness of a smoking cessation programme using television and self-help manuals but reported only 7% continuous abstinence at 12 months, admittedly utilizing stringent criteria.

It is worth reiterating at this point the general assertion that any given programme will be more effective when it is part of a general integrated programme of education and policy and when it is supported by a consistent and integrated approach within the wider community. Part at least of this requirement obtained in a reported campaign strategy for weight loss at worksites (Nelson *et al.*, 1987). As part of the Pawtucket Heart Health Program, worksite volunteers implemented a weight control campaign with 512 employees from 22 companies. At the end of the programme, a total of 1818 pounds had been lost at an average of 3.55 pounds per person and a cost of $0.81 per pound lost.

Although Chen (1984), after reviewing a sample of worksite programmes, concluded that proper experimental or quasiexperimental research design were relatively rare, the general view in North America appears to be that worksite health promotion is successful. Impact evaluation of the kinds described above is virtually non-existent in Britain. However, where a company has initiated a comprehensive programme, these seems to be a view that it was worth the effort. For instance, the personnel manager of Polaroid UK argued that for an outlay of £16 000 there had been a significant effect on people's lifestyles (Fuchs *et al.*, 1985) in relation to diet and exercise and a claimed reduction in absenteeism from 6.3% to 3.7% over a four year period.

One of the more thorough and comprehensive workplace endeavours is the Look After Yourself (LAY) programme developed by the Health Education Council. An evaluation of a pilot programme revealed evidence of effectiveness. First in relation to indirect indicators, 73% of the 60 initial recruits attended all eight sessions. Additionally various intermediate measures gave evidence of heightened awareness of stress together with a positive attitude towards and competence in controlling it. Outcome measures of changes in eating, exercise, alcohol consumption and smoking demonstrated lifestyle changes: between 26% and 89% of 85 participants recorded change in one or more of these behaviours. Changes were also observed in various physiological indicators, viz. aerobic capacity, body fat, blood pressure and lung efficiency. Programme participants also express satisfaction with and interest in the programme as a whole (Denyer, 1986).

The research designs of these programmes would doubtless not impress those favouring 'proper' experimental techniques which might allow us, in Chen's (1984) words, to '... be better able to prove that "health education indeed is worthwhile"'. However, it is worth reiterating one of the main contentions of this book, namely that although rigorous research design is often eminently desirable in order to generate internal validity, in general such designs are not essential. Indeed in the interests of external validity, process evaluation will often be more useful provided that it is based on sound theory and utilizes relevant intermediate and indirect indicators.

The bulk of the evidence discussed in this chapter leads us inexorably to the conclusion that workplace health education can work in producing behaviour change, reducing risk and even reducing costs. Cost benefit analysis, although doubtless attractive to many decision makers in the UK, is clearly of much greater relevance to North America and its peculiar system of health care delivery and payment. Nonetheless the behaviour changes which generate cost savings and increased productivity are in most cases the same changes which will enhance well-being and can thus justify both the inclusion of health promotion in Britain workplaces and the use of less rigorous measures of programme effectiveness in evaluation.

The discussion of behaviour change and economic indicators of success has, in this chapter, perhaps appeared almost obsessive! This is due to the excess of data of an economic kind and the dearth of evidence of effectiveness in other domains of a more radical nature. We will, however, finish this chapter by reporting Freudenberg's (1981) account of successful examples of consciousness raising and community action. He points out that:

Work-related diseases afflict at least 4 million people a year; as many as 400 000 Americans die annually from these diseases.

In addition, 9 million workers are injured on the job each year and 13 000 people die from these injuries. ... 20% of all cancers are related to work place exposure to carcinogens.

He cites examples of consciousness-raising health education designed to provide a radical response to the situation described above. The case of the Carolina Brown Lung Association was mentioned in Chapter 1. This radical health promotion programme provided workers with understanding and skills to monitor health hazards and take action in the case of violations. It also incorporated the broader health promotion tactics of lobbying and advocacy – for instance in order to achieve fair compensation and ensure the availability of proper health care for the victims of industrial disease.

The New York Committee on Occupational Safety and Health is also cited as an exemplar of radical health promotion. This group has sponsored educational forums on health hazards and has lobbied vigorously in order to achieve 'Right-to-Know' legislation. It also provides technical assistance and advice for trade unions and sponsors lectures at union meetings in addition to producing educational materials.

Criteria for success are readily defined: outcome indicators might include the achievement of legislation which will improve safety standards. Intermediate indicators could document the increasing level of awareness in a community and different degrees of social action. In a later article Freudenberg (1985) provides further instances of radical health promotion. Indicators of success have been extracted from these and categorized in Table 7.5.

These last examples of workplace health promotion are very different from many earlier examples: not only do they adopt a radical approach which is philosophically and ideologically distinct from the narrower individually focused and frequently 'healthist' programmes, but they also have moved us outside the bounds of the worksite and into the community. The final strategic approach which will be discussed in this book also focuses on the community. At one level of analysis it will examine the notion of

Table 7.5 Indicators of 'radical' health education

Indicators of success	Examples of process involved
Outcome	
January 1981, City of Philadelphia enacted the nation's first municipal Right-to-Know law.	Results from several years of community and workplace education by Delaware Valley Toxics Coalition.
Intermediate	
United Automobile Workers produce a handbook *A Manual for Cancer Detectives on the Job* which '... teaches members across the country how to conduct an investigation, file an OSHA complaint and bargain for health and safety'.	Stimulus from an organized coalition of tenants' associations, environmental groups and Vietnam veterans.
Tenants' Associations develop a flair for creative use of media (skills acquisition).	Learning how to produce reports; hold demonstrations; organize public meetings
A mortality study is produced by workers which identifies potential carcinogens. Improvements are made to ventilation.	Workers approach National Union for help.

community-wide approaches and consider integrated programmes which would incorporate worksite health promotion as one element in a broader but, hopefully, coherent strategy. At another level it will concern itself with a much narrower and geographically more limited approach having a very particular philosophy. This strategy is termed community development: its rationale and ideology and the methods it employs to achieve its goals have much in common with the radical formula for workplace health promotion delineated by Freudenberg.

REFERENCES

Alexander, J. (1988) The ideological construction of risk: an analysis of corporate health promotion programs in the 1980s. *Social Science and Medicine*, **26**, 559–67.

Blair, S.N., Piserchia, P.V., Wilbur, C.S. and Crowder, J.H. (1986a) Health promotion for educators: impact on absenteeism. *Preventive Medicine*, **15**, 166–75.

Blair, S.N., Piserchia, P.V., Wilbur, C.S. and Crowder, J.H. (1986b) A public health intervention model for work-site health promotion. *Journal of the American Medical Association*, **255**, 921–6.

Bly, J.L., Jones, R.C. and Richardson, J.E. (1986) Impact of worksite health promotion on health care costs and utilization. *Journal of the American Medical Association*, **256**, 3235–40.

Bosquet, M. (1977) *Capitalism in Crisis and Everyday Life* (trans. J. Howe), Harvester Press, Hassocks.

Braun, S. and Hollander, R. (1987) A study of job stress among women and men in the Federal Republic of Germany. *Health Education Research*, **2**, 45–51.

Buck, A. (1982) *Promoting Health and Safety at Work*, University of Nottingham/Nottingham Health Education Unit, Nottingham.

Chen, M.S. (1984) Proving the effects of health promotion in industry: an academician's perspective. *Health Education Quarterly*, **10**, 235–45.

Conrad, P. (1988a) Worksite health promotion: the social context. *Social Science and Medicine*, **26**, 485–9.

Conrad, P. (1988b) Health and fitness at work: a participant's perspective. *Social Science and Medicine*, **26**, 545–50.

Cooper, C.L. (1985) The road to health in American firms. *New Society*, **73**, 335–6.

Daines, J., Gralian, B., Brown,. G., Edmondson, R.E. and Atkins, M. (1986) *'Look After Yourself' 1978–86: Innovation and Outcomes*, Dept of Adult Education for Health Education Council, Nottingham.

Davis, M.F., Rosenberg, K., Iverson, D.C., Vernon, T.M. and Bauer, J. (1984) Worksite health promotion in Colorado. *Public Health Reports*, **99**, 538–43.

Denyear, B. (1986) Reducing the incidence of eye injuries. *Occupational Health*, **38**, 112–14.

Foster, A. (1983) Hearing protection and the role of health education. *Occupational Health*, **35**, 155–8.

Freudenberg, N. (1981) Health education for social change: a strategy for public health in the US. *International Journal of Health Education*, **XXIV**, 1–8.

Freudenberg, N. (1985) Training health educators for social change. *International Quarterly of Community Health Education*, **5**, 37–52.

Fuchs, J.A., Price, J.E. and Marcotte, B. (1985) Worksetting health promotion – a comprehensive bibliography. *Health Education*, **16**, 29.

Gordon, J. (1987) Workplace health promotion: the right idea in the wrong place. *Health Education Research*, **2**, 69–71.

Hollander, R.B. and Lengermann, J.J. (1988) Corporate characteristics and worksite health promotion programs: survey findings from Fortune 500 companies. *Social Science and Medicine*, **26**, 491–501.

Hopson, B., and Scally, M. (1981) *Lifeskills Teaching*, McGraw-Hill, London. Ippolito-Shepherd, J.I., Feldman, R., Acha, P.N. *et al.* (1987) Agricultural occupational health and health education in Latin America and the Carribbean. *Health Education Research*, **2**, 53–9.

Jason, L.A., Gruder, L., Buckenberger, L. *et al.* (1987) A 12 month follow-up of a worksite smoking cessation intervention. *Health Education Research*, **2**, 185–94.

Jenkins, M. and McEwen, J. (1987) *Smoking Policies At Work*, Health Education Authority, London.

Klesges, R.C., Glasgow, R.E., Klesges, L.M. Merray, K. and Quale, R. (1987) Competition and relapse prevention training in worksite smoking modification. *Health Education Research*, **2**, 5–14.

Knobel, R.J. (1983) Health promotion and disease prevention: improving health while conserving resources. *Family and Community Health*, **1**, 16–27.

Kotarba, J.A. and Bentley, P. (1988) Workplace wellness participation and the becoming of self. *Social Science and Medicine*, **26**, 551–8.

Manning, D.T. (1983/4), Suggested strategies for occupational health promotion. *Hygie*, **II**, 44–51.

McEwan, J. (1987) Health and work, in *Health Education: Perspectives and Choices*, 2nd edn, (ed. I. Sutherland), National Extension College, Cambridge.

Navarro, V. (1976) *Medicine Under Capitalism*, Croom Helm, London.

Nelson, D.J., Sennett, L., Letebvre, R.C. *et al.* (1987) A campaign strategy for weight loss at worksites. *Health Education Research*, **2**, 27–31.

Novick, M. (1987) The new work agenda into the nineties. *Work and Well-Being Quarterly*, Fall, 26–30.

Parkinson, R.S., Beck, R.N., Collings, G.H. *et al.* (eds) (1982) *Managing Health Promotion in the Workplace*, Mayfield, Palo Alto, CA.

Roman, P.M. and Blum, T.C. (1987) The relation of employee assistance programs to corporate social responsibility attitudes: an empirical study, in *Research in Corporate Social Performance and Policy*, (ed. L.E. Preston), JAI Press, Greenwich, Conn., pp. 213–35.

Roman, P.M. and Blum, T.C. (1988) Formal intervention in employee health: comparisons of the nature and structure of employee assistance programs and health promotion programs. *Social Science and Medicine*, **26**, 503–14.

Russell, L. (1986) *Is Prevention Better than Cure?* Brookings Institute, Washington DC.

Schelling, T. (1986) Economics and cigarettes. *Preventive Medicine*, **15**, 549–60.

Schenck, A.P., Thomas, R.P., Hochbaum, G.M. and Beliczty, L.S. (1987) A labor and industry focus on education: using baseline survey data in program design. *Health Education Research*, **2**, 33–44.

Shephard, R.J., Porey, P. and Cox, M.H. (1982) The influence of an employee fitness and lifestyle modification program upon medical care costs. *Canadian Journal of Public Health*, **73**, 259–63.

Sloan, R.P. (1987) Workplace health promotion: the North American experience, in *Health Promotion in the Workplace*, (ed. H Matheson), Scottish Health Education Group, Edinburgh.

Sonnenstuhl, W. and Trice, H. (1986) *Strategies for Employee Assistance Programs: The Crucial Balance*, IRL Press, Ithaca, NY.

Spilman, M.A. (1988) Gender difference in worksite health promotion activities. *Social Science and Medicine*, **26**, 525–35.

Street, C.G. (1987) Unpublished MSc dissertation, Dept. of Community Medicine, Manchester.

Symington, I. (1987) Health promotion in the workplace: legislative aspects, in *Health Promotion in the Workplace*, (ed. H. Matheson), Scottish Health Education Group, Edinburgh.

Toffler, A. (1970) *Future Shock*, Bodley Head, London.

US Department of Health and Human Services (1980) *Promoting Health/Preventing Disease: Objectives for the Nation*, Washington DC.

US Department of Health, Education and Welfare (1979) *Healthy People: The Surgeon General's Report on Health Promotion and Disease Prevention*, Washington DC.

Vojtecky, M.A., Kar, S.B. and Cox, S.G. (1985) Workplace health education: results from a national survey. *International Quarterly of Community Health Education*, **5**, 171–85.

Walsh, D.C. (1988) Toward a sociology of worksite health promotion: a few reactions and reflections. *Social Science and Medicine*, **26**, 569–75.

Warner, K.E. (1987) Selling health promotion to corporate America. *Health Education Quarterly*, **14**, 39–55.

World Health Organization (1987) *Health Promotion in the Working World*, WHO European Regional Office, Copenhagen.

This final chapter reflects the ideological discussion of Chapter 1. Its major theme is the contrast in perspectives between two approaches to working in the community. The first approach derives from the view that the community is a setting in which to deliver health education. The second approach is based on the conviction that health educators should work **with** the community and seek to facilitate the achievement of the health goals which the community itself has identified. The first approach tends to be relatively prescriptive and operates within the framework of a preventive model. The second approach is likely to have a broader, ecological perspective on health and be concered with empowerment. The former mode of working is likely to be 'top-down', the latter 'bottom-up'. We will consider both of these perspectives in this chapter, noting points of overlap as well as ideological differences and will discuss implications for evaluating effectiveness and efficiency and the meaning of success.

THE MEANING OF COMMUNITY

Before attempting to provide some insight into the distinctions between various approaches designed to foster change in underprivileged communities, we should note that while the definitions of various forms of community organization is difficult, there are also problems in deciding on the meaning of the term 'community' itself! For instance, Hubley (1985) has commented on the imprecision of the concept and cited one reviewer who had unearthed some 94 definitions. For the purposes of the present discussion, a community is distinguished from any other social aggregation in respect of its relative size, geographical contiguity and the nature of the social network and norms prevailing within this circumscribed locality. The report of the Calouste Gulbenkian Foundation (1984) would appear to provide an apt description:

> 'Community'... refers to a grouping of people who share a common purpose, interest or need, and who can express their relationship through communication face to face, as well as by other means, without difficulty. In other words, in the majority of cases we see a community as being related to some geographic locality where the propinquity of the inhabitants has relevance for those interests or needs which they share

Henderson and Thomas (1980) emphasize the focus on a relatively small geographical neighbourhood: they argue that the appropriate catchment area for community development should be between 6000 and 20 000 population. However, while the above definitions clearly apply to many varieties of community organization, the more extensive programmes such as the North Karelia Heart Disease Prevention Programme will have much larger geographical areas as their target for intervention. Again, although the potential for face-to-face communication and associated social networks are of major importance in planning 'typical' community projects, there is obviously no clear-cut distinction between a community and a geographical area of more than, say, Henderson and Thomas' upper limit of 20 000 people. In fact, MacCannell (1979) has provided an interesting continuum based on three guiding principles of 'differentiation', 'centrality' and 'solidarity'. This helps him to categorize and record key features of different social aggregates, ranging from isolated settlements to highly differentiated city communities having their own television station and other commodities of relevance for health education interventions. Such a classification system would therefore be able to incorporate the separate study towns of the Stanford Heart Disease Prevention Project, to be discussed later. Classic definitions of community development would not, however, be able to accommodate this. Neither scheme would apply, except by exclusion, to the larger rural area of North Karelia – also the location for a major heart disease prevention project.

Wellman and Leighton (1979) remark on the three major ingredients of community definitions: '... networks of interpersonal ties (outside of the household) which provide sociability and support to members, residence in a common locality, and solidarity sentiments and activities' (p. 365). They then proceed to provide an interesting critique of the way in which urban sociology has tended to focus on neighbourhoods, arguing that the notions of boundedness and density of relationships associated with this geographical concern may not in fact be as beneficial for the well-being of communities as is commonly supposed. We will revisit this point later when we consider the health benefits claimed for community development.

For the present we might usefully note Heller's (1989) acknowledgement that a community need not be defined in terms of geographical propinquity or locality. Like Wellman and Leighton, Heller observes that since modern communication systems make it possible for people to transcend geographical boundaries, it is possible to have 'relational communities'. He cites Bernard's (1973) assertion that:

> People no longer really live their lives in neighbourhoods ... [and] If the house-

keeping details of the area where they lived were properly taken care of and if security were adequate, they could scarcely care less about neighboring or social contacts with others in the area.

> (p. 7)

Having noted the geographical and relational dimensions of definitions of community, Heller adds a third: 'community as collective political power' – a point to which we will also return later in the chapter. First, though, some observations will be made about the dynamics of community change and some of the different approaches which have been espoused to achieve such change.

COMMUNITY ORGANIZATION: VARIATIONS ON A THEME

There are, as mentioned above, different orientations to community work. These differences may be largely over technique or over the means necessary to achieve commonly agreed goals. Alternatively the differences may reflect disagreements about the goals themselves and disagreement may reflect quite fundamental variations in ideology. Before considering some of the different angles taken by advocates of the importance of working in the community, we will revisit communication of innovations theory (to which reference was first made in Chapter 3) and note some of its axioms about community change.

OWNERSHIP OF INNOVATION

Rogers and Shoemaker (1971) argued that there were four basic change situations which derived from the interplay of two dimensions: (i) the origin of the innovation and (ii) recognition of the need for change. These situations are shown in Fig. 8.1.

The first point to note is that change can happen spontaneously in any social group, i.e. without any outside intervention. This

Recognition of need for change	ORIGIN OF NEW IDEA	
	Internal to social system	External to social system
INTERNAL Recognition is by members of the social system	(a) IMMANENT CHANGE	(b) SELECTIVE CONTACT CHANGE
EXTERNAL Recognition may be by change agents outside the social system	(c) INDUCED IMMANENT CHANGE	(d) DIRECT CONTACT CHANGE

Figure 8.1 Types of social change (from Rogers and Shoemaker, 1971).

situation is described by Rogers and Shoemaker as 'immanent change' and occurs where there is 'internal' recognition of the need for change; in other words, when a community has a particular 'felt need' which it recognizes. Clearly, however, immanent change will not happen unless some way of meeting that felt need is discovered. For immanent change to occur, the community itself – or some member(s) of the community – invents a solution. The origin of the new idea is internal to the social system.

The diametrically opposed situation is where some external source, for example a health authority, decides that a given section of the populace has a need, whether it knows it or not. The external source then proceeds to provide a solution to the problem it has identified. The speed of change in such circumstances is likely to be very slow or non-existent.

'Selective contact change', on the other hand, occurs when an outside source provides a solution to a problem identified by the community itself: accordingly the prognosis for adoption of the innovation is good, despite the natural tendency of people to resist apparent attempts from outsiders to tell them what to do!

The notion of 'induced immanent change' which appears in cell 'c' is an interesting one and familiar to expert sales people and disciples of Machiavelli! Those seeking to manipulate a community note that it has an unrecognized need. Taking care to avoid creating reactance, they then help individuals or community to discover that need and identify what they must do to satisfy it. Salespeople will, of course, hope that this will involve buying their product.

Although the purpose may be substantially different, the mechanism is broadly the same when community developers seek to raise community consciousness about unmet needs and then facilitate the acquisition of competences necessary for the fulfilment of those needs.

LEADERSHIP

The informal leadership function of those who succeed in inducing 'immanent change' in the manner described above is epitomized by the oft-quoted traditional Chinese poem which is reproduced below as a kind of 'ode to immanent change'!

> Go to the people
> Live among them
> Love them
> Start with what they know
> Build on what they have
> But of the best leaders
> When their task is accomplished
> Their work is done
> The people all remark
> We have done it ourselves
>
> *(Chabot, 1976)*

Rogers and Shoemaker extend the notion of leadership embodied in the poem cited above. Leadership is intimately related to the invaluable principle of homophily, an idea originated by Lazarsfeld and Merton (1964) but extended by Rogers and Shoemaker who define it thus:

> Homophily is the degree to which pairs of individuals who interact are similar in certain attributes, such as beliefs, values, education, social status and the like.

Interpersonal communication and general influence processes are more effective when individuals are homophilous. Where homophily cannot apparently exist, e.g. because change agent and client are from different social backgrounds, a functionally equivalent state is possible provided that the change agent has acquired the art of empathy – or to be more precise, the cluster of social interaction skills necessary to be empathic. The two fairly obvious implications of the homophily principle are the use of community aides in development work and the provision of appropriate social skills training for community workers.

APPROACHES TO COMMUNITY CHANGE

There are several approaches to generating change in communities and, as we noted earlier, we are emphasizing in this chapter the distinction between those approaches which seek to create change through top-down intervention and those which aim to facilitate change through bottom-up initiatives which have maximal community involvement. The generic term 'community development' (CD) is often used to describe the second of these two opposing strategies. In the USA, the phrase 'community organization' is often used synonymously. Both have a long history. For instance, Bivins (cited in Lazes, 1979) described community organization as 'an old and reliable grassroots approach to health education identified in the 1940s'.

Kindervatter (1979), in an influential book on what she terms 'non-formal education', commented that 'Community organization first appeared in US social work textbooks in the 1920s and 1930s'. However, she went on to say that '... not until the War on Poverty in the sixties did the concept and its application receive much attention'.

Croft and Beresford (1992) also comment on the expansion of community work in the 1960s, both in the US and Britain. Interestingly, though, in the light of later comments on 'colonization' and the common conviction about the ethical soundness and political correctness of CD, they remind us that such work '... had its origins in community development approaches used by the west in the developing world, first to integrate colonial territories and subsequently to support western political and economic objectives there' (p. 29).

Kindervatter (1979) suggests that community organization developed as a response to '... the conditions of poor people in western urban settings, but is now practised in a variety of forms in urban and rural locales'. Its overall purpose is '... to enable communities to improve and change their socioeconomic milieu and/or their position in that milieu'.

Croft and Beresford (1992) describe the emphasis of community development as follows.

> ... on collective rather than individual action. Its focus has been both the workplace and the neighbourhood. It has been concerned with the economic infrastructure, for example, housing and employment; with supporting people's personal growth and development, and with work performed by women in the community – often unpaid – for example, in playschemes, nurseries and carers' groups.
>
> Community development is an activity which may be undertaken by unpaid community activists, specialized community workers or other professionals adopting this approach. The objectives of community development range from encouraging self-help and mutual aid to politicization and pressure group activity; from collaboration to confrontation.
>
> *(p. 29)*

They go on to cite Twelvetrees' (1982) three overlapping approaches to community work: (i) CD itself, (ii) 'political action', i.e. a class-based approach involving coalitions and campaigns, (iii) 'social planning', i.e. the promotion of '... joint action between voluntary and community organizations and the local state to change and improve services'. Croft and Beresford then argue that two additional community 'movements' emerged in the 1970s and 1980s in response to the failure of traditional CD to address issues of sexism and racism and centring on feminist and black community action.

These various observations illustrate the variety of approaches appearing under the rubric of community work and the different interpretations which are often associated with the same or similar terminology. However, although terms may be used interchangeably, sometimes they suggest a distinctive

approach. The most common of these terms are: community organization, community development, locality development, social action, and technical or social planning. Rothman (1970) identified three separate approaches to community work: locality development, technical planning and social action. According to Nix (1970), locality development is the same as community development, community organization and the 'process approach'. Kindervatter considers locality development to be similar to community development insofar as it involves a non-directive approach to community work. She, however, views locality development, social action and 'social planning and co-ordination of services' as three different community organization approaches. Dodds *et al.* (1986), in providing a 'North American Typology' of community development/community organization, identify eight approaches which include self-help groups and 'public advocacy/pressure group tactics'. They also translate some of these terms into a British context.

While there seems to be some confusion over several of these terms, there seems to be general agreement about the nature of 'social action' which is almost universally associated with the work of Saul Alinsky (1946). According to Kindervatter, locality (community) development '... essentially enables people to co-operatively and self-reliantly solve community problems'. On the other hand:

> ... social action strategies aim to enable people to jointly challenge and change existing community power relationships. In terms of the relationship between community members and outside authorities, locality development assumes collaboration and co-operation, whereas social action assumes either competition or conflict.

According to Kirklin and Franzen (1974):

> Large numbers of people are organized to bring into being a new power aggregate ...

to force the existing political/economic power structure to change public and private policies. The battle is classically seen to be between the 'power haves' and the 'power have nots'.

For the purpose of the present chapter, only two broad categories of community intervention will be considered. The first will be generally labelled **community development** in accordance with Ross and Lappin's (1967) definition:

> ... a process by which a community identifies its needs or objectives, orders (or ranks) these needs or objectives, develops the confidence and will to work at these needs or objectives, finds the resources (internal and/or external) to deal with these needs and objectives, takes action in respect to them and in so doing extends and develops co-operation and collaborative attitudes and practices in the community.

The fundamental goal, then, is self-empowerment. This involves, in Kindervatter's words, '... people gaining an understanding of and control over social, economic, and/or political forces in order to improve their standing in society'.

Again, whether the formula is social action or community development, the goal is fundamentally political as is apparent from the following extract from the Calouste Gulbenkian Working Party Report (1984).

> We see community development as a main strategy for the attainment of social policy goals. It is concerned with the worth and dignity of people and the promotion of equal opportunity ... Community work is most needed in communities where social skills and resources are at their weakest. Community work involves working with those most affected by poverty, unemployment, disability, inadequate housing and education, and with those who for reasons of class, income, race or sex are less likely

than others to be, or to feel, involved and significant in local community life.

In the light of the discussion which follows, the reader should be able to spot three major outcome/intermediate indicators in this passage!

By comparison, what Nix (1970) has referred to as 'technical planning' and seen as equivalent to Rothman's notion of 'social planning' tends towards a top-down approach. Thus the second broad category is that of **social/technical planning** and is concerned with task rather than process goals and seeks to implement change in the community (for the good of the community) but without being concerned with the empowerment of people living therein. The assumption, of course, is that planners know what is best for the community (as indeed they may do). However the difference between a sophisticated social planning approach and more naive (top-down) programmes is that in the former case, planners are aware of the need to take account of the dynamics of change in the community. They will thus employ outreach strategies, seek to identify opinion leaders and generally apply the accumulated wisdom of studies based on communication of innovations research. They will often, therefore, look like community organization programmes, at least at first glance.

COMMUNITY DEVELOPMENT OR COLONIZATION?

In the light of our discussion of ideological differences between approaches and the associated implications for evaluation, the difference between Rothman's 'social/technical planning' approach and the other approaches described above merit some further explication.

First of all, let us remind ourselves of the 'ideal type' of the social planning model, which we might usefully characterize as a deliberate strategy to intervene in a given community in order to achieve prede-termined objectives which, if successfully achieved, will prevent disease. According to this model, either the community may be seen as whatever remains after more man-ageable settings, such as school or workplace, have been targeted or alternatively, it may be viewed as an opportunity to work less form-ally and target people in their natural habitat. Since many of the target group may be dif-ficult to reach in other settings – for instance, because they may be unemployed or because they do not respond to invitations to attend clinics or surgeries – the social planning approach may be seen as a last ditch attempt to 'get through to' disadvantaged groups or others who might be 'resistant' to change.

An alternative and often complementary orientation is that of the 'community-wide strategy'. This, as indicated earlier, may inter-pret the idea of a community programme as an integrated campaign which seeks to maximize its impact by delivering consistent and complementary health education to whatever institutions or organizations can be persuaded to embrace it. The programme may well also include less formal tactics de-signed to reach the resistants, as described above.

In seeking to achieve its goals, a sophis-ticated community programme will take full account of the psychosocial dynamics of community life and functions and use these to achieve programme goals. For instance, the importance of using opinion leaders to influence the whole social group would be acknowledged and 'community aides' might be appointed. The importance of avoiding reactance would also be recognized and various exercises in consulting the commun-ity might be undertaken. In the last analysis, though, the purpose of the programme is to achieve its preventive goals – which would, in all probability, be highly laudable and desirable.

In practice, there is often no hard and fast distinction between types of approach, espe-cially where the exercise is patently under-taken for the good of the community and seeks to meet very real problems. The dis-tinction is, however, nicely made by Hilton (1988). The example he provides is from de-veloping countries and thus especially appro-priate given the impetus which Alma Ata and primary health care gave to the recognition of the importance of creating active, particip-ating communities. Hilton provides examples of what he calls a 'community-oriented' ap-proach in which '... plans are made by out-siders and people are asked to participate'. A selection of these examples is provided below.

> Our hospital staff is overworked treating cases of malaria, dehydration and malnutri-tion that could be prevented or treated locally. Therefore we are going to build a clinic in some villages 30 miles from the hospital. We will give an employment exam to the district secondary school leavers and select the best to train as health workers to be sent to the clinics. They will learn how to treat malaria, respiratory infections, malnu-trition and other common diseases.

> We have done a survey and find very poor conditions of sanitation, hygiene and nutri-tion in all of the villages. Therefore we will train the health workers to do health edu-cation. They will teach the people that they should construct latrines and dig wells in order to prevent disease. They will have classes in nutrition for the women so that they will learn how to properly feed their children.
>
> *(p. 1)*

Hilton goes on to offer a case study in 'community-based' health promotion. This centres on the story of a primary school teacher who became a 'community organ-izer'. His training taught him 'how to listen and really hear what people are saying and feeling'. He worked on a farm but spent as much time as possible getting closely involved in the life of the community. He listened for 'generative themes' – 'topics that people have strong feelings about'. He gained the confidence of the village people and was soon invited to a number of meetings of women's groups, church meetings, etc. He prepared 'codes' on the generative themes and presented these in picture form or through story and drama. He engaged the people in dialogue about the possibilities of change. One theme was considered particularly important: the lack of money to buy vegetables from wealthy landowners. As a result the group pooled their savings and rented land on which they grew their own vegetables. 'The best product from the garden, however, was the discovery that they could work together to solve a problem.'

The process described is, of course, based on Freire's methods of adult education and further reference will be made to this when we comment on CD strategies later in the chapter. For now we will note the success of the strategy in the case study provided by Hilton. The initiative he described expanded and resulted in enhanced empowerment of local women who learned how to improve the health of their children by working as equal partners with health workers. The final stage in the process of transformation involved collaboration with other towns and villages and election of villagers to the governing council.

The CD process described above is very evidently rooted in an empowering strategy based on gaining community participation in achieving goals which the community had identified itself. It is substantially different from the 'colonizing' approach adopted by change agents who seek, with greater or lesser success, to 'plug into' community networks and utilize their dynamic to achieve predetermined preventive goals. Measures of success are primarily those which demonstrate the attainment of preventive objectives. In the case described by Hilton, success is defined in terms of the extent to which community and

individual empowerment have been achieved. It is, however, important to underline the fact that the achievement of empowerment will, in all probability, have been the most effective way of preventing the various life-threatening diseases which faced the villagers described in Hilton's case study. Whether this kind of approach might be the best way of achieving the preventive goals of those who organize community-wide preventive programmes in western contexts is clearly a matter of some interest. At all events, we will now consider these community-wide initiatives and comment on how success has been measured and also what evidence there might be to demonstrate that goals have been achieved.

COMMUNITY-WIDE INITIATIVES

As we have observed above, the characteristics of preventively driven, community-wide projects have been not only their focus on prevention but also their top-down tendency. More recent developments will cause us to modify that statement somewhat but, for now, the systematic process of programme planning central to these community programmes can be illustrated by Farquhar et al.'s (1984) discussion of the field application of 'community organization' with its three stages of 'development, implementation and maintenance'. The systematic nature of the process is evident in the following summary:

1. Development
    (a) *Goal definition.* Review of literature and baseline data to determine people's needs for information, motivation, skills, etc. in order to determine target groups and kind of programme needed to reduce their risks of disease.
    (b) *Resources definition.* Choice of appropriate resources for each risk factor.
    (c) *Community recruiting.* Identifying community leaders and enlisting

aid of organizations to achieve programme goals.

    (d) *Programme definitions*. Gaining feedback '... to fit the community's and the initiators' needs ...'; formative evaluation and design of programme are planned.

2. Implementation.

    (a) *Materials and programme development*. For example, training of leaders; pretesting materials.

    (b) *Consulting with community groups*. For example '... helping advisory boards become functioning community units ...'.

    (c) *Programme field testing*. For example redesigning and refining the programme.

3. Maintenance. This involves 'programme monitoring; programme multiplication; programme continuation'. The final goal is institutionalization and community ownership.

Bracht and Kingsbury (1990) also present a set of guidelines for community interventions. In so doing, they remind us of Rothman's three 'models' of community work: locality development (i.e. CD), social planning and social action. They also point out that Rothman viewed these models as 'analytical extremes' which would, in practice, often overlap – an observation which we will also endorse later in the chapter. It would, however, not be unreasonable to suggest that Bracht and Kingsbury's system owes more to social planning than to the other two models.

The basis for their approach may be summarized as follows.

1. Interventions must be based on a historical understanding of the community;
2. Multiple interventions are needed;
3. Health promoters should work through existing structures and take account of existing values and norms;
4. Active community participation (not tokenism) is required;

5. Intersectoral collaboration is important to maximize impact;
6. Long term needs and problems must be addressed to ensure that there will be 'life after the project';
7. The community must share responsibility for the problem and its solution.

                    (p. 72)

Planning is based on a five-stage process:

1. Community analysis;
2. Design and initiation;
3. Implementation;
4. Programme maintenance and consolidation;
5. Dissemination and reassessment.

Pancer and Nelson (1990) also provide a detailed set of guidelines for 'community mobilization' in health promotion programmes. This consists of the following ten-point plan:

1. Community involvement;
2. Planning;
3. Needs and resource assessment (health problems and available resources);
4. A comprehensive programme (dealing with multiple risk factors; utilizing several different channels; operating at different levels, e.g. families and organizations; designed to change the psychological and social factors which underpin specific disease risk factors);
5. An integrated programme;
6. Long term change (producing stable and lasting change; development of a permanent health promotion infrastructure);
7. Altering community norms (requiring participation of majority of community members);
8. Research and evaluation;
9. Sufficient resources;
10. Professional and community collaboration (especially between professionals and community leaders).

Clearly, a key issue for those designing such programmes is just how to achieve community mobilization. Rather than rely on the emergence of community involvement in accordance with pure CD principles, a more proactive process of coalition building is usually recommended.

CITIZEN PARTNERSHIP AND COALITIONS

One of the central questions in this chapter is just how people can be converted from a state of passivity into active, empowered community members. CD suggests a facilitative process which awakens felt needs and helps communities to identify and achieve their own goals. As we will see, the extent to which this is possible has been subjected to challenge and the need to gain the support of already empowered individuals or powerful groups and organizations has been articulated as a more feasible alternative.

The kinds of community-wide programmes we are considering here tend to rely on the latter strategy rather than the former. Indeed, since programme objectives will already have been stated, there is right from the start a limit to the utility of exploring felt needs! As Haglund, Weisbrod and Bracht (1990) observe, 'A core group of concerned citizens and professionals usually initiates the action process'. Five varieties of 'citizen partnership structure' are offered: 'lead' or official agency; grassroots; citizen panels; networks and consortia. In relation to the first of these, the authors point out that the 'lead agency model' is often used when a single agency has the necessary resources, authority and credibility to take the lead. They cite as an example of this situation the Pawtucket Project (to which reference will be made later) in which the local hospital took the major initiative.

The situation which Haglund *et al.* label **'grassroots'** is roughly analogous to the community development approach, i.e. it involves people who are not part of more formal structures nor represented by them. **Citizen panels**, on the other hand, work alongside official agencies. Members may be appointed or elected to these panels and, in that capacity,

be expected to contribute to policy formulation and implementation. Obviously, there will always be a danger that citizen panels become over-bureaucratized and tokenistic.

Networks refer to relatively informal and more transient operations; they tend to be triggered by single issues. The authors distinguish networks from **consortia** which feature somewhere between the loose aggregate of the network and the more formal and usually hierarchical structure which is described as a **coalition**. This key phenomenon of North American community organization merits some consideration – albeit brief.

Community coalitions

Community coalitions figure quite centrally in US community-wide initiatives (for a more extensive review, see the special issue of *Health Education Research*, 1993). Essentially they involve interorganizational collaboration directed at the attainment of common goals.

Green and Kreuter (1991), considering health promotion planning in community settings, refer to coalitions as 'groups to be reckoned with'. They identify two types of relationship within a community: exchange relationships and co-ordinative relationships. The former obtain between professionals and clients, the latter between two or more groups with common interests which collaborate to achieve common goals. Coalitions are of the latter type.

Given our discussion in this chapter of the location of power and the feasibility of changing the power and resource structure in the interests of health promotion, we will repeat here a quotation which Green and Kreuter present from Nix (1977).

Research findings suggest that reputed community leaders gain influence over others by occupying economic and governmental positions of exchange, which allow them to control, in varying degrees, the lives of other people. In order to distribute effectively this influence over community-wide affairs, community leaders must participate actively in influential organizations of a co-ordinated nature which are composed of representatives of different interest groups and organizations.

Coalitions seek to counter the substantial influence of governmental, commercial and other powerful interests subsumed in the notion of dominant ideology. We might, incidentally, note at this point that radical social action movements seeking to shift the balance of power as a primary goal would also routinely seek to establish fighting coalitions.

CITIZEN BOARDS AND TASK FORCES

The final type of citizen partnership to be considered here is that of the community or citizen board. The principle is simple and would operate in association with coalitions or other forms of structure discussed earlier. Bracht and Kingsbury list the typical representatives of various community sectors on a community board. They might include: local government officials; local media personnel; schools; commercial and business organizations; unions; health professionals; minority and voluntary groups; hospitals; churches; community groups.

The citizen board might typically be supported by a number of task forces, once a given project had been launched. The membership of the task forces might consist of professionals and lay volunteers; they would focus on particular issues such as smoking, diet, exercise or a supportive schools programme. The procedure is well exemplified by the Minnesota CHD Prevention Project, which will be discussed later.

COMMUNITY-WIDE PROJECTS: EXPECTATIONS OF SUCCESS

Before commenting on some exemplars of community-wide projects, we should note that it is undoubtedly possible to achieve evidence of success in programmes which do not meet all, or even most, of the systematic programme requirements outlined above. For instance, one of the most impressive and well evaluated health education programmes was described by Sayegh and Green in 1976. This was organized within the American University Medical Center in Beirut. Its purpose was to develop an efficient family planning intervention and, although it is perhaps more properly regarded as patient education, its focus was the community. In short an experimental group of women received education designed to promote the adoption of contraception. The baseline rate of acceptance of family planning was 4.2% but, eventually, contraceptive use settled at a steady rate of some 37%. Bearing in mind that the acceptance rate of a well known International Post-Partum Programme was 17%, there could be little doubt about the efficiency of this particular intervention. More particularly, the authors demonstrated not only behaviour change but also cost effectiveness: the programme was cheaper per success rate than alternative methods of family planning education.

Kanaaneh, Rabi and Badarneh (1976) also demonstrated the effectiveness of a properly organized and realistically targeted outreach programme in Western Galilee. The intervention occurred in a village of 3000 inhabitants and it succeeded in achieving its goal of eradicating scabies which, prior to the campaign, was prevalent in 66% of families.

More recently, Vincent, Clearie and Schluchter (1987) employed a systematic process of community organization in a programme designed to reduce adolescent pregnancies. Having raised consciousness about teen pregnancies as a social problem and performed a community assessment, the authors recruited advisory groups, developed 'community linkages', trained adult leaders and produced a joint school and community-based intervention. The evaluation demonstrated that the rate of pregnancy in the South Carolina country where the programme had been in operation had declined significantly compared with rates in comparison counties.

Green and Kreuter (1991) cite with approval an effective health promotion programme in Kentucky. A significant decline in mortality from cardiovascular disease was recorded in two intervention counties compared with one control county allegedly as a result of a properly structured hypertension control programme. In addition to the impressively hard data on mortality, a reduction in diastolic and systolic blood pressure was recorded together with improved compliance with medication.

Green and Kreuter identified 12 features of the programme which met the requirements of systematic community organization and which were responsible for the impressive results. They included: the appointment of an enthusiastic fulltime co-ordinator; the establishment of a task force (Community High Blood Pressure Control Program Council) which had membership from schools, health departments, medical society, commercial and business interests, Co-operative Agricultural Extension Service and 'interested citizens'; an existing Nutrition Aide Program to contact people at high risk identified by their doctors; development of teenage CHD prevention club using peer teaching; introduction of a school BP screening programme; establishing a volunteer BP screening and monitoring network in churches and small businesses; adding a workplace screening programme to an existing general health programme provided by local health departments; gaining general support from and involvement of local media; providing a continuing education programme for nurses; presenting health education programmes to community clubs, health fairs and large family reunions (a rural Kentucky tradition).

A QUIT SMOKING PROGRAMME IN A MINORITY COMMUNITY

Hunkeler *et al.* (1990) describe a community-wide programme which is of special interest in the context of our current discussion. First it is based on the kind of systematic community organization principles exemplified earlier and, second, it seeks to address a significant health problem in a minority community.

The main programme aim was to reduce the prevalence of smoking in the black population of Richmond, California, by 20%. Black people constituted 47.9% of the population, which would suggest that the term 'minority' is used socially rather than statistically. Forty-six per cent of men and 38% of women were current cigarette smokers. Success was to be decided in two ways: (i) an outcome indicator of smoking prevalence was to be used and smoking rates would be compared with those of a reference group composed of blacks elsewhere in the San Francisco Bay area; (ii) observations in the field would assess community reaction to programme activities and record changes in 'smoking norms, values and practices' as intermediate indicators of assumed ultimate success in outcomes.

The community analysis carried out by the team revealed some interesting features of the community. Of especial interest were strong kinship ties, an influential church presence, a history of community mobilization, a variety of voluntary organizations including a Black Chamber of Commerce, a strong sense of community pride, a high regard for families and children, 'an investment in the city's maintaining a positive public image'.

Clearly these features could be and were taken into account in planning the programme. Certain barriers to implementation were also identified from the community profile: absence of local mass media; the fact that only one third of the black population actually worked in Richmond; a suspicion of outsiders; greater public concern over crime and drug abuse than with smoking; a high level of billboard and magazine advertising of tobacco targeted at blacks.

In addition to the more general analysis of community characteristics, individual beliefs and attitudes in relation to smoking were assessed.

The programme followed the kinds of recommended procedures discussed earlier. A predominantly black working group of 20 community leaders and medical providers helped formulate activities. A Community Advisory Board was established to co-ordinate the project, consisting of 30 members from the following bodies: schools, local media and the arts, voluntary agencies, Kaiser Permanente Medical Care Program, hospitals and clinics, individual health professionals, the County Health Department, churches and religious organizations, local government and public institutions, community groups and neighbourhood organizations and representatives from the business community.

Major programme components included: provision of training in counselling and health education techniques for health professionals; an extensive media programme (including, for example, a rap music video entitled 'Stop Before You Drop'); a variety of stop-smoking materials and services; mobilization of community organizations; a number of community-wide publicity events; a school-based programme; a volunteer programme.

In the context of earlier discussions about the significance of change agents and 'lay leaders', the function of these volunteers is worth noting. In short, they were trained to:

1. Talk to family members, friends and neighbours;
2. Offer encouragement and support to young people and ex-smokers;
3. Identify smokers, e.g. in the 'contemplation stage', and provide them with stop-smoking self-help materials;
4. Maintain data on smoking cessation services and make referrals;
5. Provide a more supportive environment by setting up support groups, stop-smoking workshops, etc. and promoting education campaigns.

Reflecting on evaluation of process during the programme, the organizers identified a number of necessary strategies for successful community interventions. A summary follows.

1. Meaningful community involvement from the start.
2. Use of methods tailored specifically to the community, taking account of prevailing values and practices.
3. Locking the programme into existing social organizations and networks.
4. As well as appealing to specifically targeted groups, framing the issues so as to unite the whole community (e.g. black community leaders advised that all racial groups should be involved while maintaining a focus on blacks).
5. Designing activities to increase self-esteem and community pride in blacks.
6. Emphasizing 'winning strategies' rather than problems.
7. Utilizing influence of families, friends and fellow workers.
8. Integrating health issues with other 'felt needs' having higher priority for the black community (e.g. crime and public safety).
9. Employing black staff and spending project funds in the black community.
10. Influencing health agencies to increase resources for black people.
11. Using a variety of exciting and controversial consciousness raising activities involving large numbers of participants

but support these with 'solid' cessation services.

12. Enhancing existing community resources by bringing in external funding.
13. Including in initial planning ways of institutionalizing the programme so that it survives after the funding runs out.

At the time of writing, only an interim evaluation had been conducted. A telephone survey of 400 residents revealed a high level of awareness of the programme (70% in general, 76% in blacks). More significantly a substantial number of agencies and personnel had agreed to continue the work of the project and incorporate it into their own activities using their own funds.

HEALTH PROMOTION IN A MEXICAN–AMERICAN COMMUNITY

Amezcua *et al.* (1990) also describe a programme geared to the health needs of low socioeconomic status groups in southwest Texas. The central feature of this programme is its use of mass media supported by 'networks, organization and social reinforcement'. The organizational approach adopted was the 'lead agency model' which, as mentioned earlier, involves a single powerful organization undertaking responsibility for programme design and implementation together with any necessary coalition building. Programme goals were those of general lifestyle modification designed to achieve: reduction in incidence and prevalence of cigarette smoking, modification of dietary behaviour related to cancer risk, reduction of alcohol misuse, promotion of car seat belt wearing, increase in physical activity and fostering appropriate use of preventive services.

The theoretical basis of the programme drew heavily on social learning theory (Bandura, 1986) and, in particular, the notions of modelling and social reinforcement.

After the standard procedure of community analysis a mass media programme was devised which incorporated two sets of television productions. The first consisted of 15 programmes of five to ten minutes' duration utilizing role models presenting health 'testimonials' together with the provision of health information in a news format. The second series consisted of four half-hour documentaries featuring a health education specialist as narrator.

The community organization aspect of the programme involved two community workers supported by a number of trained volunteers working as community aides. The function of these volunteers was similar to those described in the Richmond Project and the North Karelia Project, which will be discussed in the next section. It included identification of role models in their own social networks; these models had to be people who had recently made approved changes in lifestyle.

Social reinforcement was to be provided by a coalition of the by now familiar cluster of agencies and organizations: business settings; health care providers; federal, state and local government units; education settings; religious organizations; social clubs; grassroots neighbourhood centres.

The importance of acknowledging the need for a supportive health promoting environment (again based particularly on the North Karelian experience) resulted in attempts to promote voter and consumer demand for healthier products. The process involved (i) consciousness raising to create demand, (ii) mobilization of consumers to create public pressure, (iii) consultation with political leaders, administrators and commercial producers and retailers.

The list of barriers identified by the authors is quite illuminating; some of these were also identified in the projects already exemplified here. First, the problem of change agents and volunteers competing for the public's attention with other organizations, groups and sales people. A second problem was the fact that many householders migrated to other states to harvest the fields! Third, many people seemed opposed to health professionals who were seen as too 'business oriented' rather than being interested in genuine human problems. Fourth, strained relations among neighbours due to economic depression made it hard to contact people whose 'felt needs' were frequently expressed in terms of a desire for jobs and money. Interpersonal dynamics of a different kind were also seen as problematical. For instance, community workers seemed to experience stress and feelings of helplessness when faced with the poor social circumstances and economic conditions of community members. Again, workers identified a problem associated with what they called:

> ... the small-town dynamics of social control, gossip, and suspicion of one's neighbor's motives. Husbands do not like to see their wives interacting with other women, attending meetings, or participating in social gatherings that they do not control.

There was also '... a great deal of justified fear and distrust of "official-looking" people who come around asking questions'. Accordingly, part of the educational activities involved what might be called community-building events as well as enhancing the image and public relations skills of professional workers.

Again, at the time of writing, only interim evaluation results were available centring on process evaluation of volunteer activities. Three hundred and ninety nine volunteers were interviewed, including 166 of the most active of these in greater depth. Thirty-seven per cent operated within commercial/workplace settings; 30% in neighbourhoods; 21% in religious organizations. A total of 7860 contacts was recorded: these included 6098 adults and 1762 young people. The interviewees had viewed on average 10 TV programmes featuring role models. Seventeen volunteers reported smoking cessation, five reported changes in drinking habits and 196 reported obtaining preventive care. Changes in diet were recorded by 269 volunteers and 226

reported an increase in exercise. The more active volunteers had contacted an average of over 20 people each; their contacts claimed they had seen nine TV programmes featuring role models. Moreover, of these contacts, 21 had stopped smoking, ten had modified alcohol use, 328 received preventive health care, 368 had changed their diet and 353 had increased their levels of exercise.

ASPECTS OF MENTAL AND SOCIAL HEALTH

Relatively few programmes provide evidence of successful mental health initiatives, doubtless because of a combination of problems, including difficulties in defining mental health, knowing how to tackle it and lack of funding due to the popularity of 'mainstream' preventive programmes such as the CHD prevention projects.

Hersey *et al.* (1984) did, however, demonstrate that '... an intensive combination of community activities and media exposure' could achieve desirable mental health goals. Apart from increases in knowledge and changes in attitude, respondents exposed to both media and community activities indicated '... substantial likelihood of engaging in support enhancing behaviour' compared with population groups receiving less extensive interventions.

Before considering in some detail major international CHD prevention projects, a brief description will be provided of a programme reported by Kemper and Mettler (1990) which sought to 'build a positive image of aging' and which illustrated, *inter alia*, the importance of coalition building. The context of the programme was a small American city, Boise in Idaho. A non-profitmaking health promotion research centre acted as lead agency and developed two related programmes for people over 60. These were called 'Growing Younger: A Physical Wellness Program' and 'Growing Wiser: A Mental Wellness Program'. The programmes were designed to respond to research which had provided a rather bleak consensus view of health professionals that:

1. Most older people were not interested in changing health behaviour;
2. Older people's habits were too ingrained for change to take place;
3. Even if health behaviours were improved, it was too late to do much good.

A coalition was duly established and this included: employers, Boise School District, YMCA and YWCA, the state university, two local hospitals, the District Health Department, the Idaho State Office on Aging and the Idaho Division of Health. A number of committees and task groups were set up and older people themselves were actively involved.

The aims of the first programme were not only to improve fitness and reduce risk but also to influence general community perceptions of and attitudes to ageing. A series of workshops was arranged; these emphasized positive health and included such items as improving quality of home and doctor care, dietary improvements in flexibility, strength and endurance. Successful attempts were made to sustain the impact of the programme in the form of 'neighbourhood groups' which, at the time of writing, had been meeting weekly for seven years.

During the first 30 months, 1658 older adults (12% of the target population) had participated in the programme. Subsequently, the number had grown to more than 3500 senior citizens. Pre- and post-testing indicated significant positive changes in lifestyle and utilization of services. Participants had lost weight, reduced body fat, lowered their blood pressure and lipid levels and improved flexibility. Again in relation to the programme maintenance and diffusion effects, a number of spin-off activities occurred including, for example, 'Happy Hoofers', a walking group which met twice weekly!

The mental wellness programme achieved similarly impressive results. The programme included such items as memory, mental alertness, loss and life change, choices for living and self-image.

By the end of the 18 month evaluation, 578 people had participated and a 15-question geriatric depression scale revealed a 24% improvement in risk of depression and memory performance had also improved. Again, a series of spin-offs were noted in the form of a number of 'Meeting of Minds Societies' – local discussion groups meeting weekly.

Of particular interest for the broader health promotion perspective was the evidence presented by Kemper and Mettler of the impact of the programme on public policy. Policy changes occurred within the centre for senior citizens, which increased health promotion activities, and in a regional medical centre which '... greatly expanded its services to older people and created a Senior Life Center to serve their needs better'. At the city and state level increased budgetary support was identified for older people. Moreover, the authors report the diffusion of the initiative to other states: similar programmes were sponsored in over 100 communities in 30 states at the time of writing.

INTERNATIONAL HEART HEALTH PROGRAMMES

The title of this section is something of a misnomer since the CHD prevention programmes which are described in some detail here are, with the one exception of the North Karelia Project, from the USA. This is not to say that often quite substantial programmes do not occur elsewhere. It is rather that the programmes discussed below tend to combine in the form of demonstration projects, overt application of theory, community-wide application and, typically, comprehensive and detailed evaluation. Indeed, before moving on to a consideration of these programmes, some reference will be made to certain developments in the UK.

CHD PREVENTION IN THE UNITED KINGDOM

In 1988, the National Forum for Coronary Heart Disease Prevention published a review of *Action in the UK, 1984–1987*. It commented on a number of 'special programmes' but, perhaps more importantly, noted a number of efforts both nationally and locally which involved the integration of heart health work into existing activities. One of the strengths of the UK scene compared with the USA is its National Health Service which incorporates health promotion units at district level and a primary care system which has increasingly over recent years become involved in health education and related preventive and anticipatory care activity. Clearly, if CHD prevention can be routinely incorporated within general health promotion activities as part of standard service provision, the net effect should be greater than the impact of relatively isolated, albeit high profile demonstration projects. This is, of course, provided that the delivery of health promotion is efficient; regrettably it is unlikely that anything as theoretically and organizationally sophisticated as the programmes cited so far will be readily discerned in the UK to date.

One of the best examples of a coherent and integrated approach to the development of health promotion is provided by the City of Sheffield's Strategic Plan (1990–1993). This includes a description of the 'Heart of Our City' – one of three demonstration projects. This, in turn, relates to an overall strategic programme entitled 'Healthy Sheffield 2000' which, as well as addressing major *Health of the Nation* (DoH, 1992) targets, also incorporates a philosophy consistent with the principles of health promotion outlined in Chapter 1. In the light of later discussions we might also note that the principle of a community development way of working is built into programmes wherever possible. For instance, the 'Heart of Our City' project includes in its aims: the enhancement of

personal skills, self-esteem and general well-being and the stimulation of community participation; the identification and tackling of barriers of a social, economic and environmental nature; the development and refining of evaluative techniques appropriate to community initiatives (p. 116).

The projects mentioned by the National Forum for CHD Prevention (1988) include seven 'special programmes': Oxford Prevention of Heart Attack and Stroke Project; City and Hackney Heart Disease and Stroke Prevention Project; Slough Health Habit; South Birmingham Coronary Prevention Project; Good Hearted Glasgow; Change of Heart (Northern Ireland); Heartbeat Wales (Welsh Heart Programme). Of these, only the last named, 'Heartbeat Wales', could be said to compete in rationale and scope with the international projects which we will now consider.

Farquhar *et al.* (1983) describe ten community-based multiple risk factor health education interventions. Four of these will be considered here: the Stanford Heart Disease Prevention Projects; the Minnesota Heart Health Study; the Pawtucket Heart Health Study and the North Karelia Project. A detailed review of each is beyond the scope of this chapter which will, therefore, be limited to discussing the following main features of the projects and their evaluation. First the main characteristics of the programme itself will be described. This will be followed by comments on the nature of the evaluation and, finally, observations will be made on the results of the evaluation where these are available.

As regards evaluation, it should be noted that all of the programmes reject the clinical trials model – with greater or lesser reluctance and do so for the reasons discussed earlier in this book. Some projects, however, make strenuous efforts to compensate for the lack of a true experimetal design by the introduction of various techniques to enhance the internal validity of their quasi-experiments. All projects utilize process evaluation – both to gain illumination and, in its formative mode, to monitor and improve interventions. In some instances, a true experimental design might be incorporated within a subprogramme.

Blackburn (1983) describes the main strategies which are used to mitigate the effects of what is inevitably an imperfect experiment. These are adopted by the Minnesota Project and are listed below:

1. Creation of a degree of control by matching communities for anticipated important variables such as population structure, service provision, CHD mortality, etc.
2. Staging community entry to the programme thus allowing repetition of the experimental input and the consequent strengthening of inference of cause and effect.
3. Sensitive trend measures (allowing time series analysis) by means of cross-sectional surveys of communities and repeated measures of individual change within cohorts.
4. Dose–effect measurement which looks for different degrees of response in those subjected to increasing levels of educational exposure and programme involvement.
5. Establishing links between responses to specific elements of the educational programme and subsequent changes, e.g. links between participation in a nutrition programme and subsequent change of diet/reduction in risk factors.
6. Pooling communities/groups of people exposed to education and comparing them with similar pools in control communities.

In relation to the kinds of evaluation employed, the four projects will be compared in respect of:

1. Measures of mortality/morbidity, i.e. disease related outcomes;
2. Risk factor reduction;
3. Intermediate measures of programme outcome ranging from the acquisition of knowledge, attitudes and skills to the various behaviours underpinning risk factor scores;
4. Process evaluation.

THE STANFORD STUDIES

The Stanford Three Community Study began in 1972 and has been extensively documented and described. It sought to examine the impact of two levels of intervention on two Californian towns by comparison with a control community. The populations of the towns ranged from 13 000 to 15 000. The Stanford Heart Disease Prevention Project (SHDPP) established the pattern for later schemes by building the interventions on a firm foundation of learning theory. This seems unremarkable but it is worth noting that many preventive interventions prior to this date (and many since!) had been educationally naïve, often making the assumption that providing infomation was the same as providing education. The theoretical element included an amalgam of social learning theory, attitude and communication theory and social marketing. This produced an almost standard formula which Farquhar *et al.* (1984) described as a communication–behaviour change framework. Effectively this meant ensuring a chain of events starting with agenda setting, moving on to the provision of information, enhancement of motivation, offering models, providing training and skills, offering 'cues to action' – which allowed programme participants to acquire self-management competences – and finally ensuring the availability of social and environmental support for newly acquired risk-reducing behaviours.

There were several points of special theoretical interest in the main interventions used by the SHDPP and these centre on the role of mass media. One community, Gilroy, received only a mass media programme while

Watsonville was subjected to the identical media influences and also provided with supplementary intensive instruction. For these reasons, the SHDPP found itself a kind of test case in the debate about the capabilities of mass media, a point of some interest in the light of Chapter 6. Before examining the impact of these measures, however, we should note the extent of the mass media programming employed by the Stanford team.

It consisted of some 50 television public service advertisements broadcast by four stations; three hours of television programmes; more than 100 radio spots and several hours of radio broadcasting; weekly newspaper columns, advertisements and stories; poster advertising; direct mail including calendars and cook books mailed to each household; and kits for schools. This programme was continued for nine months after pretesting in 1973 and repeated in 1974 after a second survey.

The intensive intrusion received by Watsonville was derived from social learning theory and employed a range of behaviour modification techniques. It was delivered to a group of individuals at high risk (two thirds of a random sample of individuals falling into the top risk quartile) and consisted of home counselling/group sessions for a ten week period and included spouses who were willing to be involved.

The evaluation strategy involved baseline surveys in the three towns followed by three further surveys of the same samples at one yearly intervals. Participants' knowledge and beliefs about CHD and its prevention were assessed along with relevant behaviours. The key aspect of the summative evaluation, however, was a measure of reduction in a risk score derived from an equation incorporating cardinal risk factors of age, sex, systolic blood pressure, relative weight, amount of cigarette smoking and plasma cholesterol. Process evaluation was mainly concerned with various mini surveys which monitored the impact of media, in addition to materials

pretesting and developmental testing of the intensive instruction programme. An additional interesting example of process evaluation was provided by the results of a diffusion survey using network analysis to determine the nature of interpersonal contacts stimulated by the programme. This revealed, for instance, that whereas on average an individual only receiving a mass media input might have an average number of two interpersonal contacts and a frequency of two conversations with other people about CHD, someone receiving the media programme together with screening and face-to-face education from a health educator would make contact with eight people and have 13 conversations.

The result of the Three Towns Project were convincing. After one year there was evidence of significant shifts on the baseline measures with Watsonville leading the field, presumably thus justifying the assumption of the superiority of interpersonal education. For instance, an overall improvement in knowledge about triglycerides was recorded (an increase from 18% to 45%) and belief in the statement that eating eggs could be harmful had increased from 67% to 77% in Gilroy, from 65% to 86% in Watsonville but showed no change in Tracy, the control town. As for behaviour change, there had been a decline in smoking: in Watsonville a 20% reduction was noted (44% in high risk group) but only a 3% drop had been observed in Gilroy. Of the high risk group, 31% had quit smoking during the first year of the programme. Using egg consumption as a behavioural indicator, the superiority of Watsonville at the mid-point in the intervention was again in evidence: the number of eggs eaten had declined 17% in Tracy, the control; 27% in Gilroy and 40% in Watsonville (Maccoby and Farquhar, 1975).

However, what created most interest and debate was the end-of-programme summative evaluation which demonstrated not only a significant reduction in risk but also revealed that Gilroy, the town exposed only to mass media, had virtually caught up with Watsonville. The relative risk in the control town had increased by some 6% while it had decreased by some 18% in the two experimental towns, yielding a net difference between control and treatment of between 23% and 28%. Among high-risk participants, the intensive instruction group had a 5% lower risk than the media only group (Farquhar *et al.*, 1977).

What are we to make of these results which suggest that mass media can in fact yield results virtually as good as interpersonal education? The first point to note is that the intensity and extensiveness of the media programme per head of population was very substantial. The second point is, of course, that it is impossible to know the extent to which the media campaign triggered interpersonal education by health professionals and educators. The third point to note is that the media design was based on good learning theory and approximated therefore to interpersonal communication. However, Maccoby and Solomon (1981) themselves state the case very appositely:

> We tentatively attribute much of the success of the community education campaigns to the quality of the media campaign and to the *synergistic interaction of multiple educational inputs* and to interpersonal communication stimulated by application of these inputs in a community setting (author's emphasis).

Farquahar *et al.* (1977) add:

> Intensive face-to-face instruction and counselling seem important for changing refractory behaviour such as cigarette smoking and for inducing rapid change of dietary behaviour. But we must learn how to use these methods to correct obesity, and to employ them effectively with limited resources (e.g. by training volunteer instructors). Mass media are potentially much more cost-effective than face-to-face education methods.

The Stanford Three Towns Study – despite its manifest success – was criticized on several grounds (Levanthal *et al.*, 1980). These objections may be summarized as follows. First, it was argued that the study was wrong to confuse behavioural and medical indicators (a point made in Chapter 3). For instance, health education might well produce a change in behaviour such as a reduction in dietary cholesterol, without necessarily leading to a reduction in physiological risk and community levels of CHD. This issue of the wisdom of latching on to epidemiological indicators will be mentioned again later when considering the North Karelia experience. The second objection centres on an accusation that the SHDPP was unduly wedded to a medical model and missed the opportunity of appraising a genuine community study. As Levanthal *et al.* say, 'We believe ... that the Stanford study is better described as a quasiexperimental study of individuals in a community setting and that it retains many of the failings typically ascribed to laboratory investigations'. These critics also regret the lack of sufficient process measures to describe community activities and diffusion of information. The third objection related to problems of internal validity of the kind discussed earlier and which follow failure to employ a true experimental design.

Not surprisingly the Stanford team reacted somewhat tetchily to these criticisms – and with justification (Meyer, Maccoby and Farquhar, 1980). A detailed discussion of the case is not appropriate here but we might with benefit note the impossibility of avoiding criticism on methodological grounds without the talisman of randomization! We should also note that the follow-up to the Three Towns Study sought to meet some of Levanthal *et al.*'s criticisms. This took the form of a five cities study.

The Five City Project (FCP), apart from its other goals, attempted to counter criticism of its lack of community focus and Farquhar *et al.* (1984) have described how it was established. It began in 1978 and was designed to be a genuinely community-based programme which would seek to achieve local community involvement, ownership and control. Community ownership, it was felt, might enhance the mass media components but at lower cost than the 'individualized instruction' used in the three centre study. It was also hoped that community support might maintain the long term impact of the intervention. The key features of FCP are listed below.

1. Two 'experimental' cities were to receive the health education interventions. These cities are, unlike the original three centres, quite socially complex and larger. The whole city would receive health education and this would consist of a wide range of broadcast media, print media, self-help booklets and the like.

   The community organization would involve a number of community groups and organizations and the range of settings described earlier in this chapter. Opinion leaders would be employed to act as health educators alongside more traditional and formal sources. Environmental change would be attempted; for instance, restaurants and shops would be encouraged to provide heart healthy products.
2. It was intended that FCP would run for nine years.
3. Three moderate sized cities would be used as controls; total population size would be 350 000. A wider age range would be used in surveys (ages 12–74) and repeated samples would be used to monitor programme effects. Annual rates of fatal and non-fatal cardiovascular events would be recorded.

The effects of the programme were discussed by Farquhar *et al.* in 1990. The results may be summarized as follows.

1. Knowledge of CVD risk factors increased steadily during the programme but the improvement in the 'treatment' group was significantly greater at all follow-up points.
2. Net reductions (i.e. control minus experimental groups) in cholesterol were recorded (though not substantial); average net decrease was some 2%. Net reductions of some 4% were also recorded for blood pressure.
3. A progressive reduction in smoking occurred throughout the study period, 'with declines in treatment cities always exceeding those in control cities by about 13%'.
4. Weight gain occurred in all surveys but was typically greater in control towns. However, net decrease in resting pulse rate was greater in treatment groups in most instances.
5. In the words of the authors, 'These risk factor changes resulted in important decreases in composite total mortality risk scores (15%) and coronary heart disease risk scores (16%). Thus, such low-cost programs can have an impact on risk factors in broad population groups' (p. 359).

THE MINNESOTA HEART HEALTH PROGRAM

The major difference between the Minnesota Heart Health Program (MHHP) and the SHDPP is the community organization aspect and the ways in which a wide variety of agencies and lay people are orchestrated to achieve project goals. Clearly its medical goals are identical with SHDPP and it thus represents a prime example of what we will later call a Type 4 community programme. The goals of the project are succinctly stated by Jacobs *et al.* (1985). It is interesting to observe how these have taken account of the general downward trend in cardiovascular disease (CVD) risk in their reference to accelerating the change process.

Major MHHP hypotheses are that a systematic and multiple strategy community-wide health education program is feasible and will lead to a change in the way people think about heart disease and its prevention; in behaviours related to risk for heart disease; in physiologic risk factors; and ultimately in disease rates. Some of these changes are occurring naturally. The MHHP aims to accelerate this change, and hypothesizes that an intensive education program of five years duration in a community will initiate risk factor changes leading to decreased disease rates. A further MHHP hypothesis is that the program will be taken over by the community after the researchers leave.

Three pairs of education and reference/control communities have been chosen for study and were enrolled in a phased manner (to enhance evaluation power as indicated earlier). The communities are matched and represent three different types: Mankato paired with Winona represented small free-standing towns; Fargo, North Dakota, paired with Sioux Falls, South Dakota, represented large free-standing cities; Bloomington paired with Roseville, Maplewood and North St. Paul represented large suburban areas.

The comprehensive education programme involves three major thrusts: mass media, direct education and community organization. Education is delivered through health education centres, by means of short courses, lectures, workshops and seminars and, of course, via school programmes. Target groups are community organizations and community leaders, youth, adults and health professionals. An over-riding aim is to ensure there is at least one direct contact with the majority of individuals within the community (Blackburn, 1983).

The intensity of the programme may be judged from an account of the health centre operation. This contact is designed to provide screening and 'exposure to educational and motivational messages'. It involves an audio-visual presentation for the family group to introduce them to the programme; the family rotates through various screening stations and receives further audio-visual inputs about risk factors; their physical activity level is ascertained at an interactive computer station; finally they receive a whole family counselling session.

The nature of the schools programme is well illustrated by articles by Perry *et al.* which describe a 'needs assessment' of young people's nutrition and exercise status (1985a) and the development of a 20-session heart healthy nutrition education curriculum for third and fourth grade students (1985b).

The model of community organization is described by Carlaw *et al.* (1984). It is defined as a partnership between community and the MHHP development team, and the WHO's (1983) reference to participation is cited by way of philosophical justification:

> Participation – or more correctly involvement – is a process in which individuals and communities identify with a movement and take responsibility jointly with health professionals and others concerned, for making decisions and planning and carrying out activities.

The procedures described are somewhat different from the classic grassroots bottom-up approach in, for example, disadvantaged inner city communities. The first step involves 'community analysis' by the team which consists of identifying geographical and interest sector representatives to serve on heart health boards and provision of training. It is followed by the establishment of 'task forces' which identify strategies and seek to influence their communities. Ideally this leads to the third stage, development of 'social system support' which includes skill development sessions in churches, school districts, trade unions, health clubs, etc. This hopefully leads to a 'strengthening of community norms and values'. The final stage should result in 'organizational commitment to an improved social environment' and lead to a shift in the balance of power from the initiating researchers to the community itself. However, the impression created is that the main focus is on institutions and community leaders rather than the 'hard-to-reach' targets of traditional locality development initiatives. For instance, as part of the process of 'organizational commitment', i.e. what has been described above as the final stage in the programme, the main target group consists of employers and managers who are asked to take responsibility for the provision of gentle coercion to lead the population to a healthier lifestyle. Those in authority are asked to encourage and reinforce '... consistent heart healthy behaviour through financial and other incentive systems' and 'insurance companies, banks and related organizations providing favourable rates for heart healthy families and individuals'. These last quotes point up one further way in which MHHP differs from Stanford: it incorporates many of the 'healthy public policy' aspects of health promotion. As Carlaw *et al.* (1984) state:

> A second aspect of Phase I was the development, in the community, of the opportunities to practice healthful behavior. In practical terms this translated into choices available to the consumer through services such as grocery store labelling, indexing of heart healthy menus in restaurants, improved smoking cessation services and attractive opportunities for physical activity for all age groups. Food packaging and food preparation are directed by marketing factors having little or no relationship to the health of the consumer. Considerable community initiative is needed to modify these services so that heart healthy behavior is encouraged.

Programme evaluation incorporated a wide range of measures. It is interesting to note that although the possibility existed of random allocation of communities to experi-mental or reference situations, this tactic was deliberately rejected since the small number of units involved could not guarantee equality: matching was therefore a superior strategy. Intermediate and outcome measures comprised '... *net* changes in awareness, participation, cognitions, behaviours, risk factors and disease endpoints' (Jacobs *et al.*, 1985). Process measures included 'linkage' between education components and behaviour change and 'coincidence' of community change with the staged entry of different communities to the programme.

The MHHP provides a nice illustration of three broad categories of measure representing final outcomes, intermediate indicators and indirect indicators. The final outcomes include the disease endpoints: mortality and morbidity data on CHD and cerebrovascular accident (CVA). The intermediate indicators include risk factor measures of blood pressure, smoking, total serum cholesterol and high-density lipoprotein (HDL) level together with associated behaviours relating to blood pressure control, smoking cessation, physical activity in leisure time and diet. More indirect cognitive and attitudinal measures which are related to these variables are also measured.

Jacobs *et al.* (1985) provide an excellent example of indicators occurring at an early stage on the proximal-distal/input-output chain in their 14-point list of ways in which the community might participate in the programme. These are listed in Table 8.1. The MHHP also provides a very apposite illustration of the way in which it is possible to utilize true experimental design in community studies. These do of course fall within the broader quasiexperimental framework. As Jacobs *et al.* point out, although '... it is not possible to randomly withhold from some persons television campaigns, a community walk, or a grocery store labelling program...', it is possible '... to randomly delay invitation to the MHHP Heart and Health Centre to a random group of persons'. Such

Table 8.1 Intermediate indicators of programme participation: Minnesota Heart Health Program (MHHP)

---

1. General awareness of the existence of the programme and/or its goals
2. CHD risk factor screening in the MHHP Heart Health Center
3. Exposure to general MHHP messages in the media
4. Exposure to specific MHHP messages in the media (such as television programme or a pamphlet or book)
5. Participation in the Shape-Up Challenge (a worksite physical activity programme)
6. Recognition/use of the restaurant menu labelling programme
7. Recognition/use of the grocery store labelling programme
8. Doing homework with children who participate in an MHHP school programme
9. Contact with a health professional whose practice has been influenced by MHHP
10. 'Quit and Win' smoking classes and contest
11. Participation on an MHHP task force
12. Participation in other MHHP sponsored classes
13. Social contact with the precepts and ideas of MHHP
14. Speaking at or hearing a speaker at a club or organization meeting

---

subexperiments serve to test and improve specific methods and interventions.

Process measures/formative evaluation include telephone surveys to check on particular education programmes and the use of focus groups to evaluate media messages. Blake *et al.* (1987) also describe in full detail a process evaluation of a physical activity campaign which illustrates the value of such research for programme refinement. They considered community awareness of and participation in five specific kinds of exercise opportunity using telephone surveys and observation of participation. These indicated, *inter alia*, that participation was highest for activities organized within existing organizations but awareness was highest for heavily publicized general population events.

Final evaluation results obviously await the conclusion of the programme but several encouraging indications have already been noted. For instance, Mittelmark *et al.* (1986) reported that initial objectives had been achieved. After two years, 190 community leaders were directly involved as programme volunteers; 14 103 residents (60% of adults) had attended a screening education centre; 2094 had attended health education classes;

distribution of printed media averaged 12.2 pieces per household.

One of the salient features of MHHP was the provision of medical education and training for doctors and other health professionals who would act as role models and active educators. After two years, 42 of the 65 physicians in Mankato and 728 other health professionals had participated in continuing education programmes offered by MHHP.

As regards young people's programmes, all third, fifth, sixth and eleventh grade students were involved in the MHHP heart health education teaching, and 1665 young people visited the heart health centre with their parents.

Population surveys also revealed higher levels of awareness of the various heart related risk behaviours in Mankato compared with the reference community. A telephone evaluation revealed that about one sixth of smokers watched at least one segment of a local television's five day series of cessation hints and 1% stopped smoking. A smoking cessation short course called 'Quit and Win' resulted in 5% of all smokers in the community committing themselves to give up smoking. Over 50% of those who signed up stopped for one month and 34% had not relapsed after two months (Schwartz, 1987).

Reference was made above to the inclusion of true experiments within the overall framework. One of these (Murray *et al.*, 1985) compared the level of risk of an experimental group who had received the personalized risk factor screening programme with a control group. After one year, the former group had significantly lower risk factor scores in respect of: blood cholesterol, diastolic blood pressure, reduced fat and salt consumption and increased regular exercise.

In short, Minnesota's multi-intervention community programme appears to be having a substantial impact.

THE PENNSYLVANIA COUNTY HEALTH IMPROVEMENT PROGRAM (CHIP)

This community-wide programme laid claim to developing 'a new form of social organization: the mobilization of an entire community to improve its health' (Stunkard, Felix and Cohen, 1985). Its goal was to reduce mortality and morbidity from CVD in Lycoming County, Pennsylvania. It was clearly influenced by the other CHD projects discussed in this section but allegedly differed from these in the following ways: it had considerably less than 20% of the funding of the other programmes and, as a consequence, had to utilize existing resources and facilities; it involved community participation from the outset and was designed to be owned by the community. Costs were kept as low as possible to facilitate replication.

Details of the history and planning process of CHIP may be consulted elsewhere (Stunkard, Felix and Cohen, 1985) as may details of the process of 'coalition building' which is not dissimilar to the strategies described earlier in this chapter. CHIP planners decided to operate via five 'channels'. Two of these were categorized as 'diffuse', viz. mass media and voluntary organizations, while three were 'focused': work sites, health organizations and schools.

Rather more detail will be supplied about the planning process involved in developing the workplace programme, given its relevance to Chapter 7. Fourteen steps were involved and these are listed below:

1. Introduction of programme to management including personal presentation;
2. Announcement of the programme to the employees (by company newsletter or personal letter to employees' homes);
3. Recruitment and organization of a 'Heart Health Committee' (including a broad cross-section of workers and management);
4. In-house communication planning (by newly created CHIP newsletters);
5. Employee interest and risk factor surveys;
6. Formation of risk factor subcommittees (smoking; hypertension; cholesterol; obesity; physical inactivity);
7. Exploration of communication risk factor reduction programmes (examining existing resources and assessing costs and effectiveness of various programmes);
8. Committee review and programme selection;
9. Development of a programme proposal;
10. Discussion of proposal with management (e.g. negotiation of release from work and possible financial contribution);
11. Promotion of programmes and recruitment of employees;
12. Scheduling of programmes;
13. Programme implementation;
14. Evaluation and feedback.

The evaluation of the whole CHIP programme was designed as far as possible to be compatible with the other CHD programmes discussed in this section. Whilst acknowledging the difficulties of conducting 'proper' trials, attempts were made to provide a degree of comparison by selecting Franklin County as a reference area. The major indices of effectiveness would, therefore, consist of

Table 8.2 Impact of CHIP Programme on Resource Provision (from Stunkard *et al.*, 1985)

	1980	1983
Lycoming County		
Organizations with blood pressure screening	29	52
Organizations with more extensive programmes	21	50
Total organizations with health promotion programmes	66	68
Total organizations in county	157	154
Reference county		
Organizations with blood pressure screening	29	22
Organizations with more extensive programmes	12	13
Total organizations with health promotion programmes	56	32
Total organizations in county	142	126

comparing changes in these two counties in respect of mortality, morbidity, risk factor reduction, 'community resource inventory' and cost effectiveness.

The nature of the first three measures is self-evident but the community resource inventory may need a little further explanation. Essentially its purpose is to compare changes in activity level of nine different institutions in the study area with those in the control area. It thus provides 'indirect indicators' of effectiveness. Table 8.2 describes the extent of these differences in study and control areas after three years of the programme.

Taking account of the discussion of economic indicators and cost effectiveness in Chapter 3, it is interesting to note the researcher's calculation of the likely benefit of an effective programme. The costs of CHIP were calculated at $150 000 per year. The direct and indirect costs of cardiovascular disease, on the other hand, were estimated as $33.04 million. A reduction of 10% (half that achieved in Karelia according to Stunkard *et al.*) would therefore result in savings of $3.3 million.

Additional evidence of programme effectiveness again centred on indirect indicators. For instance, the media output related to hypertension control was reported as shown in Table 8.3. Again, in relation to the evaluation of effort, 58 health promotion programmes were established in 12 different workplaces (employing more than 3800 people). On the other hand the results of two programmes of weight control in banks and retail stores provided intermediate indicators of effectiveness. Of 172 storeworkers, 34% dropped out of the programme but the remainder lost on average 7.3 lbs. There were virtually no dropouts from the banks and the average weight loss of participants in that setting was 13 lbs.

Moreover, in the context of workplace health promotion, the authors reported a decline in the proportion of people with markedly high blood pressure: a fall in workers with diastolic pressure of over 120 m.m. from 7.5% in 1981 to 4% in 1982.

Table 8.3 Media Output in One Month: CHIP Programme (from Stunkard *et al.*, 1985)

Media	Messages	Exposures
Radio	900	113 000
Television	23	45 000
Newspapers	4.5	110 000
Billboards	5.0	470 000
Pamphlet holders	190	
Pamphlets	16 500	33 000

THE PAWTUCKET HEART HEALTH PROGRAM

The special interest of the Pawtucket Heart Health Program (PHHP) in the present context is its approach to community organization and the theoretical rationale which underpins this approach. In short, this project seeks to get closer to the grassroots.

The PHHP study community is located in Rhode Island, New England. Its residents are described as predominantly blue collar. The city of Pawtucket has some 72 000 inhabitants and the population is described as very stable. For evaluation purposes it is matched with a control community of some 98 000 people. The project was planned to run from 1980 to 1991; professional guidance was provided for the first four years and thereafter the management was in the hands of a community volunteer system.

The observations made below are derived from reports by Lefebvre *et al.* (1987) and Elder *et al.* (1986). The authors, in discussing the community-level approach of PHHP, make a distinction between locality development and social planning, as discussed earlier in this chapter. Their definition of the former makes reference to the involvement of the people in goal determination and action, democratic procedures, training of indigenous leaders and educational self-help methods. Social planning is seen as an alternative view of community organization in which social change is planned by designated experts. 'Citizens are seen as being passive recipients of services ... the practitioner role of "expert" in social planning strategies contrasts markedly with the "enabler" posture of locality developers' (Lefebvre *et al.*, 1987). The PHHP is, in practice, considered to offer a blend of both of these theoretically discrete approaches together with Rothman's (1979) model of social action in which experts 'seek to organize coalitions of concerned interests to attack the problem'. Within the framework of PHHP Lefebvre *et al.* see these social action tactics as involving:

... campaign tactics; employment of facts; and persuasion within the context of voluntary association, mass media, and legislative bodies to change institutional and community policies and norms ... citizens can be either recipients or agents of action, while the practitioner role is defined more as that of a coalition builder, fact gatherer, and policy analyst.

The researchers consider that PHHP's use of churches as heart health delivery systems illustrates this social action approach within Pawtucket.

Elder *et al.* identify four principles operating within the general approach. These are:

1. the importance of local ownership;
2. the use of inexpensive resources and facilities (to make community ownership more feasible after external funding has ceased);
3. the importance of interpersonal education – with media being used as awareness-raising devices;
4. the use of multilevel programming, i.e. reciprocal contributions of community, organizational, small group and individual programmes.

Elder *et al.* also record the change in emphasis during the first 26 months of PHHP from organizations to community. During the first 11 months the focus was on worksites, churches, schools and other organizations. Progress, however, was slow and this produced a strategic shift after 11 months when an attempt was made to accelerate progress by directing the programme to the community at large in association with media publicity. By the end of this stage perhaps the most singular feature of PHHP had emerged – the 'volunteer delivery system'. Lefebvre *et al.* have argued that there are at least eight reasons for using volunteers in preventive heart health programmes: they serve as peer models (cf. the principle of homophily); they provide a support network for others who have made changes in lifestyle; their own healthy behaviour is reinforced; they promote diffusion through social networks; effective volunteers can be deliberately 'networked' to help change norms; a volunteer system helps promote community ownership; it is cost effective; it has a multiplier effect.

The goals of PHHP are similar to those of the other major cardiovascular disease prevention programmes and they are similarly 'theory-driven'. Lefebvre *et al.* summarize this aspect of the project as an 'intervention cube' where the risk factor and disease endpoints of fitness, weight reduction, fat and cholesterol control, management of blood pressure and reduction of smoking are to be attained via four programme phases. These latter involve motivating the community; providing skills training for risk factor reduction; developing support networks and finally ensuring the maintenance of ensuing change. The programmes are seen as having an impact at four levels: the individual, group, organization and the community at large.

Evaluation results to date are largely concerned with process. The general situation (Lefebvre *et al.*, 1987) is described thus:

> Children are involved in Heart Health Clubs, smoking prevention programs, and classroom heart health education;
> Parents learn to raise heart healthy children;
> People shop at grocery stores where shelf labels identify foods low in salt, fat, and calories, and eat in Four-Heart restaurants offering good-tasting menu items that are low in fat, sodium, and cholesterol;
> Senior citizens are active in Walk Jog Clubs and exercise programs;
> All residents attend community events such as Octoberfest or 'Meet us in the Park' weekends where the PHHP Heart Check trailer and van are prominently located.

Fourteen Pawtucket companies sent 23 coordinators to training sessions; 3604 of 5700 eligible employees were screened.

Twenty-one churches have been involved in social action and devoted some 2105 volunteer hours.

Trained volunteers have been accepted by both the lay community and the medical professionals. Between 600 and 1000 blood pressure readings are taken monthly at 14 Walk-In Blood Pressure Stations. In its first three years more than 30 000 hours have been invested by volunteers in the programme and the PHHP has had over 30 000 contacts with people seeking to improve their heart health.

It is, of course, too soon to look for the impact of these activities on disease endpoints. Some intermediate outcome measures have, however, been recorded. For instance, people participating in the worksite screening programme succeeded in reducing their blood pressure: prevalence of readings greater than 180/100 dropped from 34 out of 409 screened to zero.

Again, after a 'community weigh-in', 138 residents recorded a joint loss of 1061 lbs after ten weeks. Six months later, a follow-up interview of 70% of the 211 original participants revealed that 80% had lost weight and 75% were continuing to do so.

In conclusion, we can reasonably say that the PHHP has again demonstrated that a community-wide programme can achieve substantial changes. In the case of PHHP the suggestion has been made that by using a more informal community effort centring on lay workers and volunteers, changes can be produced in a lower socioeconomic status community. The methods used, however, still fall short of the 'true' community development approaches.

Whether these strategies would be effective within deprived and underprivileged inner city ghettos must remain a matter of conjecture. Again, whether the same degree of success would be achieved in a national context where healthist norms are less evident must also be a matter for speculation. Two important questions would, therefore still seem to require answers. First, whether the undoubtedly successful North American experience will generalize to disadvantaged neighbourhoods and to different national populations where health has a lower profile. Second, the question which sceptical clinicians and epidemiologists are constantly posing: will the lifestyle changes recorded by the CVD prevention projects result in a demonstrable decline in mortality and morbidity which can unequivocally be attributed to the health promotion? The final example, that of the North Karelia Project, demonstrates clear success in fostering lifestyle change in a European setting. It has also claimed to have an impact on mortality and morbidity but not without challenge!

THE NORTH KARELIA PROJECT

One of the principal features of the North Karelia Project (NKP) is its community focus and the circumstances which led to the establishment of the project are of particular significance. Indeed one of the most noteworthy features of NKP was the frequently cited popular petition to the Finnish government to deal with the problem of premature death from coronary heart disease (CHD) which had apparently forced itself on the consciousness of the population. In fact, following the Seven Countries Study of CHD mortality (WHO Collaborative Group, 1970), it became apparent that Eastern Finland held the unenviable record of heading the league table of deaths. However, it apparently took three public reports before community leaders – at the end of the 1960s – began to demand action. This coincided with Karvonen, who was leading the Finnish investigation, having a WHO advisory role and being president of the Finnish Medical Association. It is also reported that the awareness-raising effect of epidemiological data was vigorously supplemented by lobbying by the Finnish Heart Association and its volunteer task force. These somewhat serendipitous circumstances are of importance because it would be wrong to assume that the NKP was the result

of some popular upsurge of opinion. Indeed if the petition to government by community leaders had been a fundamentally grassroots eruption, the generalizability of NKP to other European countries would have been in considerable doubt. On the other hand it would be wrong to ignore the importance of community awareness: the personal exposure of community members to CHD deaths in friends and relations doubtless concentrates the mind and creates a level of perceived susceptibility which the health belief model requires as an antecedent to preventive action.

At all events the petition which was signed on 12 January 1971 by the governor, all members of parliament and representatives of official and voluntary bodies signalled the start of a ten year programme which has continued to have repercussions and has influenced the development of health promotion nationally and internationally. Again, somewhat fortuitously, the start of the project was accompanied by the establishment of a medical school at the University of Kuopio and a new public health Act which reorganized primary health care. The World Health Organization provided its support and documented the first stages of the project (WHO, 1981) and the thinking underlying the Stanford Project was incorporated.

A full description of the NKP is beyond the scope of this book. Suffice to say that its theoretical foundation – the learning theory principles – was similar to the projects discussed above and included social learning theory; communication and attitude theory; communication of innovations theory; and community organization principles. It is, however, worth noting one particular point of emphasis which distinguishes the NKP from the North American schemes and which, perhaps, reflects the different political climates of those countries. Unlike the American projects there is a more overt concern with the socioeconomic and physical environment and its effect on the individual's health choices. This is seen in item six (Puska *et al.*, 1985) in the '... seven key steps to help individuals to modify their behaviour':

1. Improved preventive services to help people to identify their risk factors and to provide appropriate attention and services.
2. Information to educate people about the relationship between behaviours and their health.
3. Persuasion to motivate people and to promote the intentions to adopt the healthy action.
4. Training to increase the skills of self-management, environmental control, and necessary action.
5. Social support to help people to maintain the initial action.
6. Environmental change to create the opportunities for healthy actions and improve unfavourable conditions.
7. Community organization to mobilize the community for broad-ranged changes (through increased social support and environmental modification) to support the adoption of the new lifestyles in the community.

The organization of the NKP was truly community-wide involving the national health service – and especially the new primary health care centres and the public health nurses – together with mass media, doctors, social workers, business leaders, voluntary organizations, administrators, trade unions, sports organizations and local political leaders. A special school and youth programme was developed (Vartiainen *et al.*, 1983) and in addition to the kinds of environmental change mentioned in, for example, the MHHP, local industry was prevailed upon to make available low-fat dairy products and a new sausage product. This latter move was apparently helped by the fact that two managers had recently experienced heart attacks (McAlister *et al.*, 1982)! Only one aspect of the many interventions described above will receive further comment: the use of voluntary groups and lay leaders.

From the start the NKP sought to gain community involvement. As with the PHHP, it utilized volunteers extensively. Local 'lay leaders' were identified by informally interviewing shopkeepers and other knowledgeable people in the community. These opinion leaders were then trained to act as models and educators. Over a four year period more than 1000 of 'the most influential members of the local communities were involved ...'. The work of these lay opinion leaders was extensively documented (Neittaanmaki *et al.*, 1980; Puska *et al.*, 1986) in the general context of diffusion theory. Measures were obtained of: participation in training; perception of relative ease of discussing the various risk factors with people; attitude to these changes; extent to which these leaders had discussed risk factors with three or more people during the preceding week; different modes of action taken (e.g. direct requests to change behaviour, provision of advice, reference to own example, etc.); frequency of discussion with different target groups; frequency of contact with health centre; perception of their effectiveness in influencing smoking, dietary behaviours and hypertension problems; involvement in the project's television programmes and involvement in general health education. The picture emerging from this evaluation is one of considerable activity with evidence of genuine influence.

In addition to the lay leader tactics, the involvement of the MARTTA Organization proved successful. This voluntary local housewives' association introduced, *inter alia*, 'Parties for a Long Life' in which women were taught how to cook heart-healthy meals and as a result of the experience came to believe that healthy cooking could be tasty! Three hundred and forty four of these sessions were recorded with 15 000 participants. At the 1976 follow-up, 9% of men and 18% of women in Karelia had been involved at least once (McAlister *et al.*, 1982).

Final observations on the NKP will be concerned with outcome measures. Before considering the customary risk factors it is worth noting an interesting finding on CHD related knowledge (Puska *et al.*, 1981). Repeated tests of total CHD health knowledge during the early phase of the NKP revealed only minimal changes (admittedly from a relatively high starting point). The net change in North Karelia (NK score minus the reference area score) was 4% for men and 2% for women. The researchers comment on interventions which have produced knowledge change but no behaviour change and others which, like SHDPP, recorded an increase in knowledge and a reduction in risk. They rightfully remark on the dubious relationship between knowledge and behaviour change by comparing the minimal shift in knowledge in North Karelia with the 17% and 12% respective decrease in risk factor levels during the same period.

In relation to behaviour change, changes in self-reported dietary behaviours were recorded which indicated a decline in fat consumption. The influence of the programme on smoking was also extensively analysed (Koskela, 1981). Puska *et al.* (1985) report a net change in North Karelia of 28% in amount of reported daily smoking by men and 14% for women over the period 1972–82. Elsewhere, in a comparative report of the results of various community projects (Schwartz, 1987), the decline in male smokers in North Karelia is recorded as a shift from 44% to 31% compared with 39% to 35% in the rest of the country. By the fifth year, the net percentage decline in prevalence was 2.5% for men and 6.1% for women (bearing in mind that a general decline was also occurring in the reference area and in the country as a whole).

With regard to risk factors generally, a decline was noted in mean serum cholesterol. This decline occurred in both the study and the reference areas but was greater in North Karelia. The net decline was 3% in men and 1% in women for the period 1972–1982. Again, a significant net decline in both systolic and diastolic blood pressure was observed in the experimental area. The net change between 1972 and 1982 was 3% in systolic blood pressure (SBP) and 1% diastolic blood pressure (DBP) for men and 5% and 2% respectively for women. As with other measures an overall decline was also occurring in the reference county and the net decline was greater during the first five years of the programme, suggesting a general diffusion effect.

The NKP also evaluated its programme in terms of late primary and secondary prevention. For instance, Salonen *et al.* (undated) state that a higher proportion of men recovering from heart attacks in North Karelia did not resume smoking compared with a similar sample from the reference area. McAlister *et al.* (1982) noted an increase in the proportion of hypertensives receiving medication from a level of 13% in both Karelia and the reference area to 45% in the study area and 33% in the reference county. The proportion of hypertensives was also alleged to be lower in the intervention area.

Before reporting on disease endpoint measures, we should consider an outcome measure which did not figure in the North American CHD prevention projects described above and which serves to illustrate the comprehensiveness and thoroughness of the NKP. The survey questionnaires included questions which attempted to assess the psychosocial consequences of the programme. In addition to items checking perceptions of health status, questions were also asked about stress, psychosomatic symptoms and the like with a view to checking the possibility that the interventions might have generated hypochondria or other negative side effects. There was in fact no evidence of this and a statistically significant shift for both men and women in the direction of improved subjective health status was reported. The increase was greater in North Karelia than in the reference area while a greater decline in the 20-variable survey of 'complaints' about stress, etc. was noted in the experimental area. It seems then that subjective well-being was enhanced without creating negative effects, all of which was taken to indicate a greater degree of satisfaction with health enhancement in the intervention county.

MORTALITY AND MORBIDITY: THE LAST FRONTIER?

The North Karelia Project, along with the other interventions discussed in this chapter, has demonstrated unequivocally that it is possible to mobilize community resources, both professional and lay, and generate changes in knowledge, beliefs and attitudes. Skills can be provided and lifestyle can be influenced such that the risk of premature death and morbidity from contemporary diseases can be reduced. And yet the most important question remains to be answered. Is it possible to demonstrate that the changes wrought in a community like North Karelia will actually reduce the numbers of deaths and the amount of illness caused by the factors which the programme is designed to prevent? The NKP certainly has something to say on the matter and, as the longest running project which has recorded mortality and morbidity events, it would seem to be in a good position to comment. Unfortunately the issue remains clouded, a situation which is due to the quasi-experimental status of the intervention and the fact that a general decline in CVD is occurring in the country as a whole.

It has been quite clear that there has been a decline in mortality from CHD in Finland as a whole and, as Salonen *et al.* (1983) have shown, the decline in North Karelia was greater still. This reduction, between 1969 and 1979, was 24% in men and 51% in women compared with a decline of 12% and 24% respectively in other counties of Finland. McAlister *et al.*, writing in 1982, commented on the implications of this relative reduction when they observed that there had been a comparable reduction in cardiovascular dis-

ease pension payments in North Karelia. As they put it, 'Estimates from pension disability data already suggest that payment of over $4 million dollars in disability payments may have been avoided by the less than $1 million expended on the project's intervention activities.'

Tuomilehto *et al.* (1986) described the mortality trends in Finland from 1969 to 1982. They remarked that the annual decline in CHD mortality in men was 2.9% in Karelia whereas in the rest of Finland it was 2.0%. For women the respective annual declines were 4.9% and 3.0%. The net decline in North Karelia was 100 deaths per 100 000 men. On the face of it it seems reasonable to ascribe the substantial progress in North Karelia to the NKP. Indeed, Tuomilehto *et al.* were moved to comment 'As we cannot think of any reason for the greater decline of mortality from ischaemic heart disease in North Karelia other than the prevention programme it is reasonable to argue that it was a consequence of the project.' Others, however, could think of alternative explanations and Salonen in 1987, one of the principal investigators, felt obliged to produce a disclaimer which acknowledged four potential sources of bias ranging from differential rates of decline in different regions of Finland to the possible effect of general unspecified changes in Finnish society.

Needless to say, this retraction was greeted with barely disguised pleasure by more conservative clinicians (Oliver, 1987) who could not see the logic of changing risk factors unless they have an aetiological role in disease reduction. However, in the last analysis – and given the undesirability/impracticability of using randomized controlled trials for community studies – the implementation of such programmes involves an act of faith. The act of faith is however based on a mass of supportive if not conclusive evidence, not least of which is the Oslo study (Holme *et al.*, 1985) which was a randomized controlled trial and demonstrated a 47% reduction in incidence of the first major CHD event after health education about diet and smoking in a group of 1232 high risk middle-aged men. Perhaps the single most important piece of advice which could be offered to those seeking to measure the success of health education programmes is to avoid 'premature evaluation', i.e. taking the risk of measuring educational success by using clinical outcome measures when the links between educational outcomes and disease endpoints are by no means clearcut.

The project 15 years on

The debate about whether or not the North Karelia Project has produced more substantial and directly attributable effects in the 'treatment' area than in the reference area – or indeed than in Finland as a whole – is in the last analysis a matter of mainly academic interest. As Pietinen *et al.* (1989) commented:

> The original idea to have a reference area for the comparison of trends in risk factor levels and mortality rates has now lost much of its original meaning and importance because the development in all parts of the country quickly became almost identical.
>
> *(pp. 1022–3)*

It is, in fact, probably not worth the effort of trying to produce a replica of the randomized controlled trial in community programmes – a point which will be made somewhat more forcibly in the next section in this chapter. Apart from the ethical issue and the problems of different baselines and time scales which Salonen (1987) was obliged to address, it is remarkably difficult to prevent 'leakage' from one area to another. Indeed, the knock-on effect of a successful community or regional project should be considered as a definite indicator of success and such an effect has been clearly shown in Finland.

In 1989, Puska *et al.* reflected on the project 15 years after its launch. They noted the level of risk factors in North Karelia, Kuopio (the reference county) and south west Finland between 1972 and 1987. The smoking rates in North Karelia were lower than elsewhere although the serum cholesterol and blood pressure levels were still high (and higher than in south west Finland). An analysis of mortality trends showed an initial steep decline in North Karelia (in the 1970s) but slowing down in the 1980s. By the mid-1980s the decline in Finland as a whole had reached that of North Karelia. However, a bigger decline seemed to have occurred in North Karelia between 1974 and 1978. Moreover, during the nine years from 1974 to 1983, a significant decline in cancer mortality was observed in North Karelia, considerably more than the reference area and more substantial than the rest of Finland.

These observations reveal the difficulties (mentioned earlier in this book) of assessing the effectiveness of health promotion by means of mortality and morbidity data. They also remind us of the truism incorporated in communication of innovations theory: it can take a long time before the large majority of the community adopts health innovations!

Interestingly, Puska *et al.* demonstrate the continuing rise in reported levels of subjectively perceived health status. In all areas there was an increase in the percentage of the population rating subjective health as 'very good' or 'good'. The increase varied between men and women (with women reporting higher levels). Between 1972 and 1987 the average increase was from around 33% to 46% for men and from 32% to 51% for women. Puska *et al.* rightly argue that the programme as a whole should be considered a success.

Throughout the 15 year period the feasibility of the programme has been good. This has been so despite the fact that – at least in the early years – health service resources were scarce, society's traditional norms militated against change and the diffusion of innovations in lifestyle. Local health services and their staff have co-operated well, thus forming the back bone for the activities. The local population has readily participated in the activities and various community organizations have contributed in various ways to the aims of the project in the area. Because the project aims were integrated with the existing health services and broad community participation was a key feature, the overall costs of the programme have been modest.

A major task in North Karelia was how to influence people's health related lifestyles. This is not easy. Even when the hazards of unhealthy habits are well known, many intervention activities meet with limited or no success. The results and experiences presented here indicate major changes and show that, at least in favourable conditions, comprehensive, determined and well planned action can lead to substantial favourable changes.

(p. 172)

Similar observations might well be addressed to other community ventures involving attempts to introduce often problematical changes into individual behaviours and community practices.

Reflection on the variety of community-based projects discussed here has revealed a considerable consensus on organization, methods and evaluation. What is much less clear is the extent of ideological consensus. In particular, many researchers and programme planners endorse community participation, even if this is occasionally somewhat formulaic. We described earlier programmes which are built on the principle of participation, which emphasize the need to work from people's felt needs and which urge community workers first of all to address issues of inequality and imbalance of resources between the 'haves' and 'have nots'. Clearly there will be some sort of divide between programmes of this sort and those which

have been rather scathingly defined in terms of 'colonization'. By definition, of course, the various projects we have just described cannot be considered as 'pure' community development since they have a 'top-down' disease prevention agenda – even if health workers try to operate in a 'bottom-up' way. Even so, many if not all of these programmes have demonstrated considerable concern to achieve community ownership of the project. Obviously this concern may stem from ideological conviction or, alternatively, the recognition that the preventive goals of the programme are more likely to be achieved if maximal community participation can be achieved.

We will now return to the subject of community development and give some further consideration to these matters. We will, in doing so, suggest that a neat division into 'politically correct' CD versus ethically dubious colonization cannot easily be made in practice. We will also consider some of the more problematic features of CD and the question of evaluation.

PARTICIPATION, EMPOWERMENT AND COMMUNITY DEVELOPMENT

We will open this section of the chapter by recalling WHO's manifesto for primary health care and health promotion. At its heart is the ultimate goal of a socially and economically productive life which is to be achieved through the creation of the active, fully participating community. This too is the holy grail of community development.

Before further exploring CD, we should clarify a few points. First, empowerment is not synonymous with participation despite their constant and reiterated association. As we noted in Chapter 1, an empowered person is more likely to engage in active community participation than someone who is helplessly apathetic. On the other hand, participation may contribute to empowerment. Self-empowerment, as we have seen, has to do with beliefs about control and the possession efficacy-creating competences which contribute to the acquisition of power, i.e. a degree of control over environmental circumstances and other people. Again in Chapter 1 we distinguished self-empowerment from community empowerment. Although in an important sense an empowered community may be said to be the sum of the self-empowered individuals it contains, there are those who view empowered communities as rather more than that, though this distinction is probably a matter of definition.

A second assertion should be made at this point: empowerment and community participation (CP) may be conceived as goals in their own right or as having an instrumental function. The WHO philosophy seems to include both of these. The instrumental function is evident in more recent definitions of health, i.e. empowerment and health are means to the end of achieving a socially and economically productive life. More precisely, an empowered participating community is not only necessary to galvanize individuals into looking after themselves but is also a prerequisite for achieving equity and remedying inequalities which are, in turn, the single most important barrier to achieving health goals. At the same time, WHO retains its fondness for its earlier broad definition of health as some positive state (not merely the absence of disease) having mental and social dimensions as well as physical attributes. Empowerment and its component parts provide as good an example as any (and better than most) of well-being or positive health, especially in the mental and social domains.

Fortunately for those whose employment obliges them to address their energies to the prevention of disease, it is possible to have the best of both worlds since, as indicated earlier, the achievement of preventive goals is best achieved through empowerment.

In Chapter 1 we noted that it is possible to produce a typology of individual control ranging from a kind of cursory and token consultation to the possession of real power.

DEGREES OF ACTUAL POWER	Control
	Delegated power
	Partnership
DEGREES OF TOKENISM	Placation
	Consultation
	Informing
NON-PARTICIPATION	Therapy
	Manipulation

Figure 8.2 Arnstein's ladder of participation (Arnstein, 1971).

In the same way we can define degrees of community participation. Arnstein (1971) makes this point in the form of an oft-quoted 'ladder of participation' which is reproduced in Figure 8.2.

Maximal participation is located at the top of the ladder – the community has some degree of genuine control; at the bottom we have zero participation – complete manipulation. At the mid point there are various degrees of tokenism. We are reminded of the Paris students' declension of the verb 'to participate' during the period of unrest: 'I participate, you participate, they profit'!

Brager and Specht (1973) devised an equally well known scheme to describe this 'spectrum of participation' which is shown in Figure 8.3.

This particular scheme has the additional advantage of providing an illustration of typical interactions between a community and an organization, such as a health department or health project management body. It needs no further explication.

While on the subject of degrees of participation, it would be remiss not to mention the issue of consumerism. At first glance one of the few points of contact between radical–conservative ideology and the principles of health promotion is the apparent concern of the former to give the consumer a better deal, for instance in the form of patients' charters and curbs on professional power. While such

Degree	Participants' action	Illustrative mode
Low	None	The community is told nothing.
	Receives information	The organization makes a plan and announces it. The community is convened for informational purposes; compliance is expected.
	Is consulted	The organization tries to promote a plan and develop the support to facilitate acceptance of, or give sufficient sanction to, the plan so that administrative compliance can be expected.
	Advises	The organization presents a plan and invites questions. It is prepared to modify the plan only if absolutely necessary.
	Plans jointly	The organization presents a tentative plan subject to change and invites recommendations from those affected.
	Has delegated authority	The organization identifies and presents a problem to the community, defines the limits and asks the community to make a series of decisions which can be embodied in a plan which it will accept.
High	Has control	The organization asks the community to identify the problems and to make all the key decisions regarding goals and means. It is willing to help the community at each step accomplish its own goals, even to the extent of administrative control of the programme.

Figure 8.3 A spectrum of participation (Brager and Specht, 1973).

moves should doubtless be applauded, they are different from CP. Croft and Beresford (1992) explain this point concisely:

> The emergence of consumerist thinking on health and welfare services has coincided with the expansion of commercial provision and political pressure for a changed economy of welfare. Service users or clients are now conceived of as consumers. Now the discussion of participation is overlaid with the language of consumerism and the concerns of the market (Ward, 1990). Consumerism starts with the idea of buying the goods and services we want instead of making collective provision for them. Two competing meanings underpin the idea of consumerism: first, giving priority to the wants and needs of the 'consumer' and second, framing people as 'consumers' and commodifying their needs into markets to be met by the creation of goods and services. ... In the debate about user-involvement, while the consumerist approach has tended to come from service providers and to address the concerns and needs of services, for example, improving management to achieve greater economy, efficiency and effectiveness, the democratic approach has largely been developed by service users and their organizations. What distinguishes these organizations from traditional pressure groups is that they seek to **speak for themselves** instead of other groups speaking on their behalf. Here the primary concern has been with empowerment, the redistribution of power and people gaining more say and control over their lives. (*Campbell, 1990*)

We will now return to consider a point made at the end of the last section when it was suggested that there might be a quite considerable gulf between top-down 'colonizing' community programmes and the 'pure type' of bottom-up initiative which is epitomised by CD. Figure. 8.4 suggests that programmes might, in fact, be categorized into one of five types. Type 1 would be represented by CD and the leadership would be concerned only to raise consciousness about felt needs and provide the community with the wherewithal to bring those felt needs to fruition. The priority of Type 1 programmes would be to achieve empowerment and an improvement in socioeconomic status. On the

Type 5 Limited 'outreach' programmes; limited community participation but uses mix of agencies, e.g. media plus schools, plus drop-in centres and delivery of services directly to housing estate or workplace.

Type 4 Innovators' goals are primarily those of preventive medicine. This type is epitomized by the various CHD prevention programmes. It is more top-down than Types 1–3 but it emphasizes the importance of enlisting the support of the community and utilizing community dynamics such as networks.

Type 3 Characterized by 'community health projects'. Innovators' goals are to enhance health and prevent disease. They aim to do this by raising the profile of health but are prepared to help the community work through other more pressing 'felt needs' prior to their acknowledging a need to improve cardiovascular health, for example.

Type 2 As with Type 1 but during the process of developing a community profile and identifying felt needs, the community itself acknowledges needs which are consistent with standard preventive medicine goals, e.g. a need for better primary care services, accident prevention, dealing with child health problems.

Type 1 Innovators' goal for the community is primarily self-empowerment and improvement in socioeconomic status. Self-empowerment = Health.

Figure 8.4 Categories of community organization by levels of participation.

other hand, the priority of Type 5 programmes would be the achievement of preventive medical targets and their associated epidemiological outcomes. The major CHD prevention programmes discussed earlier would be categorized as Type 4 programmes.

It is not difficult to imagine the circumstances in which Type 2 projects might emerge. The community worker conducts a survey of felt needs and a disease related issue arises; for example, child accidents or problems with the medical services. The community itself has acknowledged the issue and the worker then acts as a facilitator. Programme objectives would probably be

acceptable to the managers of the health service. It is, of course, possible that a disease related issue may be generated which is not acceptable because it does not fit into current priorities. For instance, it is highly likely that a disadvantaged urban community would identify damp housing as a problem. While this is clearly a mental health issue, it might not be compatible with health authority goals for mental health, either because they had been marginalized in the face of problems such as AIDS or CHD or because they did not quite fit the prevailing mental illness model. Furthermore, because of lack of clear epidemiological proof that damp housing caused significant respiratory illness, the issue might again be relegated. The health worker may then have to compile evidence to demonstrate that felt need was in fact a genuine medical problem. This might well prove to be an unpopular measure since the cost implications of modifying housing stock would be politically threatening (see, for instance, Martin *et al.*, 1987).

As indicated earlier, community developers do not infiltrate a community without an ideological agenda: their overt purpose is at the very least to remedy inequalities and gain better and fairer distribution of resources for the community in question. We might therefore suggest – albeit a little mischievously – that if a community refuses to identify with the facilitator's political agenda and the facilitator insists on persevering with that agenda, then the programme becomes a Type 3 intervention. Type 3 programmes more typically refer to what are often called 'community health projects'.

COMMUNITY HEALTH PROJECTS

The term 'community health project' is used here to refer to projects which utilize strategies of community development in order to address recognizable health issues, many of which would be congruent with preventive goals. There are many such projects in the UK (for instance, the London Health Action Network listed almost 200 such schemes in 1984). More recently, the Community Projects Foundation (1988) has provided a critical appraisal of a number of such projects, as have Smithies *et al.* (1990). The projects do, however, differ from a 'colonization' approach in several ways. Rosenthal (1983) lists their characteristics as follows.

1. They are firmly based outside the health professions;
2. They are concerned with addressing inequalities in health and health care provision;
3. They are concerned to promote collective awareness of social causes of ill health;
4. They assert that the monopoly of information about health and ill health by professionals must be challenged both individually and collectively;
5. Activities centre on work with small groups of local people;
6. Projects have a catalyst function in stimulating local health, social and education services.

Simmons (1976) edited a series of reports from a workshop which according to her represented '… the first effort to present an overall picture of how health education principles were applied in the past decade to health programmes serving low-income and minority groups'. Six of these community health projects which Simmons presented and analysed demonstrate the importance of community participation and run almost the whole gamut of types of intervention described in Figure. 8.4. The communities in question ranged from hospital patients and staff to isolated villages in Alaska. One study in particular, the 'Forty Family Pilot Study' epitomizes the broader community organization programme which is more representative of Type 2 community interventions than Type 3. The importance of locating medical goals within a broader framework and subordinating them to more fundamental socioeconomic

targets is highlighted by the project's philosophy which is reproduced below:

Poverty is more than a lack of economic resources. It also includes a set of values and states of existence which exclude the poor from the opportunities offered middle-class persons.

Citizens in the low-income group must be brought from the periphery of social living into the structure of the community. Nothing that the community does for the poor can be durably effective until the poor are a functioning part of the community.

There is a need not only for medical, educational and occupational assistance for low-income people, but especially for a system of touching the lives and attitudes of the poor so that they can take advantage of all resources available to them.

The impact of the Forty Family Pilot Study project which applied the community education principles discussed above was dramatic. The various indicators listed below reveal not only standard epidemiological/clinical measures but much broader (and arguably more important) testimony of success.

1. Eighty-five per cent of families received dental and physical examinations during the first year compared with less then 5% previously.
2. Mothers became aware of nutritional aspects of meal planning; there was an improvement in general health knowledge.
3. The number of adults receiving the General Education Diploma increased by 19% in one year.
4. All but 0.9% of children were in school compared with a previous drop-out rate of 19%.
5. Thirty-two per cent of people were now buying their own homes compared with 20% the previous year.
6. Average family income increased from $3900 in July 1972 to $4960 in July 1973.

THE HEALTHY COMMUNITY

We have already noted that participation and/or empowerment might legitimately be viewed as a desirable end in itself or a means to an end. For many sociologists and advocates of community development, the mere existence of a community as defined earlier is healthy. In the late 19th century, Tonnies' (1955) theory of *gemeinschaft* is consistent with this view. That is to say, the 'traditional' community, in which people act together to achieve common goals, is intrinsically healthy. Clearly there is an element of tautology here and a not uncommon tendency to equate 'healthy' with 'good', i.e. whatever is consonant with any individual's or group's predominant value system.

For many people the idea of 'sense of community' would be seen as part and parcel of *gemeinschaft* and for some, would form an integral part of the definition of community empowerment. McMillan and Chavis (1986) consider that a clear definition of a sense of community is a necessary prerequisite for the development of policy measures designed to create or preserve the intrinsically beneficial features of 'community'. They argue that a sense of community has four elements:

1. Membership – a feeling of belonging;
2. Influence – a sense of mattering, '... of making a difference to a group and of the group mattering to its members;
3. Integration and fulfilment of needs – '... a feeling that members' needs will be met by the resources received through their membership in the group';
4. Shared emotional connection – '... the commitment and belief that members have shared and will share history, common places, time together, and similar experiences'.

The definition they propose is, 'Sense of community is a feeling that members have of belonging, a feeling that members matter to one another and to the group, and a shared faith that members' needs will be met through their commitment to be together' (p. 9).

Raeburn (1986) also endorses the importance of *gemeinschaft* arguing that:

'... when people do enjoyable and worthwhile things together at a local level, positive bonds will form between them. This, in turn, leads to residents' overall awareness of local talents, issues and values, so that there is less tendency to look outside one's place of residence for a satisfactory life experience.

(pp. 392–3)

Raeburn describes the use of 'comprehensive community projects' and 'community houses' to achieve this 'oldfashioned' sense of community in Maori communities.

Allen and Allen (1987) considered that a sense of community was one of three 'core enabling factors' for achieving health promoting 'culture change' – for instance, in organizations. The other two components were 'shared vision' and 'a positive culture'. This latter notion indicates positive commitment to one's social group and its goals and might well have figured as a component of sense of community in McMillan and Chavis' definition. A sense of community proper is considered by Allen and Allen to be definable by responses to five questions:

1. Is there a sense of community between people involved in your programme?
2. Do people feel related to and supportive of one another?
3. Do people know each other as multidimensional people?
4. Do people care about each other's successes?
5. When people drop out, do others contact them to show their concern and interest?

Using questions such as these, the authors describe the effectiveness of what they see as a health promotion programme designed to deal with worksite problems such as high accident rates, alcoholism, absenteeism and (of course) worker productivity and company profits! After the introduction of a 'culture change process', '... the creativity and talents of the organization's members were unleashed in new ways so that seemingly "unsolvable" problems of the past could be addressed'. The result? A reduction in ill health and a rise in profits.

These rather cosy views of sense of community and the value of *gemeinschaft* are challenged in an astringent article by Wellman and Leighton (1979). They comment on the tendency of many urban sociologists to lament the loss of the traditional community in its transformation into a more modern and alienated form. As they put it, 'Lost scholars have seen modern urbanites as alienated isolates who bear the brunt of the transformed society on their own' (p. 369). And so, if the traditional community is 'healthy' the modern community would appear to be sick. The characteristics of this sick 'community lost' are listed by Wellman and Leighton as follows: 'urbanites' are no longer full members of 'solidary communities'; they are limited members of **several** social networks. Primary contacts with people are fewer and more narrowly defined. These ties '... tend to be **fragmented** into isolated **two-person** relationships rather than being parts of extensive networks'. Relationships are weaker in intensity and those networks which do exist are 'sparsely knit', i.e. interfacing with only a small proportion of potential contacts. Networks are 'loosely bounded' having few separate clusters or primary groups. Little structural support is provided for '**solidary activities** or **sentiments**'. As a result of these features, the 'modern' community is less able to provide support and assistance for network members.

The authors point out that a major goal of many community workers and sociologists has been to use CD and other techniques to save the traditional community (or rather recreate it). The characteristics of 'community saved' are the obverse of 'community lost'. As Wellman and Leighton put it, 'Many saved social pathologists have encouraged the nurturance of densely knit, bounded communities as a structural salve for the stresses of poverty, ethnic segregation and physical and mental diseases'.

There is, however, according to the authors a third category of community – 'community liberated'. In short, they have the temerity to challenge the healthgiving qualities of *gemeinschaft*. They argue that the focus of community analysis should not be so much on geographical neighbourhood but rather on networks. At a theoretical level, this makes it easier to identify both 'communities without propinquity' and the existence of 'urban villages'. Moreover, they argue that in terms of the mobilization of support, being able to move among a number of social networks may be more beneficial than being limited to those existing within the confines of a neighbourhood. Indeed, modern communication systems render this close geographical contact irrelevant. The authors do concede that the 'liberated community' may be particularly suited to more affluent sectors of (? American) society insofar as it places a premium on '... a base of individual security, entrepreneurial skills in moving between networks, and the ability to function without the security of membership in a solidary community'. They do, on the other hand, caution that solidarity does not necessarily mean egalitarianism: '... not all of the community's resources may be gathered or distributed equally'. Moreover, there may actually be disadvantages for working class and ethnic minority communities in the 'community found' situation:

Concerns about conserving, controlling and efficiently pooling those resources which the beleaguered community possesses also resonate with its members' inability to acquire additional resources elsewhere. A heavy load consequently is placed on ties within the saved community.

NETWORKS AND HEALTH PROMOTING SOCIAL SUPPORT

A considerable number of studies have focused on the beneficial effects of social support for a number of health outcomes. A review of this area is beyond the scope of the present chapter but we may seize upon one or two key points. First, Gottlieb and McLeroy (1992) view social support as one of three features of social health. They noted that early definitions of social health focused on the integration of the individual into the community, their participation in community activities, conformity to social norms and appropriate performance of social roles. A more appropriate conceptualization, in their view, includes 'social integration or involvement' (quantity and quality of relationships); 'social support' (e.g. functional content of relationships such as emotional support); 'social networks' (the structure of relationships with other people within a social system). All three aspects constitute 'social participation' – which is, to all intents and purposes, synonymous with community participation.

Gottlieb and McLeroy remind us of the wealth of literature on these various aspects of social participation: they note that Current Contents (the journal abstracting service) listed about 100 articles per year from 1989–1991 on the effects of social support and social networks. A number of studies have provided quite clear evidence of the direct beneficial effects of participation (as defined above). Gottlieb and McLeroy summarize these for us as follows:

1. The impact of social relationships on physical health is non-specific and is related to all-cause mortality rather than to certain specific causes of death.
2. Risk of dying is increased with very low levels of social relationships (social isolation).
3. The impact of social interaction on health varies with community size and with gender; it is stronger in urban than in rural areas.

The indirect effects on health of social participation must be many and varied. Indeed the first task is to consider the nature and mechanism whereby social participation exerts its instrumental effect on health promotion and/or the prevention of disease. Various theories have been propounded but we will limit ourselves here to acknowledging the important work of Israel (for instance, 1982, 1987). In 1982, after a review of the literature on the effects of social support and networks on physical and mental well-being, she concluded that five different types of support could be provided through interpersonal relationships. The first of these was affective support which provided respect and comfort. The second, instrumental support, included material help such as money, food or child care assistance. Cognitive support, on the other hand, was beneficial in providing the information and advice needed to make decisions. A fourth kind of support was referred to as maintenance of social identity and provided 'validation of a shared world view' (cf. Lewis' notion of existential control which was cited in Chapter 1). Finally 'social outreach' provided access to social contacts (see also House, 1988).

Before moving on, one interesting example of programme success will be provided in this social support context. It refers to a study by Sosa *et al.* (1980) cited by Gottlieb and McLeroy. It concerns 40 pregnant women in Guatemala City who were randomly assigned to treatment and control groups. The former group of women were provided with continuing support from lay women from admission to the birth of the child. The control group, by contrast, underwent the normal delivery process. The length of delivery time for the group which had received social support was 8.7 hours compared with 19.3 hours for women in the control group.

COMMUNITY DEVELOPMENT: PRINCIPLES
AND PRACTICE

The philosophical basis of CD and its major
purpose have already been discussed. Those
who wish to consult an early review of the
principles of CD are referred to Dunham
(1963) who reviewed 11 compilations of

principles or 'value judgements' which were
intended to provide 'guidelines to sound or
effective practice'. The 11 sets of principles
included 142 statements of individual principles. The reader will doubtless be relieved
that these will not be reproduced here! It is
sufficient merely to recall that the major value
judgements concern the mobilization of an

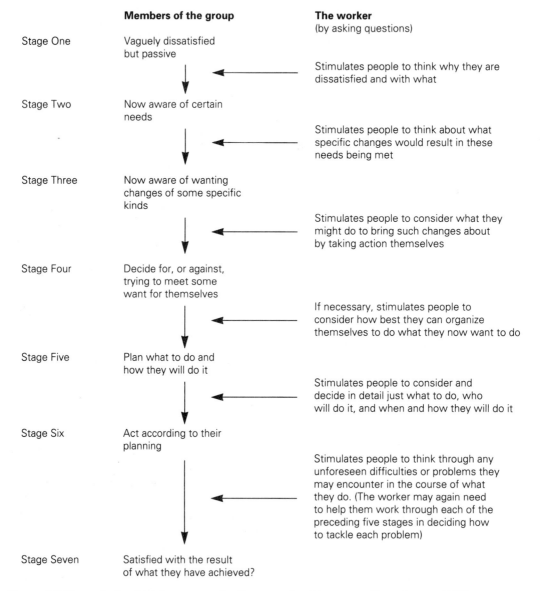

Figure 8.5 Stages in the thinking process leading to action by a group (from Batten, 1967).

active participating community to address its felt needs with the assistance of a facilitator who, in turn, is motivated by a desire to remedy inequalities.

A discussion of detailed tactics is not possible here but Figure 8.5 is doubly interesting. First, it provides a fairly general set of guidelines for the facilitator and signals a series of stages through which a community might be expected to move before the programme goal had been achieved. Second, and in this latter context, we are provided at a stroke with a framework for process evaluation!

As we commented earlier, there are a number of alternative and competing approaches to community programmes which share the goal of empowering and/or tackling problems of inequality. Freire's approach has been seen by some (e.g. de Kadt, 1982) as such an alternative. On the other hand, many would regard critical consciousness raising as the method of choice for alerting the community to its felt needs and subsequently getting community members to develop feelings of indignation at the circumstances in which they find themselves. Key features of

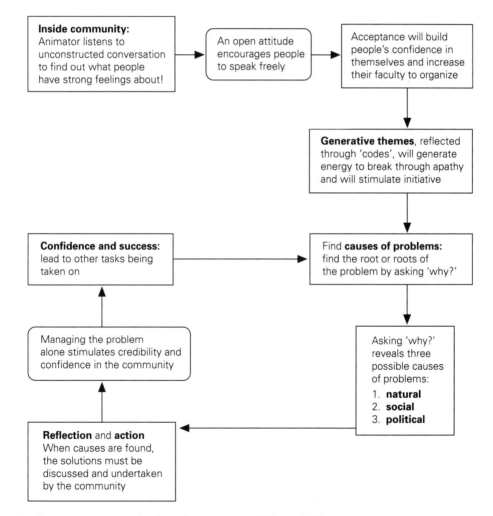

Figure 8.6 Summary: community-based programme (Hilton, 1988).

Freire's approach have already been mentioned in Chapter 1 but will be repeated here in the form of Figure 8.6.

Hilton (1988) has already been cited in this chapter when we made the distinction between genuine participative community action and colonisation. Figure 8.6 is from the same issue of *Contact* (a bimonthly publication of the Christian Medical Commission) and it describes a process of consciousness raising by a village 'animator' as part of the broader process of creating community participation (Paruvani, 1988). Again from the same article, Hope and Timmel (1988) describe the use of Freire's methods as 'training for transformation'.

Hopefully, this discussion and earlier illustrations will now allow us to look a little more critically at CD and the whole notion of community participation and consider some of its problematic areas prior to reviewing evidence of its successful application.

PROBLEMATIC ASPECTS OF COMMUNITY DEVELOPMENT

Various criticisms have been levelled at both community participation and community development. De Kadt (1982), commenting on the success or otherwise of CD initiatives in developing countries, observed that it:

> ... hardly ever faced up to the differences in interest that could exist between different members of the 'community' that was to be 'developed', notably in terms of their control over opportunities to make a living. Neither did it have an eye for the unequal (class) relations prevalent within many 'communities'. It thus failed to understand the fundamental social – and political – dynamics of communities in many parts of the world.
>
> (*p. 574*)

On the other hand, he suggests that Freirean approaches may not have made that mistake since they started from an assumption of the existence of socioeconomic inequalities due to the nature of capitalist economic systems. Whereas the community developers achieved little because they disregarded inequality, conflict and power relations, the '... *conscientisadores* ... had over-optimistic, some would say naive, views on the political reaction which their activities were likely to provoke, and on the people's power, or lack of it, to overcome them' (p. 574).

As for the process of CP, he cites a review by David Werner of 40 rural health projects in Latin America:

> ... when it came to the nitty-gritty of what was going on in the field, many of these ambitious 'king-sized' programmes actually had a minimum of effective community participation and a maximum of handouts, paternalism and superimposed initiative-destroying 'norms'.
>
> (*Werner, 1980, p. 94*)

Now it is clear we cannot assume that all CD programmes follow an identical pattern. Indeed, as we have stated, the key feature of recent western, urban CD programmes has been a recognition of the existence of inequalities and a determination to tackle it. However, it may well be the case that even if CD manages to achieve proper community participation, it may be unable to do very much in the face of oppressive environments and socioeconomic circumstances. It may, in fact, be true that as Moynihan (cited by Hubley, 1985) said, community work will '... promise a lot; deliver a little. Lead people to believe that they will be better off but let there be no dramatic improvement. Try a variety of programmes, each interesting, but marginal in impact and severely underfinanced'.

Heller (1989), in defining communities, acknowledged both their geographical and relational elements but insisted that a community should also be defined in terms of 'collective political power'. He distinguished empowerment from collective power. He commented that empowerment means the process of giving power or authority to an individual or group whereas '... in actuality, meaningful power must be **taken**. Ultimately, power is in the community of like-minded individuals who come together to form political coalitions.'

In a very different context, Gruber and Trickett (1987) discussed the possibility of empowering parents and students in an American public school. They defined empowerment as the 'extent of decision making power that people actually wield in an organization'. They concluded that membership of the policy council (or governing body) of the school was not sufficient to achieve this end due to the real power invested in the key members of the institution. They remarked that '... there is a fundamental paradox in the idea of people empowering others because the very institutional structure that puts one group in a position to empower also works to undermine the act of empowerment' (p. 353).

A thorough review of this important question of the locus of power cannot be undertaken here and readers are referred to Dixon's (1989) review. We might, however, provide a reminder of our reiteration in this book of the importance of the process of 'reciprocal determinism' of individual action and environmental constraint or facilitation.

There are a number of other problems with CD and it is worth summarizing an interesting review by Constantino-David (1982) who provided a detailed and thoughtful critique of community organization. First she cautions against the members of a community becoming dependent on the workers so that the project collapses once the workers withdraw. Second, she warns of the possibility of creating a new elite of community aides/ indigenous workers. Third she notes the dilemma for workers whose major self-empowering goal is to facilitate self-empowered choice and promote long term outcomes such as literacy, autonomy or healthy lifestyles and yet find they must concentrate on specific felt needs – issues which may

catch the community's imagination but which may be relatively insignificant in the longer term. She also highlights the 'facilitation vs. manipulation' dilemma in which there is a temptation for the worker to manipulate the attitudes and behaviour of the community to conform to the values and political motivation of the worker rather than facilitate empowered choice in the community members. Constantino-David also emphasizes the political paradoxes and problems which are usually greater in community organization than in other health promotion programmes which are more likely to be congruent with the dominant power structure in society. Loney's (1981) analysis of the British Community Development Projects makes a similar point. The potential for initiating radical action may be limited when funding comes from central government. As Loney says, 'It is rather like pacifists suddenly finding they have army funding.' He does, however, note in his reference to the Community Development Project report, *Gilding the Ghetto* (1977), 'That such a document could emerge from a state sponsored programme and could be printed at government expense must itself encourage a more cautious approach to summary dismissals of the possibilities of working in the state apparatus'. This is doubtless cheering news for many workers faced with the issue of programme evaluation. They might, however, be excused for a degree of scepticism since community programmes are more likely than most to give rise to a significant gap between the aspirations of funders and those of the workers themselves – to say nothing of the aspirations of the community! As the next section shows, there are other difficulties with evaluating community organization programmes.

EVALUATING COMMUNITY ORGANIZATION

In keeping with the aims of this book, no attempt will be made here to provide specific guidelines for evaluating community organi-zation. Good practical texts are readily avail-able (Feuerstein, 1986; Hedley, 1985). It is, however, essential to acknowledge the major issues. Voth (1979) suggests that there are five main problems associated with evaluating community work:

1. Ambiguity of goals;
2. Absence of a model of the community development process;
3. Inability of the researcher to control assignment to treatments;
4. Weak effects, crude measurement, and small samples;
5. Political problems.

Although there are, as we have seen, difficulties over definition, the absence of a theoretical model hardly seems a major pro-blem. It is clear that several detailed sets of suggestions for achieving community organ-ization have been provided by many of the authors cited above. It may be the case that workers are not aware of them or prefer to reject theory, but that is a different issue. The question of political difficulties has already been explored, both in general in Chapter 2 and more specifically above. No further dis-cussion is necessary here. On the other hand the remaining issues do need further consider-ation: they have to do fundamentally with goal setting and the writing of objectives and with the matter of experimental design.

First, with regard to goal setting, it is un-doubtedly true that community organization suffers from a tendency to state vague and/or overambitious aims or even to refuse to state any aims at all! There are probably two main reasons why there is frequently a reluctance to carry out the essential task of operational-izing general aims. First, it is often argued that because genuine community development must be based on community-defined goals, i.e. felt needs, it is neither possible nor desir-able to state programme objectives other than as general statements of intent such as

'empowering the community' or 'producing a shift in power'. Second, there may be an ideological objection to evaluation derived from a misconception that evaluation is inevitably associated with a logical–positivist approach and the much maligned medical model. These reasons or rationalizations are patently false. As we have said, community organization has broad goals such as reduc-ing disadvantage and enhancing empower-ment and these can readily be operationalized into a series of process measures. One of these is, of course, to produce a 'needs assessment' of the community. Now while it may not be possible or desirable to establish objectives before this step has been taken, it is perfectly possible, not to say essential, to develop objectives after establishing felt needs. Success may then be judged by the extent to which these needs are met or modified in the light of subsequent education and consciousness raising. With regard to the ideological objec-tion to evaluation *per se*, this is either a counsel of despair, an attempt at obfuscation or a decline into anarchy! It is, however, reasonable to challenge certain paradigms of evaluation. Indeed, as indicated earlier, this chapter is asserting that the clinical trials paradigm is inappropriate and damaging, as is its educational equivalent. Voth's remain-ing issues are in fact related to this matter and will therefore be considered now.

It is interesting to observe that Voth's sug-gestion that community developers need to combat the problem of 'weak effects, crude measurement and small samples' derives from an assumption that an experimental or quasi-experimental design cannot be expected to work in non-formal community settings. There seems to be an assumption that this is rather unfortunate. The approach adopted here, however, is that the alternative quali-tative research designs discussed in Chapter 2 are not merely appropriate but more pro-ductive than their more quantitative counter-parts. The reasons for the inappropriateness of the latter paradigm may be summarized as follows (and considered in the light of general comments made in Chapter 2).

1. Classic research design requires both experimental intervention and comparison or control groups. It is often inappropriate to utilize controls because of both the difficulty of avoiding cross-contamination in community interventions and the ethical issue of not depriving the community of a beneficial input.

2. More importantly, because of the great complexity of the intervention, evaluators will need to use equally complex factorial research designs. These in turn will result in an unacceptable sacrifice of external validity to internal validity.

   Parlett and Hamilton (1972) make this point graphically: 'To attempt to simulate laboratory conditions by "manipulating educational personnel" is not only dubious ethically, but also leads to gross administrative and personal inconvenience. Even if a situation could be so unnervingly controlled, its artificiality would render the exercise irrelevant; rarely can "tidy" results be generalized to an "untidy" reality.'

3. Community programmes must take account of the different needs of various stakeholders: community, funders, workers, health professionals, etc., and utilize an evaluation design which can record these various goals.

4. Community development is above all concerned with action research: it is inappropriate for evaluators to maintain an Olympian detachment and merely report on whether or not certain programme objectives have been achieved. Innovatory programmes require a continual flow of information in order to better change course in pursuit of relevant goals and react to changing circumstances.

5. Participatory evaluation is also a key element in the empowering process.

In general, then, formative rather than summative evaluation is needed: with a complex community programme, merely to be told that objectives have or have not been achieved is likely to leave the worker bemused and wondering why (s)he has failed or, paradoxically, why (s)he has been successful. This is not of course to disparage the clinical trials model or what, in education, Parlett and Hamilton have referred to as the 'agricultural–botanical paradigm'. They are both powerful tools when used in the right circumstances. Although clinical trials might be excellent for avoiding placebo effects in testing the efficacy of a drug or single clinical intervention, complex health promotion programmes require illumination rather than the double blind.

It should be noted that the use of formative and process evaluation is not only the method of choice for community development, it is also equally appropriate for medically oriented programmes of the social/technical planning variety. As Means and Smith (1988) have argued, there needs to be a pluralistic approach to evaluation. They apply this to the complex requirements of a community alcohol education programme whose goal is fundamentally one of prevention.

The arguments ranged against the clinical trials model should, of course, not be used to justify sloppy thinking and a refusal to develop objectives. Although it is important, through process evaluation, to accumulate evidence which illuminates the reasons for success or failure and provide guidance for more effective action, it is equally important to examine whether or not objectives have been achieved. It is equally possible to utilize experimental design within a programme to check a hypothesis or to compare the relative effectiveness of alternative approaches to achieving a given objective. Typically the objectives in question would give rise to indirect or intermediate indicators of performance. The literature on CD and many of the examples provided in this chapter provide ready-made indicators of this kind. For instance, we have already noted how Batten's

(1967) seven stages could provide a useful basis for process evaluation as the community moves from passivity to self-empowered action (or not, as the case may be!).

No further observations will be made about the evaluation of CD. There are specialist texts in this area (see, for instance Hedley, 1985; Feuerstein, 1986; Rifkin *et al.*, 1988). Clearly it would be reasonable to expect to see some element of participatory research (Tandon, 1981), a point which has been explored in Chapter 2 along with other ideological and theoretical precepts of relevance for CD work.

By way of concluding this chapter, we will consider one or two examples of apparently successful programmes which utilize CD principles or emphasize the importance of participation.

COMMUNITY PROJECTS: SOME EXAMPLES OF SUCCESS

While it is probably true to say that many community workers are more concerned with achieving success than with measuring it, there are several examples of project evaluation in the development literature. Kindervatter (1979), for example, describes a series of youth and village development workshops in Thailand. Although at first glance these would not seem to have great relevance for planning and evaluating community health projects in western inner city areas, the fundamental principles are identical and many parallels can be drawn. For instance, the goal of the organizers of the Thai workshops (which they acknowledged as deriving from them rather than from felt needs) was encapsulated in the concept of 'khit pen'*. This notion is directly compatible with Freire's (1972) pedagogical aims and is consonant with the aims of self-empowerment as described in Chapter 1. The methods adopted by the 'facilitators' are akin to those recommended for use in various UK schools' health and life skills teaching – e.g. analysis of felt needs, team building, goal setting, problem solving, etc. The goals of the Thai project, however, proved to be more tangible and immediate and included the acquisition of occupational skills which might be used to help the community by, for example, putting into practice a village project such as building a water drainage system. In other words, we have a scheme which incorporates the two classic goals of community organization/development: first the 'ideological' and all-embracing aim of self-empowering individuals and community; second the more specific objectives which emerge from the 'felt needs' of the participants.

As for the evaluation, planners utilized a number of simple tools to determine (i) a process effect – participants' and facilitators' responses to the programme, (ii) intermediate indicators of participants' learning – attitudes and behaviours, and (iii) longer term outcome indicators. The process evaluation indicated, for instance, that '... outside resource people tended to present boring lectures'! This fact was taken into account when revising the programme along with various positive recommendations – that the occupational skills sessions were effective as were the morning calisthenics. With regard to intermediate indicators, various changes in attitude were recorded such as a greater awareness of village problems and a recognition that the individuals' abilities could be used to improve their lives. At the same time ambivalent results were noted in respect of such items as 'I am

---

* 'Some people translate "khit pen" as critical thinking, others as rational thinking, still others as problem-solving. It is, in fact, the combination of these processes and more. A man (or woman) who has mastered "khit pen" will be able to approach problems in his life systematically ... If due to outside circumstances or lack of certain necessary knowledge or skills, the solution of his choice can not be implemented right away, a "khit pen" man will not become frustrated. Instead, he will adopt a lesser solution while preparing to make the solution of his choice possible ... In other words, this philosophy encourages people to change, but not to destroy themselves physically and mentally doing so.' Dr Kowit Vorapipatana, Thai Adult Education Division, July 1975, pp. 7–8, cited by Kindervatter (1979).

confident of my abilities' and 'I think my life will be better five years from now'. Clearly self-empowerment had been tempered by a recognition of the real social and environmental contraints.

As for outcome indicators, participants were reported to have become more active in discussion and had acquired increased skills in working in small groups (again it is interesting to note the parallel with school-based life skills evaluation measures). More importantly, perhaps, for the good of the community and the experience of success by the participants, most of the planned projects had been completed by the end of three months (e.g. raising $300 for village development projects; establishing a day care centre; preparing a village learning centre; construction of three roads and the repair of a public hall).

Reference was made earlier to Raeburn's (1986) discussion of community projects designed to enhance participation and create a sense of community with its concomitant health benefits. Raeburn reported that the resources had not been available to carry out large scale evaluation but reported evidence of the social impact of 'comprehensive community projects' in the Birkenhead Community Project. He provided the following details:

After six years, the annual participation rate was 8000–10 000 people in a total community of 21 000.

A random survey done in Birkenhead three years after the BCP started showed that about 18% of residents were involved and that 77% of these had found their contact with the BCP 'very satisfactory' or 'satisfactory'.

The same survey showed that 90.3% of adult residents said that they liked living in Birkenhead and 80% said that they got on well with their neighbors.

A 1982 telephone well-being survey commissioned by the Auckland evening

newspaper found that Birkenhead was one of two best-liked suburbs in Auckland – a far cry from the 'social volcano' of ten years before.

In the same ten-year period, the local police noted that Birkenhead had gone from having the highest juvenile crime rate in the district they served to the lowest, a phenomenon they ascribed directly to the BCP.

Gordon (1985) described an interesting community development project which was implemented in communities providing labour for a timber-producing company in a rural area of South Africa.

Programme goals were to promote community participation by setting up 'an infrastructure of decision making bodies in the villages'; to develop a social and recreational programme to foster community solidarity; to increase income levels by 'enabling residents to participate in informal income generating activities'.

Within a 12 month evaluation period, the following indicators of success were reported:

Community committees were functioning autonomously and further elections organized by the committees were held.

They organized a number of corporate ventures, such as plowing fields and hiring cattle herders.

Equipment for sport and recreation was jointly purchased by the company and the communities.

By the end of the year, soccer and netball clubs were operating smoothly and two competitions had been supported with great enthusiasm.

(The Community Development Officer) organized hearings of two cases in which employees claimed that they had been unfairly dismissed by their supervisors. As a result of the hearings both complainants were rehired. Labor turnover dropped from 80% to 40% over the 12 months of study.

(p. 334)

Another useful set of exemplars of certain possible indicators of the success of CD programmes is provided by Fawcett *et al.* (1984). The authors presented seven case studies, each of which illustrated success in at least some of the processes necessary for empowering people. These processes were described as follows:

1. Increasing **knowledge of community problems** from the perspective of those most affected by the problems.
2. Increasing **knowledge of solution alternatives** generated by those most affected by the problems.
3. Increasing **knowledge of the possible consequences** of projects proposed by persons outside the affected community.
4. **Involving consumers** in the redesign of social programmes to fit local needs and resources.
5. **Training new behaviours** for increasing the effectiveness of individual citizens.
6. **Training new behaviours** for increasing the effectiveness of leaders of community groups.
7. **Developing and communicating research information** to increase the likelihood of actions taken regarding problems affecting the poor or disadvantaged.
(pp. 148–9)

N.B.   Phrases shown in bold represent our emphasis and indicate potential programme objectives within the overall empowerment aim.

The seven separate community studies discussed by Fawcett *et al.* are listed below:

1. Development of pressure to ensure allocation of scarce resources for social services for areas of need.
2. Identification of community concerns as part of a process of establishing consumer advisory committees for people with disabilities.
3. Helping people disseminate information about the possible impact on neighbourhoods of proposed new road development schemes.
4. Using study circles to generate community participation in decisions about technologies which might affect their neighbourhood.
5. Provision of training for community members to equip them to chair meetings.
6. Development of ways of helping communities influence public decisions.
7. Development and communication of information in relation to charging lower rates for winter heating for vulnerable groups.

It may be recalled that we have previously commented that community empowerment may well be conceptualized as the sum of the number of empowered individuals in that community. We also observed that, logically, the way to community empowerment was therefore to provide individuals with empowering skills and competences, including such 'community' skills as how to organize effectively and how to seek support from networks. To work with individuals in this way is not to indulge in victim blaming provided that the limitations imposed by the environment are recognized and additional steps are taken, where necessary, to address any such oppressive environmental factors. Indeed, following criticisms which we reported earlier of the limitations of community development, we might need to argue that CD should always be supplemented by, say, advocacy for healthy public policy and, perhaps, the organization of powerful coalitions as recommended by the CHD prevention projects. At all events, Fawcett's analysis illustrates nicely the provision of the various health and life skills needed to empower people once consciousness has been raised. Note, for instance, the specification of precise skills in the context of developing ways of helping communities influence public decisions (item 6 above) to the extent that people were taught how to write protest letters.

Despite caveats about expecting too much from a CD mode of working – without the sorts of supplementary help to which reference was made above – it is clear that CD can empower. For instance, O'Sullivan *et al.* (1984) described how a small American Indian community was faced with the loss of their homeland as a result of a proposal to build a dam. The results of such a move would have been to damage the physical, psychological, economic and social well-being of that community. Over a number of years a coalition of environmental interest groups (including environmentalists, religious leaders, antigovernment advocates, pro-Indian supporters and river recreationists) took up the Indians' cause. Apart from various exercises in lobbying and advocacy, a deliberate attempt was made to gain maximal community participation. Subsequently the tribe (the Yavapai) '… engaged in an effective, consistent, and intensive media campaign, culminating in a three day march from the reservation to the state capital. They presented a signed petition with an alternative to the proposed dam.' As the authors put it, '… the tribe publicly demonstrated opposition … that was **forceful, skilful and credible**. To use Bell's (1975) lexicon of political linguistics, the Fort McDowell tribal community entered a power position by communicating to their opponents that they could and would tie up … (the dam project) … for so long that it could not be built in the foreseeable future.'

According to the authors, one of the results of this community action (which was more akin to 'social action' in its use of coalitions and conflict than to CD) was that the tribe changed its perception of itself as powerless. One tribal elder stated '… it was the first time the Yavapai had ever won a battle with the government, and we beat the white man at his own game'. The community had moved towards self-empowerment – and the dam was not built!

As we have seen, community development involves working from a social group's 'felt needs', raising consciousness about their physical and social circumstances, providing support and skills to enable them to achieve the goals they have identified with their new-found consciousness – and then to withdraw. As we noted earlier, this process was described by Batten (1967) in relation to the 'thinking process' leading to action by a group and identifying the ways in which community workers would, by asking questions, move a community from stage one (vaguely dissatisfied but passive) through to stage six (acting according to planning) and the final stage seven, evaluating the results of action.

We also described in Figure 8.6 above a different but related developmental process derived from Freire which, naturally, focused in on the development of critical consciousness raising.

Kieffer (1984) provides a particularly valuable insight into the developmental nature of the empowering process. Unlike Batten, he does not report the process of empowerment from the point of view of the facilitator but rather from the perspective of the individual member of the community. We will conclude this chapter with quotations from some of these actors who describe the changes they are undergoing. In so doing we will also demonstrate the way in which a qualitative research method can provide rich insights into such changes.

Kieffer considered that community members moved through four stages on their journey to empowerment. Following a process of consciousness raising, an initial 'era of entry' is followed by an 'era of advancement'. This stage is in turn succeeded by an era of 'incorporation' and, finally, an 'era of commitment'. The era of entry is characterized by an emergent feeling of 'commitment to self-reliance and feelings of attachment and support within a caring community …'. Kieffer describes the feeling of powerlessness which can exist prior to this first stage in the words of an American living in Harlem.

It would never have occurred to me to have expressed an opinion on anything ... It was inconceivable that my opinion had any value ... that's lower than powerlessness ... You don't even know the word 'power' exists. It applies to them ... I didn't question that that's the way the world was ... It was their world ... And I was an intruder, you know?

and Emily ...

People like us ... have a hard enough time copin' with every day livin'. When you have to work every day for your basic food, shelter, clothes, and safety, you're not very much apt to have a lot of energy left to go to meetin's ... People ... are so busy earnin' a livin' they don't really stop and think about ... what real impact they may have as a citizen.

The 'era of entry' involves a kind of awakening. Kieffer, however, describes this as happening from a basis of 'felt-rootedness in a community' and '... feelings of attachment and support within a caring community of peers'. Moreover, the initial reaction, he argues, is not fostered by mere consciousness raising but rather by the 'immediate and physical violation of the sense of integrity ...'. Through a kind of 'trial and error' process they start to develop a 'sense of themselves as active political beings'.

Individuals hopefully progress to this second developmental stage. According to Kieffer there are three necessary conditions for satisfactory progress. These are 'a mentoring process', '... supportive peer relationships within a collective organizational structure, and the cultivation of a more critical understanding of social and political relations'. This process requires at least a year of '... intensive engagement and reflection'.

The role of the 'enabler' or mentor is nicely illustrated by Lucinda:

When I first got involved ... the (facilitators) all saw beyond me ... they just didn't see

me. They saw what I was capable of, what I could be ... It was so important that somebody cared enough to be there encouraging me, pushing me ... coming back after me ... no matter how afraid I was.

The third 'era of incorporation' reflects the maturing of 'self-concept', 'critical comprehension' and 'strategic ability'. Emily describes the experience:

I've changed ... I think I'm understanding more of the structure of our society and understanding more of how people operate within our society. But I've still not gotten it straight in my mind where is my little niche. Or do I have one? And what can I really do? One thing's for sure, I won't ever be the same self as I was when this thing first started.

According to Kieffer, 'The fundamental empowering transformation ... is in the transition from sense of self as helpless victim to acceptance of self as assertive and efficacious citizen.' Clearly this goal is eminently desirable in its own right and it is hard to imagine such an empowered individual within an empowered community not responding positively to the narrower preventive objectives of more orthodox health educators and public health specialists.

The attainment of empowerment, as we have seen, is essentially problematic and different tactics and strategies have been proposed to achieve such goals in a continuing battle with environmental forces. It is a major assertion in this book that the effort is worthwhile and that it is not incompatible with values espoused by other health educators – with the exception of those whose perspective on people is essentially from top downwards! The different strategies are not mutually exclusive. Indeed, as is the case with the CHD prevention projects, a coherent and integrated approach to empowerment is desirable, whether this be in the hospital or surgery, in the school or workplace or, less formally, in the broader community. The words of Lucinda provide us with the kind of performance indicator to which we might well aspire:

> What I've learned in the past four years, I'm applying to **all** my life. It's changed my whole life – personal, professional, everything. My values have changed. My priorities have changed. Everything has changed.

REFERENCES

Alinsky, S.D. (1946) *Reveille for Radicals*, Vintage Books, New York.

Allen, R.F. and Allen, J.A. (1987) A sense of community, a shared vision and a positive culture: core enabling factors in successful culture based health promotion. *American Journal of Health Promotion*, **6**, 40–7.

Amezcua, C., McAlister, A., Ramirez, A. and Espinoza, R. (1990) A Su Sulad: health promotion in a Mexican-American border community, in *Health Promotion at the Community Level*, (eds N. Bracht *et al.*) Sage, London.

Arnstein, S.R. (1971) Eight rungs on the ladder of citizen participation, in *Citizen Participation: Effecting Community Change*, (eds S.E. Cahn and B.A. Passett), Praeger Publications, New York.

Batten, T.R. (1967) *The Non-Directive Approach in Group and Community Work*, Oxford University Press, Oxford.

Bell, D.V. (1975) *Power, Influence and Authority: An Essay in Political Linguistics*, Oxford University Press, New York.

Blackburn, H. (1983) Research and demonstration projects in community cardiovascular disease prevention. *Journal of Public Health Policy*, **4**, 398–421.

Blake, S.M., Jeffery, R.W., Finnegan, J.R. *et al.* (1987) Process evaluation in a community-based physical activity campaign: the Minnesota Heart Health Program Experience. *Health Education Research*, **2**, 115–21.

Bracht, N. and Kingsbury, L. (1990) Community organization principles in health promotion: a five stage model, in *Health Promotion at the Community Level*, (eds N. Bracht *et al.*) Sage, London.

Brager, C. and Specht, H. (1973) *Community Organising*, Columbia University Press.

Calouste Gulbenkian Foundation (1984) *A National Centre for Community Development: Report of a Working Party*, Gulbenkian Foundation, London.

Campbell, P. (1990) *Self-advocacy: Working Together for Change*. Presentation to MIND Conference, 10th October, Survivors Speak Out.

Carlaw, R.W., Mittlemark, M.B., Bracht, N. and Luepker, R. (1984) Organization for a community cardiovascular health program: experiences from the Minnesota Heart Health Program. *Health Education Quarterly*, **11**, 243–52.

Chabot, J.H.T. (1976) The Chinese system of health care. *Tropical Geographical Medicine*, **28**, 87–134.

Community Development Project (1977) *Gilding the Ghetto*, CDP Inter-Project Editorial Team, Mary Ward House, 5 Tavistock Place, London WC1H 9SS.

Community Projects Foundation/HEA/SHEG (1988) *Action for Health: Initiatives in Local Communities*, CPF, London.

Constantino-David, K. (1982) Issues in community organization. *Community Development Journal*, **17**, 190–201.

Croft, S. and Beresford, P. (1992) The politics of participation. *Critical Social Policy*, **26**, 20–44.

De Kadt, E. (1982) Community participation for health: the case of Latin America. *World Development*, **10**(7), 573–84.

Department of Health (1992) *Health of the Nation*, HMSO, London.

Dixon, J. (1989) The limits and potential of community development for personal and social change. *Community Health Studies*, **XII**(1), 82–92.

Dodds, J., Fraser, W. and Rendall, M. (1986) *Community Development Approaches to Health Promotion in North America: Comparative Underinvestment and Untapped Potential in the United Kingdom?* Health Education Council, London.

Dunham, A. (1963) Some principles of community development. *International Review of Community Development*, **11**, 141–51.

Elder, J.P., McGraw, S.A., Abrams, D.B. *et al.* (1986) Organizational and community approaches to communitywide prevention of heart disease: the first two years of the Pawtucket Heart Health Program. *Preventive Medicine*, **15**, 107–17.

Farquhar, J.W., Maccoby, N., Wood, P.D. *et al.* (1977) Community education for cardiovascular health. *Lancet*, **i**, 1192–5.

Farquhar, J.W., Fortmann, S.P., Maccoby, N. *et al.* (1984) The Stanford Five City Project: an overview, in *Behavioural Health: A Handbook of*

Health Education and Disease Prevention, (eds J.D. Matarazzo *et al.*), John Wiley, New York.

Farquhar, J.W., Fortmann, S.P., Flora, J.A. *et al.* (1990) Effects of communitywide education on cardiovascular risk factors: The Stanford Five City Project. *Journal of the American Medical Association*, **264**(3), 359–65.

Farquhar, J.W., Fortmann, S.P., Wood, P.D. and Haskell, W.L. (1983) Community studies of cardiovascular disease prevention, in *Prevention of Coronary Heart Disease: Practical Management of Risk Factors*, (eds N.M. Kaplan *et al.*), W.B. Saunders, Philadelphia.

Farquhar, J.W., Maccoby, N. and Solomon, D.S. (1984) Community applications of behavioural medicine, in *Handbook of Behavioural Medicine*, (ed. W.D. Gentry), Guildford Press, New York.

Fawcett, S.B., Seekins, T., Whang, P.L., Muiu, C. and Suarez de Balcazar, Y. (1984) Creating and using social technologies for community empowerment, in *Studies in Empowerment: Steps Toward Understanding and Action*, (eds J. Rappaport, C. Swift and R. Hess), Haworth Press, New York.

Feuerstein, M.T. (1986) *Partners in Evaluation*, Macmillan, London.

Freire, P. (1972) *Pedagogy of the Oppressed*, Penguin, Harmondsworth.

Gordon, A. (1985) Learned helplessness and community development: a case study. *Journal of Community Psychology*, **13**, 327–37.

Gottlieb, N. and McLeroy, K.R. (1992) Social health, in *Health Promotion in the Workplace*, 2nd edn, (ed. M.P. O'Donnell), Delmar Publishing, New York.

Green, L.W. and Kreuter, M. (1991) *Health Promotion and Planning: An Educational and Environmental Approach*, Mayfield, Palo Alto, CA.

Gruber, J. and Trickett, E.J. (1987) Can we empower others? The paradox of empowerment in the governing of an alternative public school. *American Journal of Community Psychology*, **15**(3), 353–71.

Haglund, B., Weisbrod, R.R. and Bracht, N. (1990) Assessing the community, its services, needs, leadership, and readiness, in *Health Promotion at the Community Level*, (eds N. Bracht *et al.*), Sage, London.

Health Education Research, special issue on community coalitions, 8(3), 1993.

Healthy Sheffield 2000: Health Promotion Programme Strategic Plan, 1990–1993, Programme Steering Group, Sheffield Health Promotion Unit, Sheffield.

Hedley, R. (1985) *Measuring Success*, ADVANCE, 14 Bloomsbury Square, London WC1.

Heller, K. (1989) The return to community. *American Journal of Community Psychology*, **17**(1), 1–15.

Henderson P. and Thomas, D.N. (1980) *Skills in Neighbourhood Work*, Allen and Unwin, London.

Hersey, J.C., Klibanoff, L.S., Lam, D.J. and Taylor, R.L. (1984) Promoting social support: the impact of California's 'Friends Can be Good Medicine' campaign. *Health Education Quarterly*, **11**, 293–311.

Hilton, D. (1988) Community-based or community-oriented: the vital difference. *Contact*, **106**, 1–4.

Holme, I., Hermann, M.D., Helgeland, A. and Leren, P. (1985) The Oslo Study: diet and anti-smoking advice. *Preventive Medicine*, **14**, 279–92.

Hope, A. and Timmel, S. (1988) Training for transformation. *Contact*, **106**, 4–7.

House, J.S. (1988) Structures and processes of social support. *Annual Review of Sociology*, **14**, 293–318.

Hubley, J.H. (1985) *Papers on Community Development* (mimeo), Leeds Polytechnic.

Hunkeler, E.F., Davis, E.M., McNeil, B., Powell, J.W. and Polen, M.R. (1990) Richmond quits smoking: a minority community fights for health, in *Health Promotion at the Community Level*, (eds N. Bracht *et al.*), Sage, London.

Israel, B.A. (1982) Social networks and health status: linking theory, research and practice. *Patient Counselling and Health Education*, **4**, 65–79.

Israel, B.A. and Rounds, K.A. (1987) Social networks and social support: a synthesis for health educators. *Advances in Health Education and Promotion*, **2**, 311–51.

Jacobs, D.R., Luepker, R.V., Mittelmark, M.B. *et al.* (1985) *Community-Wide Prevention Strategies: Evaluation Design of the Minnesota Heart Health Program*, University of Minnesota, Minneapolis.

Kanaaneh, H.A.K., Rabi, S.A. and Baderneh, S.M. (1976) The eradication of a large scabies outbreak using community-wide health education. *American Journal of Public Health*, **66**, 564–7.

Kemper, D.W. and Mettler, M. (1990) Building a positive image of aging: the experience of a small American city, in *Health Promotion at the Community Level*, (eds N. Bracht *et al.*), Sage, London.

Kieffer, C.J. (1984) Citizen empowerment: a developmental perspective, in *Studies in Empowerment: Steps Towards Understanding and Action*, (eds J. Rappaport, C. Swift and R. Hess.), Haworth Press, New York.

Kindervatter, S. (1979) *Nonformal Education as an Empowering Process*, Center for International Education, Anherst, Mass.

Kirklin, M.J. and Franzen, L.E. (1974) *Community Organization Bibliography*, Institute on the Church in Urban Industrial Society, Chicago, Ill.

Koskela, K. (1981) *A Community Based Antismoking Programme as a Part of a Comprehensive Cardiovascular Programme (The North Karelia Project)*, University of Kuopio, Finland.

Lazarsfeld, P. and Merton, R.K. (1964) Friendship as social process: a substantive and methodological analysis, in *Freedom and Control in Modern Society*, (eds M. Berger *et al.*), Octagon, New York.

Lazes, P.M. (ed.) (1979) *Handbook of Health Education*, Aspen Systems Corp., Maryland.

Lefebvre, R.C., Lasater, R.M., Carleton, R.A. and Peterson, G. (1987) Theory and delivery of health programming in the community: the Pawtucket Heart Health Program. *Preventive Medicine*, **16**, 80–95.

Leventhal, H., Cleary, P.D., Safer, M.A. and Gutmann, M. (1980) Cardiovascular risk modification by community-based programs for lifestyle change: comments on the Stanford study. *Journal of Consulting and Clinical Psychology*, **48**, 150–8.

Loney, M. (1981) The British Community Development Projects: questioning the state. *Community Development Journal*, **16**, 55–67.

MacCannell, D. (1979) The elementary structures of community: macrostructural accounting as a methodology for theory building and policy formulation, in *Community Development Research*, (ed. E.J. Blakely), Human Sciences Press, New York.

Maccoby, N. and Farquhar, J.W. (1975) Communication for health – unselling heart disease. *Journal of Communications*, **25**, 114–26.

Maccoby, N. and Solomon, D. (1981) Experiments in risk reduction through community health education, in *Health Education by Television and Radio*, (ed. M. Meyer), K.G. Saur, Munchen.

Martin, C.J., Platt, F.D. and Hunt, S.M. (1987) Housing conditions and ill health. *British Medical Journal*, **294**, 1125–7.

McAlister, A., Puska, P., Salonen, J. *et al.* (1982) Theory and action for health promotion: illustrations from the North Karelia Project. *American Journal of Public Health*, **72**, 43–55.

McMillan, D.W. and Chavis, D.M. (1986) Sense of community: a definition and theory. *Journal of Community Psychology*, **14**, 6–23.

Means, R. and Smith, R. (1988) Implementing a pluralistic approach to evaluation in health education. *Policy and politics*, **16**, 17–28.

Meyer, A.J., Maccoby, N. and Farquhar, J.W. (1980) Reply to Kasl and Leventhal *et al. Journal of Consulting and Clinical Psychology*, **48**, 159–63.

Mittelmark, M.B., Luepker, R.V., Jacobs, D.R. *et al.* (1986) Community-wide prevention of cardiovascular disease: education strategies of the Minnesota Heart Health Program. *Preventive Medicine*, **15**, 1–7.

Murray, D.M., Luepker, R.V., Pirie, P.L. *et al.* (1985) *CHD Risk Factor Screening and Education: A Community Approach to Prevention of Coronary Heart Disease* (mimeo), University of Minnesota, Minneapolis.

National Forum for Coronary Heart Disease Prevention (1988) *Coronary Heart Disease Prevention: Action in the UK 1984–1987*, Health Education Authority, London.

Neittaanmaki, L., Koskela, K., Puska, P. and McAlister, A.L. (1980) The role of lay workers in community health education: experiences of the North Karelia Project. *Scandinavian Journal of Social Medicine*, **8**, 1–7.

Nix, H.L. (1970) *The Community and Its Involvement in the Study Planning Action Process*, US Dept of Health, Education and Welfare, Atlanta, Georgia.

Oliver, M.F. (1987) Letter to the Editor. *Lancet*, **ii**, 518.

O'Sullivan, M.J., Waugh, N. and Espeland, W. (1984) The Fort McDowell Yavapai: from pawns to powerbrokers, in *Empowerment: Steps Toward Understanding and Action*, (eds J Rappaport, C. Swift and R. Hess), Haworth Press, New York.

Pancer, S.M. and Nelson, G. (1990) Community-based approaches to health promotion: guidelines for community mobilization. *International Quarterly of Community Health Education*, **10**(2), 91–111.

Parlett, M. and Hamilton, D. (1972) *Evaluation as Illumination: A New Approach to the Study of Innovatory Programmes, Occasional Paper 9*, Centre for Research in the Educational Sciences, University of Edinburgh.

Paruvani, C. (1988), Bringing people together. *Contact*, **106**, 10–13.

Perry, C.L. Griffin, G. and Murray, D.M. (1985a) Assessing needs for youth health promotion. *Preventive Medicine*, **14**, 379–93.

Perry, C.L., Mullis, R.M. and Maile, M.C. (1985b) Modifying the eating behaviour of young children. *Journal of School Health*, **55**, 399–402.

Pietinen, P., Vartiainen, E., Korhonen, H.J. *et al.* (1989) Nutrition as a component in community control of cardiovascular disease (The North Karelia Project). *American Journal of Clinical Nutrition,* **49**, 1017–24.

Puska, P., Vienda, P., Kottke, T.E. *et al.* (1981) Health knowledge and community prevention of coronary heart disease. *International Journal of Health Education,* **XXIV**, (Supplement).

Puska, P., Nissinen, A., Tuomilehto, J. *et al.* (1985) The community-based strategy to prevent coronary heart disease: conclusions from the ten years of the North Karelia Project. *Annual Review of Public Health,* **6**, 147–93.

Puska, P., Koskela, K., McAlister, A. *et al.* (1986) Use of lay opinion leaders to promote diffusion of health innovations in a community programme: lessons learned from the North Karelia Project. *Bulletin of the World Health Organization,* **64**, 437–46.

Puska, P., Tuomilehto, J., Nissinen, A. *et al.* (1989) The North Karelia Project: 15 years of community-based prevention of coronary heart disease. *Annals of Medicine,* **21**, 169–73.

Raeburn, J.M. (1986) Toward a sense of community: comprehensive community projects and community houses. *Journal of Community Psychology,* **14**, 391–8.

Rifkin, S.B., Muller, F. and Bichmann, W. (1988) Primary health care: on measuring participation. *Social Science and Medicine,* **26**(9), 931–40.

Rogers, E.M. and Shoemaker, F.F. (1971) *Communication of Innovations,* Free Press, New York.

Rosenthal, H. (1983) Neighbourhood health projects: some new approaches to health and community work in parts of the United Kingdom. *Community Development Journal,* **13**(2), 122–31.

Ross, M.G. and Lappin, B.W. (1967) *Community Organization: Theory, Principles and Practice,* Harper and Row, New York.

Rothman, J. (1979) Three models of community organization in practice, in *Strategies of Community Organization,* (eds F. Cox *et al.*), F.E. Peacock, Chicago.

Salonen, J.T. (1987) Did the North Karelia Project reduce coronary mortality? Letter to the Editor. *Lancet,* **ii**, 269.

Salonen, J.T., Hamynen, H. and Heinonen, O.P. (undated) *Impact of a Health Education Programme and Other Factors on Stopping Smoking after Heart Attack* (mimeo), University of Kuopio, Finland.

Salonen, J.T., Puska, P., Kottke, T.E. *et al.* (1983) Decline in mortality from coronary heart disease in Finland from 1969 to 1979. *British Medical Journal,* **286**, 1857–60.

Sayegh, J. and Green, L.W. (1976) Family planning education: programme design, training component and cost effectiveness. *International Journal of Health Education,* **19**, (Supplement).

Schwartz, J.L. (1987) *Smoking Cessation Methods: The United States and Canada, 1978–1985,* US Dept of Health and Human Services, Washington DC, pp. 62–71.

Simmons, J. (ed.) (1976) *Making Health Education Work,* American Public Health Association, Washington DC.

Smithies, J., Adams, L., Webster, G. and Beattie, A. (1990) *Community Participation in Health Promoion,* Health Education Authority, London.

Sosa, R., Kennel, J. and Klaus, M. (1980) The effect of a supportive companion on perinatal problems, length of labor, and mother–infant interactions. *New England Journal of Medicine,* **305**, 597–600.

Stunkard, A.J., Felix, R.J. and Cohen, R.Y. (1985) Mobilizing a community to promote health: the Pennsylvania County Health Improvement Program (CHIP), in *Prevention in Health Psychology,* (eds J.C. Rosen and L.J. Solomon), University Press of New England, Hanover, New Hampshire.

Tandon, R. (1981) Participatory research in the empowerment of people. *Convergence,* **XIV**(3), 20–9.

Tonnies, F. (1887; 1955) *Community and Association,* Routledge and Kegan Paul, London.

Tuomilehto, J., Geboers, J., Salonen, J.T. *et al.* (1986) Decline in cardiovascular mortality in North Karelia and other parts of Finland. *British Medical Journal,* **293**, 1068–71.

Twelvetrees, A. (1982) *Community Work,* Macmillan, London.

Vartiainen, E., Pallonen, V., McAlister, A. *et al.* (1983) Effect of two years of educational intervention on adolescent smoking (the North Karelia Youth Project). *Bulletin of the World Health Organization,* **61**, 529–32.

Vincent, M.L., Clearie, A.F. and Schluchter, M.D. (1987) Reducing adolescent pregnancy through school and community-based education. *Journal of the American Medical Association,* **257**(24), 3382–6.

Voth, D.E. (1979) Problems in the evaluation of community development efforts, in *Community Development Research: Concepts, Issues and Strategies,* (ed. E.J. Blakeley), Human Sciences Press, New York.

Ward, C. (1990) Product minded. *New Statesman and Society*, 12 October, 31.

Wellman, B. and Leighton, B. (1979) Networks, neighbourhoods, and communities: approaches to the study of the community question. *Urban Affairs Quarterly*, **14**(3), 363–91.

Werner, D. (1980) Health care and human dignity, in *Health: The Human Factor: Readings in Health, Development and Community Participation*, (ed. S.B. Rifkin), CONTACT Special Series No. 3, World Council of Churches, Geneva.

World Health Organization (1981) *Community Control of Cardiovascular Diseases: The North Karelia Project*. WHO European Regional Office, Copenhagen.

World Health Organization (1983) *New Approaches to Health Education in Primary Health Care, Technical Report Series 690*. WHO, Geneva.

World Health Organization Collaborative Group (1970) Multifactorial trial in the prevention of coronary heart disease. *European Heart Journal*, **1**, 73–9.

CONLUSION

The Introduction set the scene for the book and provided some updating observations on its key themes. In this final section we will return briefly to 'effectiveness', 'efficiency' and also to the new theme in its title – 'equity'. In addition we will provide concluding comments on evaluation and note some prevailing impressions gained of the literature in the process of producing this second edition. Finally, we will look forward and make some suggestions for health education and its evaluation.

It has been indicated at numerous points in the book that there is good evidence of effective activities linked to the outcomes of the various ideological positions on health education. In conclusion we need to comment on the extent and magnitude of successes with respect to individual outcomes, specific client groups and specific settings. As we have noted in earlier chapters, the different aspects of health have not received equal attention from evaluators. In addition some of the more complex indicators associated with the empowerment approach are under-represented in the literature by comparison with some simpler outcome measures associated with the preventive model. While it is conceptually useful to identify different ideological positions on health education it does not necessarily follow that programmes are constituted solely in line with a particular position. Many of the relatively complex interventions in the drugs prevention area contain, for example, variable mixes of indicators which can be linked to preventive, educational and empowerment approaches.

Evaluations which have sought to demonstrate effectiveness by the use of experimental methods have tended to focus on psychological variables with some limited consideration of social influences. In some topics, smoking education in school settings being a key example, sophisticated combinations of psychosocial approaches have been developed in pursuit of behavioural change and a degree of satisfaction recorded with the results achieved. The early optimism that such approaches might readily transfer to other areas of health has been modified. The relative lack of success of psychosocial approaches in alcohol education, for example, may in part be due to failure properly to appreciate the nature of the social contexts in which alcohol use occurs and the patterns of social influence on alcohol related behaviours – although we also noted in the schools chapter a challenge to the whole psychosocial approach to this aspect of health. Meta-analyses of studies in the drugs prevention area have illustrated the wide variety of elements used and the numbers combined in specific interventions. On the basis of common sense we might assume that as long as activities are complementary an increased number might be associated with increased success over and above what ensues from greater time investment. Where anything from 5–9 distinct components may be involved we need better understanding of their separate and interactive contributions to overall success. With such knowledge, programmes can then include not only what is necessary for success but also what is sufficient, thus making better use of scarce resources.

While the pursuit of ever more sophisticated methodological approaches carefully tailored to specific areas may be one way forward, an alternative and probably more widely applicable strategy is to focus on the quality of the educational process. As noted in the Introduction, given enough time and variety success may probably be achieved with most methods. This point was endorsed by Mullen *et al.* (1985) in concluding from a number of meta-analyses in the area of patient education that effectiveness was not determined by a specific educational technique but by the quality of the planning of the intervention. The criteria for estimating this quality were noted earlier, i.e relevance, individualization, feedback, reinforcement and facilitation.

Effective and efficient activities have been noted in each of the settings discussed in earlier chapters. The new emphasis on health promoting settings promises to be a good stimulus to increased health education activity and there is also, at global level, plenty of evidence of support for health education, particularly in school and community settings, but to date progress in achieving institutionalized successes has been slow. This is due to multiple reasons – some global, some country and some setting specific. They include economic constraints; shortcomings in professional motivations and skills; difficulties in achieving sustainability; and problems associated with the management of change and dissemination of good practice. A few points can be made, in turn, about each of these.

In most countries and settings, health education has to compete for scarce resources. Ideological shifts in some countries towards the broad welfare sector have led to further economic constraints. In the schools setting, for example, these shifts have been associated with a renewed emphasis on basic subjects and demands for greater accountability with consequences for the development of health education. Taking England as an example, there has been a reduction of advisory support staff and specialist health education co-ordinators within local education author-

ities, leading to a reduction in inservice training and other curriculum development activities. The pressures for accountability in basic areas of the curriculum also make it difficult for time and resources to be given to health education except in the case of the limited content which is included within the statutory orders for other subjects in the curriculum. At the same time the change to schools having responsibility for the management of their limited budgets will have implications for achieving health promoting schools across the whole of a local authority.

We also noted the threat from economic pressures within hospital settings, in particular to the patient education co-ordinators in the USA. Such pressures are not necessarily negative forces. As Green (1990) noted, they may also serve to stimulate the identification and use of effective approaches. A major problem associated with acute economic pressures is that scarce resources may have to be used for those interventions which have been shown to be effective and which are also cheap. These may not be in line with consumer needs, with commitments to equity or with other preferences.

While official statements on health education continue to note the importance of initial and inservice training for professionals, progress towards incorporation of core courses which provide effective preparation is again slow. With the growth of the emphasis on development of health education within health promoting settings which in turn form alliances with other settings, the training requirements are also broadened. In addition to enabling professionals to incorporate effective health education within their own area of practice they also need, for example, to be able to work with other professionals within and across sectors. If we also support the view that research and evaluation should be a routine part of a health education practitioner's role rather than an externally initiated and managed activity, further training is required.

Where developments have been initiated, achieving sustainability remains a difficulty as we noted in discussing the School Health Evaluation Study in the USA. McLeroy *et al.* (1992), in an editorial for *Health Education Research*, called for papers which addressed the problems of programme maintenance within community-wide and multiorganizational settings. Many positive evaluations come from specially resourced projects often built around enthusiasts. Given the withdrawal of additional project resources and the moving on of people, achievements may go into reverse. Identifying the most appropriate ways to initiate and support health education development and change merits closer attention. A small change that is acceptable to the majority in a context and can be institutionalized may be more important in terms of measurable outcomes at population level than a highly complex and highly effective programme which depends on particularly skilled and enthusiastic practitioners and is not easily institutionalized. While there may, for example, be good sense in advocating comprehensive, integrated and co-ordinated health education activities within settings this can be seen as an essentially top-down emphasis if sufficient resources are not available to allow for the participatory learning required to ensure that practitioners identify with and wish to 'own' such a model.

In some settings support for small scale initiatives built around felt needs may in the end be a more effective strategy for achieving institutionalized development. The discussion of the development of the patient education co-ordinator role in the Netherlands provided a nice example of reaching wider development goals through working with a felt need. The process of developing a patient education leaflet became a stimulus to the wider goals of organizational change; in short, an amalgam of bottom-up and top-down change strategies.

In the first edition we made the point that although there was still much to learn about achieving effectiveness in relation to specific outcomes, there was enough known which, if applied, could bring measurable improvements. What is needed, therefore, is wider dissemination of effective strategies and the development of the necessary skills to implement them. While there has been a tendency to give attention to professional researcher led evaluations equal importance needs also to be given to the routine reporting of practitioner evaluation. At the same time the dissemination of information about ineffective activities and also those with negative impacts needs to be emphasized. McLeroy *et al.* (1992) noted the paucity of articles in the professional literature on unsuccessful programmes from which we might learn as much as from successful ones. Reports on unsuccessful ones needed to provide reflections, they suggested, on the reasons for lack of success whether this be failure of theory, failure to understand target populations or failures in implementation in the shorter or longer term.

While much health education does take place within workplace, educational and health care settings the community is the context through which significant proportions of people need to be reached. Within this all-embracing setting many groups can be particularly difficult to reach and in many respects can be outwith the standard social community networks tapped in community oriented health education. We have noted a recognition of needs of such groups as street children, homeless young people, sex workers, nomadic peoples, refugees, etc. It is vital that the fashion for working within settings does not detract from further development of activities with such groups.

The HIV/AIDS issue has been one stimulus to specific initiatives with the more difficult-to-reach groups. Aggleton and Kapila (1992) see outreach and detached work as providing opportunities for meeting the sexual and reproductive health needs of such groups as the young homeless, young unemployed, young people who inject drugs and those who sell sex. Disengaged from mainstream social networks, such young people may need special help in responding to HIV/AIDS. It is also worth suggesting that work in informal settings may be the more effective approach to health education with those young people who can also be reached through schools.

In Chapter 3 we noted the growing attention to the assessment of quality, the precise indicators of which are debated but equity appears, alongside effectiveness and efficiency, in various quality statements. Inequalities in health between and within countries have been extensively documented as have the difficulties in achieving significant reductions. Efforts to reduce inequalities in health have been central to the health promotion movement as reflected in WHO and other key documents. Because of the differing understandings about health inequalities – for some including all differences but for others only those that may be defined as unjust and unfair – recent WHO documents preferred to use the term equity. Equity in health means (WHO, 1986) that ideally everyone should have a fair opportunity to attain their full health potential and, more pragmatically, that no one should be disadvantaged from achieving this potential if it can be avoided. In pursuit of equity we would not, it is suggested by Whitehead (1991), be looking for equality of outcomes which would be unrealistic but for availability of equal opportunities and the reduction of the barriers to achieving health.

Achievement of equity involves all elements of health promotion. As far as health education is concerned it involves providing health education in response to defined needs, ensuring provision reaches all to whom it is relevant, the use of acceptable methods and, where resources are limited, the use for areas of greater need. In this respect, as we have previously noted, there has been growing attention in discussions at global level to the need to ensure that health education reaches all sections of communities – those easily reached but also those who are reached with difficulty. What does a goal of equity mean for health education at the practice level? Assuming that there is existing provision it may mean a more differentiated approach to planning and implementation beginning with an acknowledgement that need ought to be assessed in ways that take felt needs fully into account and guard against assuming homogeneous experience for large sections of communities. This has been emphasized with respect to work with children and young people by Kalnins *et al.* (1992) and by Aggleton and Kapila (1992) who have said with reference to sexual health (although the comments would be generally applicable) that:

> Particular attention should be given to identifying ways in which the views of disadvantaged and vulnerable young people can be elicited, including those of ethnic and sexual minorities. This may be especially challenging in those societies not renowned for acceptance of social difference.

They go on to discuss priorities for health education and emphasize that health educators should be sceptical of conventional claims about the nature and universality of adolescent experience. The transition from childhood to adulthood varies considerably within as well as between societies: young heterosexual men experience it differently from young heterosexual women: young people who are disabled differently from the ablebodied, and young lesbians from gay men. Equity may mean much more emphasis on bringing health education nearer to where people are and identifying and using the strategies that have proven effective in specific contexts.

Where the activity of evaluation is concerned views about approaches to it and the actual activities undertaken reflect the diversity within health education – further complicated if we also refer to the wider framework of health promotion. Primarily it is important that evaluation does in fact take place. In many disciplines there is a tradition of evaluation being externally planned and implemented with the evaluators having varying degrees of independence from funders and from practitioners. At the same time there has been a growing move towards seeing evaluation as an integral part of practice undertaken by practitioners themselves and including variable commitment to collaboration with programme participants. While there is clearly room for both externally and internally managed evaluation if our real concern is to ensure effective health education across institutional contexts the development of professional motivation and skills in carrying out evaluation needs full support. Kok and Green (1990) have noted shortcomings in this respect in commenting that 'health promotion practitioners and administrators are not always interested in, or receptive to, evaluation research and furthermore they are often unaware of the conditions that must be fulfilled for valid research'. In Chapter 2 we noted a further reluctance of practitioners to undertake evaluation, part of what Campbell described as the dilemma of the 'trapped administrator' (Stevenson and Burke, 1991). Trapped administrators 'are so committed to their projects that they cannot afford a rigorous programme evaluation that might point to failure'.

In Chapter 2 we also noted within health education the same debates about research methodology which exist in other areas of the social sciences and similar resolutions of these debates. While there are strong advocates for the use of more sophisticated experimental styles of evaluation and emphasis on enhancing skills in experimental and survey methods there are equally those who are in strong opposition to anything which reflects positivist methodology and who wholeheartedly embrace the phenomenological tradition. This is seen to generate more egalitarian ways of working with people and more valid health education knowledge. We can caution against

adoption of doctrinaire positions. For example, the forswearing of positivist research may be to the detriment of communities with whose health we are concerned.

Hunt's studies of housing and health (1993), while modelling good practice in achieving community participation and collaboration, were not confined to qualitative research methods. The careful use of survey methods established a dose response relationship between levels of mould in houses and symptoms in children – a relationship independent of a range of other factors. In effectively challenging the typical victim blaming statements on housing and health the evidence acquired was arguably more valuable than qualitative data would have been in achieving responses by authorities.

This study offers an example of the emerging consensus in support of methodological pluralism – not necessarily in the context of one study or in the work of particular individuals – but in the discipline as a whole. The adoption of pluralism seems most appropriate in seeking to answer the range of questions with which health education is concerned. Moreover, where evaluation of programmes is concerned it facilitates the production of fully comprehensive pictures of both process and outcomes. Within any particular evaluation, while the particular methodological preferences of those directly involved are of importance they need to be seen alongside consideration of the characteristics of a particular project, the specific questions that need to be addressed, the requirements of any sponsors of a programme and the uses to which evaluation findings will be put. Ultimately, philosophical, pragmatic and political considerations need to be carefully balanced.

Some evaluations address limited interventions and are narrowly focused on a restricted range of outcome indicators. By contrast others address comprehensive programmes taking place over extended periods of time where full attention needs to be given to process and outcomes. In the case of the former the research approach may stimulate no great debate while in the latter the various stakeholders may have very different views about the content and the approach to evaluation. We noted earlier the constraints that can be imposed by fundholders and others on the process of evaluation and on the publication of findings. A relevant discussion has recently been offered by Smithies and Adams (1993) of such difficulties encountered in the evaluation of community participation within the English Health Education Authority.

Most evaluation is carried out with the goal of assessing, and ultimately improving, specific programmes and not with a view to developing generalizable precepts. As Robottom and Colquhoun (1992) have commented on their action research programme with young people in Australia:

> It is important that the research outcomes are useful in improving participants' self understandings in relation to their own social contexts, and while hopefully they will be useful to people in a range of contexts, our commitment as participatory investigators is restricted to those people who are participants in the study.

At the same time much of the literature on which we have drawn has been describing experimental and survey styles of evaluation from which it is hoped to garner recommendations for wider applicability.

We have noted in the broader field of health promotion evidence of efforts to develop a particular philosophical position on research influenced by postmodern theorizing and the drawing of parallels between health promotion and other social movements. This designation of health promotion as a social movement is usefully challenged by Stevenson and Burke (1991) in noting the contradictory character of the health promotion movement – 'sharing the discourse but not the social base of new social movements with a resultant contradictory or incoherent outlook on research'. The literature on health promotion research combines, they say, 'the phenomenological relativism and sociological pluralism of the postmodern discourses of new social movements with the positivist logic and abstract universalism typical of enlightenment social theory and bureaucratic rationalism'. They argue against embracing uncritically postmodern theory and phenomenological methodology in that movement in the direction of postmodernism can lead to confused and unfocused research practice and to a profound depoliticization of the struggle for health.

Throughout the book various references have been made to facilitating active participation in health education activities, including research and evaluation. Participation is not uniformly conceptualized. It may range from limited involvement through to participation as part of an empowerment process. Where evaluation is concerned in moving from the former to the latter questions arise about the sharing of what may be seen as professional skills. Advocacy for such sharing is made by Smithies and Adams (1993) and while there may be broad support for their position the difficulties of achieving it in large scale projects have to be clearly recognized. A caution has also been offered by Stevenson and Burke if undue participation in the research process is to the exclusion or discounting of other kinds of popular activity. While recognizing the importance of community involvement in research if this is confined simply to the process of conducting research the 'potentially transformative project of empowering is rendered politically innocuous'. Much more consequential, they say, 'is the kind of power that enables communities to implement the results of research, to use research to gain resources, to overcome barriers to health, and effect social change'. Difficulties in facilitating a process of participation are also addressed by Robottom and Colquhoun (1992) in reporting work with young people where 'attempts to transfer the locus of control over the research to those young people actually creates

a form of insecurity, rather than empowerment as they learn to deal with their new
found lack of direction'.

LOOKING FORWARD

At a basic level we would be looking for
continuation of the existing diversity of
evaluation activities which characterize contemporary health education. By undertaking
activities informed by the range of methodological positions we can best answer the
variety of questions which need to be addressed and develop a knowledge base that
can be used to further Health for All. There is
a place, therefore, for further developments of
experimental and survey style interventions
leading to more detailed knowledge of effectiveness and efficiency. Since it is unrealistic to
expect that all health areas can be subjected to
detailed research particular attention to the
identification of transferable findings would
be encouraged. At the same time equal or
even greater importance should be attached
to enhancing the routine evaluation by practitioners of ongoing health education using a
variety of methods as appropriate and with
careful attention to ensuring that core values
of health education are not contradicted in
research and evaluation activities.

Evaluation will involve equal attention to
both process as well as outcome indicators. The
importance of process measures is expressed
by Engelkes (1993) in her discussion of the
evaluation of primary health care programmes:

> Quantitative monitoring of output, in terms
> of coverage and health practice is easy but
> has little relevance if the underlying pro-
> cess is not measured. The nature of this
> process varies from project to project but
> it must be defined and analysed. In a
> Columbian case study it was found that
> process evaluation carried out as participa-
> tory evaluation and review gave the most
> relevant information on quality, accept-
> ability and relevance of interventions.

The importance of theory in planning and
guiding health education research and practice
has been variously emphasized within the
book. Various shortcomings have been noted
in the range of theories drawn on as well as
the use of theory in formulating research and
evaluation questions. While many postgraduate health education training courses
now give parity to social and psychological
theory and analysis this has not always been
so and published research and evaluation
continues to reflect the longer relationship
with psychology.

While there are demands for refinements
and further developments in the use of psychological theory, of equal if not greater importance is the need to expand the use of
social theory. A few examples of shortcoming
in use of theory can be noted. Roter and Hall
(1991), in discussing the shift to active patient
participation and increased consumerism,
claim that 'health education as a field has not
developed a well articulated consumerist
perspective nor a theoretical base to guide
research and practice'. They reinforce Steele
et al.'s view (1987) that research in the particular field of patient participation should be
driven by theory rather than advocacy. In
commenting on health promotion, Pederson
et al. (1989) have noted the 'failure genuinely
to engage the literature of the social sciences'
while Bunton *et al.* (1991) argue that models
of behavioural change informing health promotion have relied on underdeveloped conceptions of social structure and cultural
process due to a bias towards individually
based behavioural change. They call for more
specific analyses and accounts of the social
processes of groups and their interaction with
social structure.

Comments have also been made about the
misuse of theory. Wallston (1991) has recorded the heavy use of Health Locus of Control
scales as measures of beliefs but also their
heavy misuse. He emphasizes that measures
of HLC beliefs should be within the context
of a larger theoretical framework and that

taking one construct – HLC – out of that context leads to an overabundance of false negative conclusions.

Stevenson and Burke may be given the last word on this issue. They argue that the way ahead:

> requires close engagement with developments in political and social theory, the specification of coherent theoretical models of health, and a systematic and rigorous research practice. Only this kind of articulation of theory and research will provide an explanation of community health experiences and illuminate the kinds of social forces impeding healthy change.

Finally we should be looking for enhanced dissemination of existing knowledge on achieving effective, efficient and equitable health education complemented by education and training programmes that would lead to high quality institutionalized health education in line with community needs.

REFERENCES

Aggleton, P. and Kapila, M. (1992) Young people, HIV/AIDS and the promotion of sexual health. *Health Promotion International*, **7**(1), 53–60.

Bunton, R., Murphy, S. and Bennett, P. (1991) Theories of behavioural change and their use in health promotion: some neglected issues. *Health Education Research*, **6**(2), 153–62.

Engelkes, E. (1993) What are the lessons from evaluating PHC projects? A personal view. *Health Policy and Planning*, **8**(1), 1–18.

Green, L.W. (1990) Hospitals and health care providers as agents of patient education. *Patient Education and Counselling*, **15**, 169–70.

Hunt, S.M. (1993) The relationship between research and policy: translating knowledge into action, in *Healthy Cities: Research and Practice*, (eds J.K. Davies and M.P. Kelly), Routledge, London.

Kalnins, I., McQueen, D., Backett, K., Curtice, L. and Currie, C.E. (1992) Children, empowerment and health promotion: some new directions in research and practice. *Health Promotion International*, **7**(1), 53–9.

Kok, G. and Green, L.W. (1990) Research to support health promotion in practice: a plea for increased cooperation. *Health Promotion International*, **5**(4), 301–8.

McLeroy, K.R., Steckler, A.B., Goodman, R.M. and Burdine, J.R. (1992) Editorial: Health education research: theory and practice – future directions. *Health Education Research*, **7**(1), 1–8.

Mullen, P.D., Green, L.W. and Persinger, G.S. (1985) Clinical trials of patient education for chronic conditions: a comparative meta-analysis of intervention types. *Preventive Medicine*, **14**(6), 753–81.

Robottom, I. and Colquhoun, D. (1992) Participatory research, environmental health education and the politics of method. *Health Education Research*, **7**(4), 457–69.

Pederson, A.P., Edwards, R.K., Kelner, M., Marshall, V.W. and Allison, K.R. (1989) *Coordinating Healthy Public Policy: An Analytic Literature Review and Bibliography*, Ministry of National Health and Welfare, Ottawa.

Roter, D.L. and Hall, J.A. (1991) Health education theory: an application to the process of patient–provider communication. *Health Education Research*, **6**(2), 185–94.

Smithies, J. and Adams, L. (1993) Walking the tightrope: issues in evaluation and community participation in Health for All, in *Healthy Cities: Research and Practice*, (eds J.K. Davies and M.P. Kelly), Routledge, London.

Steele, D.J., Blackwell, B., Gutmann, M.C. and Jackson, T.C. (1987) The activated patient: dogma, dream or desideratum? *Patient Education and Counselling*, **10**, 3–23.

Stevenson, H.M. and Burke, M. (1991) Bureaucratic logic in new social movement clothing. *Health Promotion International*, **6**(4), 281–90.

Wallston, K.A. (1991) The importance of placing measures of health locus of control beliefs in a theoretical context. *Health Education Research*, **6**(2), 251–2.

Whitehead, M. (1991) The concepts and principles of equity and health. *Health Promotion International*, **6**(3), 217–28.

World Health Organization (1986) *Social Justice and Equity in Health*, Report on a WHO meeting, Leeds, United Kingdom, 1985, WHO European Regional Office, Copenhagen.

APPENDIX: THE 38 TARGETS FOR WHO EUROPEAN REGION

1. By the year 2000, the actual differences in health status between countries and between groups within countries should be reduced by at least 25%, by improving the levels of health of disadvantaged nations and groups.
2. By the year 2000, people should have the basic opportunity to develop and use their health potential to live socially and economically fulfilling lives.
3. By the year 2000, disabled persons should have the physical, social and economic opportunities that allow at least for a socially and economically fulfilling and mentally creative life.
4. By the year 2000, the average number of years that people live free from major disease and disability should be increased by at least 10%.
5. By the year 2000, there should be no indigenous measles, poliomyelitis, neonatal tetanus, congenital rubella, diphtheria, congenital syphilis or indigenous malaria in the region.
6. By the year 2000, life expectancy at birth in the region should be at least 75 years.
7. By the year 2000, infant mortality in the region should be less than 20 per 1000 live births.
8. By the year 2000, maternal mortality in the region should be less than 15 per 100 000 live births
9. By the year 2000, mortality in the region from diseases of the circulatory system in people under 65 should be reduced by at least 15%.
10. By the year 2000, mortality in the region from cancer in people under 65 should be reduced by at least 15%.
11. By the year 2000, deaths from accidents in the region should be reduced by at least 25% through an intensified effort to reduce traffic, home and occupational accidents.
12. By the year 2000, the current rising trends in suicides and attempted suicides in the region should be reversed.
13. By 1990, national policies in all member states should ensure that legislative, administrative and economic mechanisms provide broad intersectoral support and resources for the promotion of healthy lifestyles and ensure effective participation of the people at all levels of such policy making.
14. By 1990, all member states should have specific programmes which enhance the major roles of the family and other social groups in developing and supporting healthy lifestyles.
15. By 1990, educational programmes in all member states should enhance the knowledge, motivation and skills of people to acquire and maintain health.
16. By 1995, in all member states, there should be significant increases in positive health behaviour, such as balanced nutrition, non-smoking, appropriate physical activity and good stress management.
17. By 1995, in all member states, there should be significant decreases in health-

damaging behaviour, such as overuse of alcohol and pharmaceutical products; use of illicit drugs, dangerous chemical substances; dangerous driving and violent social behaviour.

18. By 1990, member states should have multisectoral policies that effectively protect the human environment from health hazards, ensure community awareness and involvement, and effectively support international efforts to curb such hazards affecting more than one country.

19. By 1990, all member states should have adequate machinery for the monitoring, assessment and control of environmental hazards which pose a threat to human health, including potentially toxic chemicals, radiation, harmful consumer goods and biological agents.

20. By 1990, all people of the region should have adequate supplies of safe drinking water, and by the year 1995 pollution of rivers, lakes and seas should no longer pose a threat to human health.

21. By 1995, all people of the region should be effectively protected against recognized health risks from air pollution.

22. By 1990, all member states should have significantly reduced health risks from food contamination and implemented measures to protect consumers from harmful additives.

23. By 1995, all member states should have eliminated major known health risks associated with the disposal of hazardous wastes.

24. By the year 2000, all people of the region should have a better opportunity of living in houses and settlements which provide a healthy and safe environment.

25. By 1995, people of the region should be effectively protected against work related health risks.

26. By 1990, all member states, through effective community representation, should have developed health care systems that are based on primary health

care and supported by secondary and tertiary care as outlined at the Alma Ata Conference.

27. By 1990, in all member states, the infrastructures of the delivery systems should be organized so that resources are distributed according to need, and that services ensure physical and economic accessibility and cultural acceptability to the population.

28. By 1990, the primary health care system of all member states should provide a wide range of health promotive, curative, rehabilitative and supportive services to meet the basic health needs of the population and give special attention to high risk, vulnerable and underserved individuals and groups.

29. By 1990, in all member states, primary health care systems should be based on co-operation and teamwork between health care personnel, individuals, families and community groups.

30. By 1990, all member states should have mechanisms by which the services provided by all sectors relating to health are co-ordinated at the community level in the primary health care system.

31. By 1990, all member states should have built effective mechanisms for ensuring quality of patient care within their health care systems.

32. Before 1990, all member states should have formulated a research strategy to stimulate investigations which improve the application and expansion of knowledge needed to support their national 'Health for All' developments.

33. Before 1990, all member states should ensure that their health policies and strategies are in line with 'Health for All' principles and that national legislation and regulations make their implementation effective in all sectors of society.

34. Before 1990, member states should have a managerial process for health development geared to the attainment of 'Health

for All', actively involving communities and all sectors relevant to health and, accordingly, ensuring preferential allocation of resources to health development priorities.

35. Before 1990, member states should have health information systems capable of supporting their national strategies for 'Health for All'.

36. Before 1990, in all member states, the planning, training and use of health personnel should be in accordance with 'Health for All' policies with emphasis on the primary health care approach.

37. Before 1990, in all member states, education should provide personnel in sectors related to health with adequate information on national 'Health for All' policies and programmes and their practical application to their own sectors.

38. Before 1990, all member states should have established a formal mechanism for the systematic assessment of the appropriate use of health technologies and of their effectiveness, efficiency, safety and acceptability, as well as reflecting national health policy and economic restraints.

AUTHOR INDEX

SUBJECT INDEX

Numbers given in italics represent tables, those given in bold represent figures.

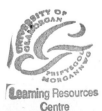